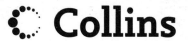

Health and Social Care
Level 2 Diploma Candidate Handbook

Mark Walsh • Eleanor Langridge • John Rowe
Ann Mitchell • Elaine Millar • Lois Greenhalgh

Published by Collins Education
An imprint of HarperCollins Publishers
77-85 Fulham Palace Rd
Hammersmith
London
W6 8JB

Browse the complete Collins Education catalogue at
www.collinseducation.com

10 9 8 7 6 5 4 3 2 1

ISBN 978-0-00-743051-2

British Library Cataloguing in Publication Data. A Catalogue record for this
publication is available from the British Library.

Commissioned by Charlie Evans
Edited by Tim Satterthwaite
Picture research by Erdinch Yigitce and Matthew Hammond
Design and typesetting by Q2A Media
Cover design by Angela English

Index by Indexing Specialists Ltd

Printed and bound by L.E.G.O.S.p.a

Welcome to the Level 2 candidate's handbook for the Diploma in Health and Social Care (Adults) award.

How is the book organised?

Each chapter of the book covers a specific level 2 unit. You will see that the chapters are divided into different sections, which are exactly matched to the specifications for the level 2 qualification. Each section provides you with a focused and manageable chunk of learning and covers all of the content areas that you need to know about in a particular unit.

There is a strong work-related focus to the materials in this book, using case studies, a range of practice-focused activities and realistic examples to develop your interest in and understanding of professional practice within the Adult health and social care workplace.

How is assessment covered?

In order to achieve your level 2 award, you will need to provide evidence of your knowledge and understanding as well as your practical competence in the real work environment. Each chapter of this handbook begins with a summary of 'What you need to know' and 'What you need to do' in order to successfully complete the unit. The checklist at the end of the each chapter will help you to keep track of your progress.

The suggested assessment tasks in each chapter will help you to gather the evidence you need for each unit. Your tutor or assessor will help you to plan your work in order to meet the assessment requirements.

Which units should I choose?

The material in this book covers all nine mandatory units of the level 2 diploma, together with a range of optional units. You must achieve a minimum of 46 credits to gain the Level 2 Diploma in Health and Social Care (Adults) award. To do this you must achieve:

▶ 24 credits from the mandatory units (chapters 1 to 9)

▶ a minimum of 2 and a maximum of 7 credits from the optional context and specialist knowledge units (chapters 10, 11 and 15)

▶ at least 15 credits from the optional competence units (chapters 12 to 14 and 16 to 20)

If you wish to claim a specialist dementia pathway award you must complete chapter 10 (DEM 201) and either chapter 16 (DEM 204) or 17 (DEM 210) found on the CD-ROM. Social care workers in Wales must complete chapter 20 (SS MU 2.1) Introductory awareness of sensory loss, to gain their award. Other candidates in Wales, Northern Ireland and England have a free choice of optional units.

We hope that the material in this book is accessible, interesting and inspires you to pursue a rewarding career caring for and supporting adults in health and social care settings. Good luck with your course and your future career!

Mark Walsh

1 | Introduction to communication in health, social care or children's and young people's settings (SHC 21)

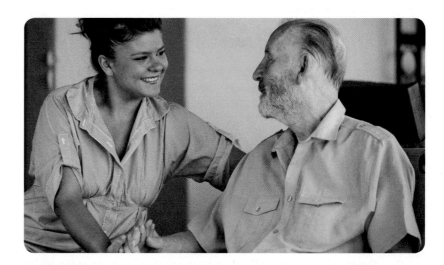

Assessment of this unit

This unit introduces you to the central importance of communication in health and social care work. It focuses on the reasons why people communicate in health or social care settings, the methods they use and the importance of ensuring that communication in care settings is effective. You will need to:

▶ understand why communication is important in the work setting

▶ be able to meet the communication and language needs, wishes and preferences of individuals

▶ be able to reduce barriers to communication

▶ be able to apply principles and practices relating to confidentiality at work.

The assessment of this unit is partly knowledge-based (things you need to know about) and partly competence-based (things you need to do in the real work environment). To successfully complete this unit, you will need to produce evidence of both your knowledge and your competence. The charts opposite outline what you need to know and do to meet each of the assessment criteria for the unit.

Your tutor or assessor will help you to prepare for your assessment and the tasks suggested in the chapter that follows will help you to create the evidence that you need.

AC What you need to know

1.1 Identify the different reasons people communicate

1.2 Explain how effective communication affects all aspects of your work

1.3 Explain why it is important to observe an individual's reactions when communicating with them

AC What you need to do

2.1 Show how to find out an individual's communication and language needs, wishes and preferences

2.2 Demonstrate communication methods that meet an individual's communication needs, wishes and preferences

2.3 Show how and when to seek advice about communication

3.1 Identify different barriers to effective communication

3.2 Demonstrate ways to reduce barriers to effective communication

3.3 Demonstrate ways to check that that communication has been understood

3.4 Identify sources of information and support or services to enable more effective communication

4.1 Explain the term 'confidentiality'

4.2 Demonstrate confidentiality in day-to-day communication in line with agreed ways of working

4.3 Describe situations where information normally considered to be confidential may need to be passed on

4.4 Explain how and when to seek advice about confidentiality

Assessment criteria 2.1, 2.2, 2.3, 3.2, 3.3 and 4.2 must be assessed in a real work environment.

Understanding why communication is important in the work setting

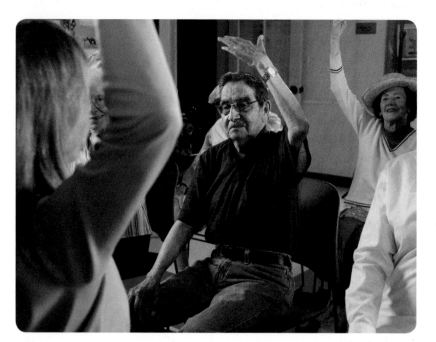

Effective communication is needed to motivate people and build relationships in health and social care settings

Your assessment criteria:

1.1 Identify different reasons why people communicate

Key terms

Verbal: forms of communication that use (spoken or written) words

Non-verbal: ways of communicating without using words (for example, through body language)

What is 'communication'?

People who work in health and social care settings need to develop effective communication skills in order to make and maintain relationships. Health and social care practitioners communicate with adults for a number of different reasons. This unit will help you appreciate the importance of this aspect of your own work. You must understand:

▶ what communication involves

▶ the different reasons for communication

▶ the way communication affects how practitioners work.

Communication is about making contact with others *and* being understood. When communicating, people send and receive 'messages'. We all communicate continuously by sending messages. Figure 1.1 describes how this happens through a communication cycle.

The communication cycle is a way of showing that communication involves a two-way process of sending and receiving messages. These messages can be:

▶ verbal, using spoken or written words

▶ non-verbal, using body language such as gestures, eye-contact and touch.

Discuss

Why do you think communication is an important part of care practice? Share some ideas with your work or class colleagues, noting the different ways people communicate in their work roles.

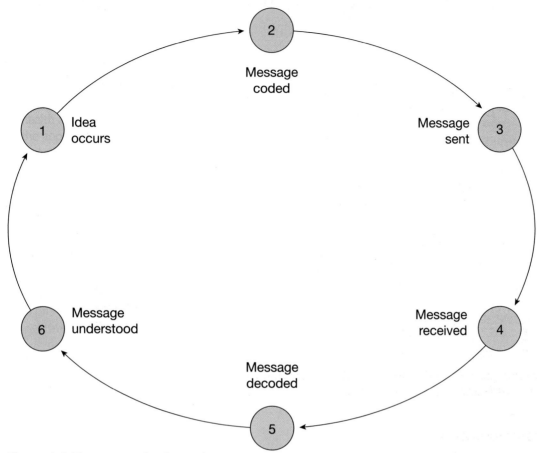

Figure 1.1 The communication cycle

People who work in health and social care settings may communicate with the people they are caring for, with relatives and visitors, with colleagues and with practitioners from other care agencies, and for a variety of different reasons.

Case study

Charlie is 32 years of age. He has very limited speech due to a brain injury he sustained in a motorcycle accident. He now lives in supported accommodation. Charlie enjoys helping out in the kitchen when Clare, his support worker, is making a meal. When she says 'Can I get some fruit for you, Charlie?', he puts his thumb up, makes a noise in the back of his throat and smiles at her. Clare responds by passing him a bowl of fruit, saying 'Okay, help yourself this time, Charlie'.

1. How does Charlie's support worker communicate with him in this example?

2. How does Charlie communicate non-verbally with Clare in response to her question?

3. Describe how a cycle of communication occurs in this example.

Reflect

Think about a recent conversation that you had with a service user or colleague. Can you see how it followed the communication cycle?

Why do people communicate in work settings?

Your assessment criteria:

1.1 Identify different reasons why people communicate

A lot of communication happens in health and social care settings: many different kinds of conversations occur, as well as a variety of meetings, activity and treatment sessions and consultations with medical and other practitioners that also involve communication. A closer look at these activities will show you that service users, practitioners and other adults **interact** and communicate with each other for a variety of different reasons in your workplace (see Figure 1.2).

Key terms

Interact: relate to another person

Making relationships

People communicate to make new relationships. In health and social care settings these relationships may be with service users, visitors or colleagues. Positive verbal and non-verbal communication skills, such as being friendly, smiling and shaking hands when greeting the person, are needed to make a good first impression in a relationship.

Developing relationships

Health and social care practitioners develop relationships with service users, their relatives or carers and colleagues, by maintaining a friendly, supportive approach, and by being interested in what other people are doing and feeling. This enables service users to feel comfortable and secure, and that they can trust and rely on professionals.

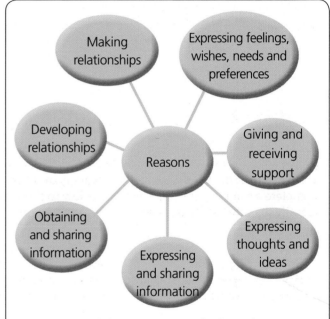

Figure 1.2 People communicate for lots of different reasons

Obtaining and sharing information

Health and social care practitioners may need to obtain and share information about service users with colleagues and other professionals to ensure the team is fully informed. A practitioner may also need to communicate with a service user or a family member about the care and support they receive, or about the kinds of services and facilities that are available in a care setting.

Expressing thoughts and ideas

A health or social care practitioner may need to share their thoughts about care issues or about aspects of practice with colleagues. Effective communication skills are also needed to encourage service users to talk about what they are feeling, to say what they think or to express their needs, wishes or preferences.

Giving and receiving support

Users of health and social care services and their relatives often seek reassurance from practitioners as a way of developing their self-confidence. In response, practitioners use praise and touch, and give time and attention as a way of rewarding a person's efforts and achievements and to reassure them. Some care settings also use support groups, staff meetings and appraisals as ways of providing practitioners with support and reassurance about their work performance.

Expressing feelings, wishes, needs and preferences

Health and social care practitioners need to find ways of encouraging service users to express their feelings and to talk about how they wish to be treated, as well as to say what they like and dislike. People will communicate in this way if they trust, and have a secure relationship with, a practitioner.

Reflect

Think about a day at work. Why did you need to communicate with others? Reflect on the different reasons for your communication.

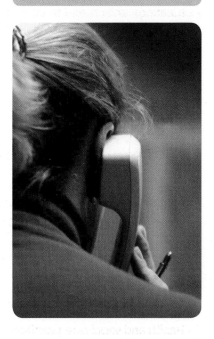

Knowledge Assessment Task   1.1

You will communicate with service users, visitors, colleagues and other professionals, in the setting where you work or are on placement, in a number of different ways and for a variety of different reasons. Complete a summary sheet like the one below to show that you can identify the different reasons why people communicate.

Who took part in this example of communication?	What happened? Describe the communication you observed.	What were the reasons for this episode of communication?

How does effective communication impact on your work?

Effective communication is a central part of the work that happens in care settings. You will need to develop a range of communication skills and be able to use them effectively to carry out the various aspects of your work role. You will need to be able to communicate effectively with service users, their relatives and your colleagues, as well as colleagues from other agencies.

Figure 1.3 identifies a variety of people with whom you may need to communicate in your care setting. Knowing about the communication cycle and being able to send and receive messages appropriately is the key to communicating well. In general, you will use communication effectively as part of your work role if you:

▶ get the other person's attention before you begin talking to them

▶ speak clearly and directly so that you get your message across

▶ adapt the way you talk so that the child or adult you are talking to is able to understand you

▶ use **empathy** to try and understand the other person's point of view or the way they might be affected by what you are saying to them

▶ listen carefully to what the child or adult says to you

▶ use your own non-verbal communication skills effectively

▶ summarise what the other person has said as a way of checking and confirming your understanding of that they mean.

Your communication skills will develop and become more effective as you gain experience in your work role, and learn by observing more experienced colleagues. Learning from others, seeking advice and using support are all part of this process.

Your assessment criteria:

1.2 Explain how effective communication affects all aspects of own work

Key terms

Empathy: understanding another person's feelings as if they are your own

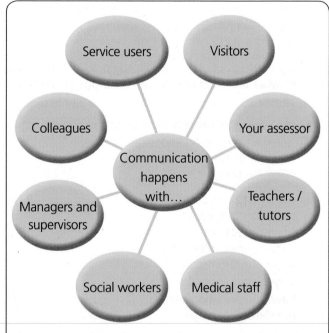

Figure 1.3 Who will you need to communicate with?

Effective communication with service users

People who work in health or social care settings are expected to be able to communicate effectively with the adults who receive care in the setting. This is not always easy or straightforward. Communication with the people with whom you work is more likely to be effective if you:

▶ get the individual's attention before you start talking, making eye contact at the person's own level

▶ use simple language, short sentences and a friendly tone of voice

▶ give the person time to understand what you are saying and enough time to respond to you

▶ are patient and attentive when an individual is talking to you, give them time to express themselves and don't rush them or interrupt to speed things up

▶ listen carefully and use simple questions to clarify what the person is telling you if you are not sure that you fully understand their communication

▶ are aware of your own body language and also take note of what the other person's body language is communicating to you

▶ use your facial expression in an active, positive way to support what you are saying and as a way of responding to what the person says to you

▶ use pictures, colourful posters or displays to express ideas or to communicate information in easy to understand ways. This might involve having information leaflets translated into other languages.

▶ summarise what the other person has said as a way of checking and confirming your understanding of that they mean.

Being respectful, consistent in your approach, and patient in the way you listen and respond to people in your work setting, will encourage them to trust and communicate with you.

Reflect

What are your own communication strengths and weaknesses? Review the list opposite and think about what you do well, and how you could develop your communication skills further.

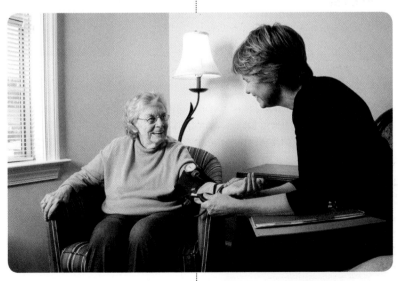

Good eye contact and appropriate body language make communication more effective

Effective communication with relatives and visitors

Health and social care service users and their relatives need to be able to trust you and have confidence in your ability to support and care for them. Communication with relatives and visitors is more likely to be effective if you:

▶ establish a good rapport with each individual

▶ show people respect by using their preferred names (e.g. 'Mrs Griffiths' not 'Jenny', if preferred) and recognise that they should always be consulted about anything that affects their care

▶ speak directly and clearly, using positive body language and good eye contact

▶ give each individual enough time to understand what you are saying and listen carefully to what they say to you

▶ respond quickly and in an appropriate way to an individual's communication by phone, email or in person

▶ respect confidentiality by communicating personal, sensitive or private information about individuals in an appropriate, private area of the care setting

▶ adapt your communication skills to meet the needs of a people who have hearing or visual impairments or whose first language is not English.

Your assessment criteria:

1.2 Explain how effective communication affects all aspects of own work

Key terms

Confidentiality: ensuring information is only accessible to people who are authorised to know about it

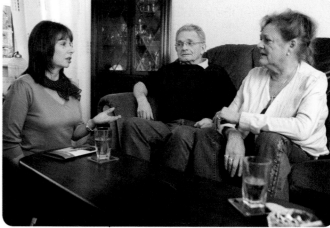

People will trust and respect you if you adopt a consistent, professional and respectful approach when you communicate with them. They need to be confident that you value them as a person and that you are able to communicate with them about their particular needs, wishes and preferences relating to care.

Care practitioners often need to consider when, whether and how they should communicate with the relatives of people they provide care for

Effective communication with colleagues

Effective communication with colleagues is an essential part of your work role in a team-working environment. Communication with colleagues is more likely to be effective if you:

▶ establish an appropriate work-related rapport with each of your colleagues

▶ show that you respect your colleagues' skills, abilities and professional approach towards their work role

▶ talk to your colleagues clearly and directly, using positive body language and giving them enough time to absorb what you are saying

▶ always listen to your colleagues' point of view, making sure you are polite and constructive where you disagree

▶ check that colleagues understand what you are trying to communicate when you are passing on important information

▶ clarify any points or ask questions where you don't fully understand what you have been told or are being asked to do

▶ demonstrate that you understand and respect confidentiality and the feelings of your colleagues by communicating about sensitive, personal or private issues in an appropriate private place

▶ ask someone to check any emails, letters or notes that you write on behalf of the care setting to ensure your language and presentation are appropriate and professional.

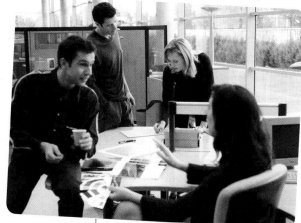

Effective communication with work colleagues is based on establishing a friendly but professional working relationship where you can give and receive support. Communication with colleagues should revolve around your shared goal of promoting the health and wellbeing of the people you provide care and support for.

Knowledge Assessment Task   1.2

You will need to communicate with service users and colleagues on a one-to-one basis and in groups as part of your health or social care work role. You should understand and be able to explain how effective communication affects all aspects of your work. Complete a table like the one below to explain how effective communication with others affects aspects of your work role.

Focus of communication	Identify a reason why you need to communicate	Explain how effective communication affects your work role
Communication with service users		
Communication with service users, visitors or relatives		
Communication with colleagues		

Why is it important to observe feedback?

Effective communication is a two-way process: when you are listening you are not just waiting for your turn to speak! To be an effective communicator, you have to notice how other people *respond* to your communication. People react non-verbally both to the *way* that you are communicating with them and to the *content* of your communication (see Figure 1.4). So, being able to read non-verbal feedback is very important. Indeed, this may be the only kind of response you receive from some people who are not confident enough or who are too unwell to speak to you. Observing feedback is a way of assessing:

▶ whether the person has understood your communication

▶ the person's feelings about what you said to them

▶ the effectiveness of your method of communication

▶ the appropriateness of the language you used.

Bear in mind that an individual's cultural background, disabilities, health status, religious beliefs, stage of development and personality may affect the way they react to you and use non-verbal methods of feedback.

Your assessment criteria:

1.3 Explain why it is important to observe an individual's reaction when communicating with them

Reflect

How do you make use of touch and eye contact when you communicate with service users? Think about what you do and what the purpose of this is.

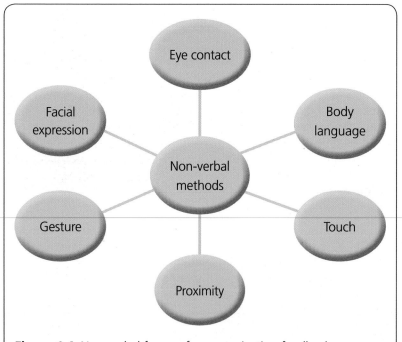

Figure 1.4 Non-verbal forms of communication feedback

Knowledge Assessment Task   1.3

As a health or social care practitioner you need to develop the ability to observe the reactions of others to your communication in one-to-one and group situations. These reactions may be expressed verbally (what the other person says in reply) or non-verbally (through their body language). Complete a table like the one below to explain why it is important to observe an individual's verbal and non-verbal reactions when you are communicating with them.

Focus of observation	What should you observe?	Why is it important to observe this?
Verbal response		
Non-verbal response		

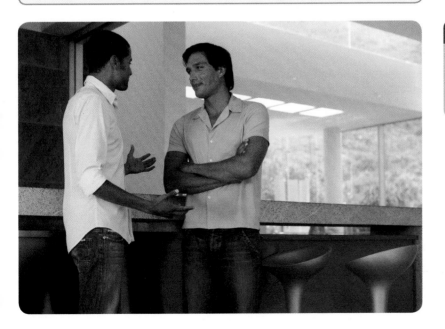

Reflect

How are these two men communicating non-verbally? What do you think each person's body language is 'saying'?

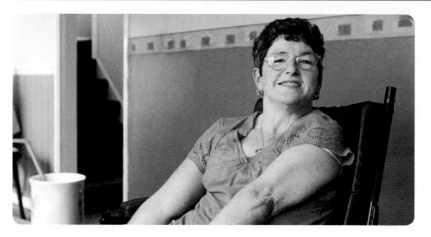

It is always important to find out about each individual's particular communication and language needs, wishes and preferences

How can you find out about individual's communication and language needs and preferences?

Effective communication happens when the right method is used to send a message, so it can be received and understood. Health and social care practitioners need to know about a range of communication methods. They should also be skilled at identifying the communication and language needs, wishes and preferences of the people with whom they work and interact.

Health and social care settings are used by people from a diverse range of backgrounds who will want to communicate in different ways. Finding out about each individual's language needs, wishes and preferences is an important part of your role. You can do this by:

▶ asking people whether they or their relatives have particular language or communication needs

▶ reading reports and notes about service users that provide information on speech and language issues, learning difficulties, disabilities (e.g. hearing or visual impairment) or physical conditions (e.g. stroke, cleft palate) that may affect their ability to communicate

▶ being aware that an individual's culture, ethnicity and nationality may affect their language preferences and needs

▶ observing the people who use your setting to see how they use their communication and language skills

▶ asking your supervisor/mentor, senior staff and specialist professionals such as speech and language therapists, occupational therapists and social workers for information, advice and support about how best to communicate with adults who have special communication needs.

You may need to communicate with people who have special communication needs as a result of a hearing or visual impairment, or because English is not their first language. General guidance on communicating with adults with hearing and visual impairments is provided in Figure 1.5.

Figure 1.5 Adapting to meet special communication needs

Hearing impaired people	Visually impaired people
• Make sure that your face can be seen clearly. • Face the light and the person you are speaking to at all times. • Speak clearly and slowly – repeat and rephrase if necessary. • Minimise background noise. • Use your eyes, facial expressions and gestures to communicate, where appropriate. • Do not be tempted to shout into a person's ear or hearing aid.	• Speak in the same way as you would to a sighted person – not louder or more slowly! • Say who you are in your greeting as your voice won't necessarily be recognised even if you have met the person before. • Always introduce other people who are with you and explain what is going on if a visually impaired adult joins you in a group. • Let the visually impaired person know when you are about to do something that is likely to affect communication (such as leave the room or move away). • End conversations clearly and let the person know that you are leaving – do not just walk away. • Ask the person if they need any particular help – to sit down or to move about, for example – but do not assume that this is always necessary or wanted.

Case study

Danielle, a 27-year-old learning disabled woman, was admitted to a hospital medical ward for observation during the night. On admission, Danielle was confused and disorientated following a series of epileptic seizures. Since waking early this morning Danielle has been concerned about her money and her coat. She thinks that the care staff have forgotten to give these things back to her and she is becoming increasingly upset about this. Danielle has taken to sitting on a chair outside of the ward office and is trying to get the attention of the ward manager, who is inside, as well as that of people who pass by.

1. How would you go about identifying Danielle's communication needs in this situation?
2. What factors might be affecting Danielle's ability to communicate effectively with members of staff?
3. Suggest two things that you would do to adapt to Danielle's communication needs in this situation.

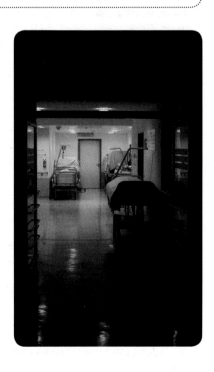

How can you use verbal and non-verbal communication?

Health and social care practitioners use two main types of communication as part of their work roles. These are verbal and non-verbal communication. Verbal communication is based on the use of words. Health and social care practitioners need effective verbal skills to:

Your assessment criteria:

2.2 Demonstrate communication methods that meet an individual's communication needs, wishes and preferences

▶ obtain information from colleagues, service users and others who use the setting

▶ respond to questions

▶ contribute to team meetings

▶ give feedback and report observations about service users

▶ provide support to service users, relatives and colleagues

▶ deal with problems and complaints

▶ write notes and reports

Non-verbal communication occurs when a person uses their body, behaviour and appearance to communicate with others. For example, an individual's body language may tell a health or social care practitioner that they are uncomfortable or need to go to the toilet even when they say they're okay. Important forms of non-verbal communication are outlined in Figure 1.7.

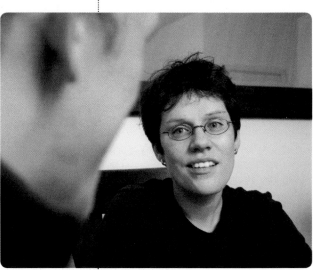

Paying attention is an important part of active listening

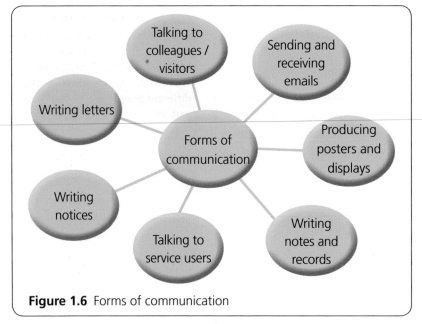

Figure 1.6 Forms of communication

Forms of communication:
- Talking to colleagues / visitors
- Sending and receiving emails
- Writing letters
- Producing posters and displays
- Writing notices
- Talking to service users
- Writing notes and records

Investigate

Use the internet to locate websites relating to the communication needs of people who are hearing impaired or visually impaired. Find out how people with these problems overcome their communication difficulties.

Figure 1.7 Forms of non-verbal communication

Non-verbal communication	What does it involve?	Examples
Eye contact	Looking another person directly in the eyes	Short or broken eye contact can express nervousness, shyness or mistrust.
		Long unbroken eye contact can express interest, attraction or hostility.
Touch	Physically touching or holding a person	Holding someone's hand
		Placing a hand on a person's arm or shoulder to reassure them
Physical gestures	Deliberate movements of the hands to express meaning	Thumbs-up gesture to show agreement or pleasure
		Shaking a fist to show anger or aggression
Body language		
Facial expression	Movements of the face that express a person's feelings	Smiling
		Frowning
Proximity	The physical closeness between people during interactions	Being very close may be reassuring and may be seen as accepting the person. It might also make the person feel uncomfortable and threatened. People need less personal space (increased proximity) when they have a close, trusting relationship.

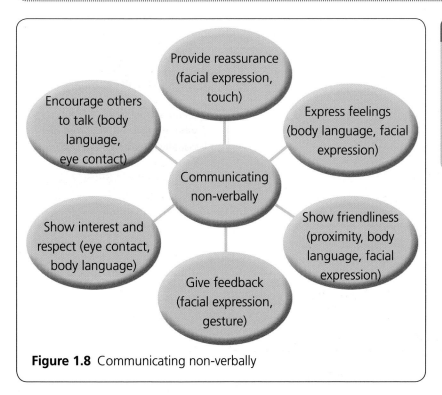

Figure 1.8 Communicating non-verbally

Investigate

Observe the way service users, visitors or your colleagues use their bodies to communicate during a group activity in your workplace. Try to work out what different people are 'saying' non-verbally.

How can you choose the right communication method?

To be an effective communicator in your work setting, you need to be able to use methods of communication that meet each individual's needs, wishes and preferences. Your goal is always to ensure that the messages you send can be received and understood. To achieve this you may sometimes need to change or adapt the form of communication you are using. Figure 1.9 identifies some of the issues you might consider when thinking about the best way to communicate with others.

Figure 1.9 Thinking about communication methods

Method	When might you use it?	Issues to consider
Talking face-to-face	• Asking or answering questions • Providing information or feedback • Receiving information or feedback • Making and maintaining work relationships • Providing support for service users, relatives or colleagues	• Does the individual understand English? • Is my choice of words appropriate to the person's language ability? • Does the person have any hearing impairment? • Will the person need support from an interpreter or signer? • Have I chosen an appropriate place to talk with the person? • Are there any cultural, religious or gender issues that might affect my communication with the other person?
Talking on the telephone	• Asking or answering questions • Providing information or feedback • Receiving information or feedback • Ordering resources • Arranging meetings	• Does the other person have any hearing impairment? • Are the other person's English language skills good enough for a telephone conversation? • What is the best time to call the person? • Would it be appropriate (and avoid breaching confidentiality) to leave a message for them?
Writing	• Writing letters, notes or notices for service users to read • Writing letters, reports, memos or minutes of meetings for colleagues or other professionals to read • Writing notices, displays or signs for relatives, visitors or colleagues to read	• Is the language I'm using appropriate, clear and direct? • Will the person be able to read and understand what I've written? • Does the intended reader have dyslexia, learning difficulties or problems with reading? • How will I make sure the person actually receives or sees what I'm writing?

continued...

Method	When might you use it?	Issues to consider
Email, text message	• Writing replies or brief notes to service users, relatives, other professionals or colleagues • Sending newsletters or information to colleagues, service users, their relatives or other professionals	• Do I have the email or phone details for everybody who wants or needs the information? • Is the language I'm using appropriate and easy to understand? • Have I removed any confidential information from emails sent to groups of people?
Non-verbal communication	• Talking face-to-face with an individual (using appropriate eye contact, body language, proximity and facial expression) • Explaining or providing support for a service user (using appropriate use of gestures and touch) • Talking face to face or on the telephone (using appropriate tone of voice and pitch)	• Is my non-verbal communication appropriate to the situation? • How can I use non-verbal communication to support what I am saying? • Are there any cultural, religious or gender issues that might affect the way others understand my non-verbal communication? • Does the person have a visual impairment or learning difficulty that might mean they don't notice my non-verbal communication?

Health and social care practitioners who use their communication skills effectively are able to think about the different ways in which they might communicate with each individual. The key is to choose the method of communication that is most suited to the situation.

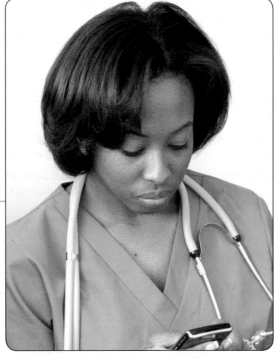

Health and social care practitioners increasingly use a variety of communication devices and methods, including mobile phones, and other new media

When should you seek advice about communication?

Your assessment criteria:

2.3 Show how and when to seek advice about communication

There may be situations in which you feel unsure about how you should communicate with a service user or another person in your work setting. Perhaps you will be aware that you are struggling to communicate effectively with somebody. In situations like these, you should seek advice and obtain support. You can do this by:

▶ talking to your supervisor, mentor or line manager about the difficulty – ask for their advice about how to deal with the problem

▶ talking to communication or language support specialists (teachers, psychologists or speech and language therapists) who work at or spend time in your work setting.

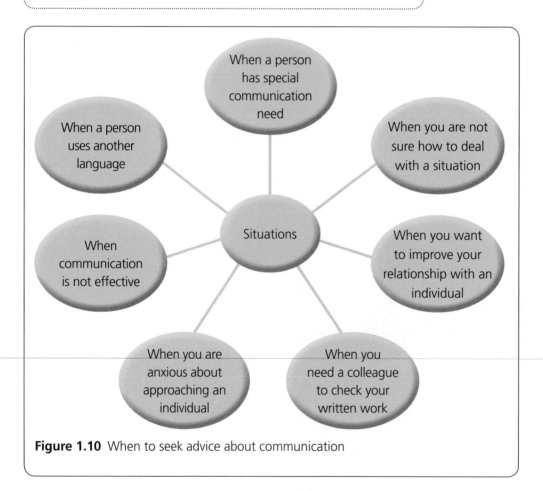

Figure 1.10 When to seek advice about communication

Practical Assessment Task

2.1 **2.2** **2.3**

Your first meeting with a service user or one of their relatives is an ideal opportunity to find out about the individual's communication and language needs, wishes and preferences. To complete this assessment task you need to demonstrate that you are able to do this competently. You will need to produce evidence based on your practice at work which demonstrates that:

▶ you can find out about an individual's communication and language needs, wishes and preferences

▶ you can use communication methods (verbal and non-verbal) that meet the individual's communication needs, wishes and preferences

▶ you know how and when to seek advice about communication.

Your evidence must be based on your practice in a real work environment and must be witnessed by, or be in a format acceptable to, your assessor.

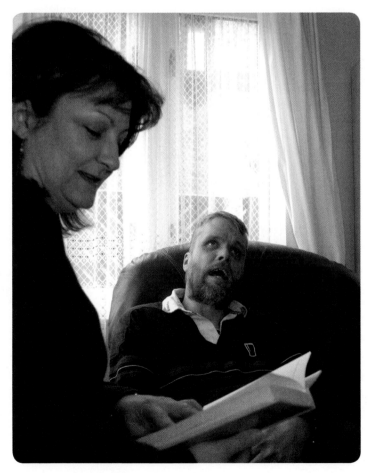

A range of specialist communication support and assistance is available for people who have sensory impairments

أهلاً وسهلاً
WELCOME

Your assessment criteria:

3.1 Identify barriers to effective communication

What barriers can reduce the effectiveness of communication?

Despite your best efforts, you may sometimes find that you are unable to communicate effectively with another person in your work setting. There are a number of possible reasons why this might happen. Knowing about different barriers to effective communication will enable you to avoid potential difficulties and adapt your communication approach where this is necessary. Barriers to communication are things that interfere with a person's ability to send, receive or understand a message. These may include the following:

▶ *environmental factors* – noise impairs listening and concentration. Poor lighting can prevent a person from noticing non-verbal communication and could reduce a hearing impaired person's ability to lip read. Environments that are too hot or cold cause discomfort and those that lack privacy discourage people from expressing their feelings and problems.

▶ *developmental stage* – a person's developmental stage could limit their ability to communicate and may be a barrier to effective communication if you don't take this into account when choosing your words or way of talking to them. Don't use long sentences, complex words or unusual phrases with young children, for example.

▶ *sensory deprivation and disability* – visual impairment may reduce a person's ability to see faces or read written signs and leaflets. Hearing impairment may limit conversation. Conditions such as cerebral palsy, stroke, cleft palate, Down's syndrome and autism tend to limit a person's ability to communicate verbally and non-verbally; difficulties interpreting non-verbal communication are typical of autism.

▶ *language and cultural differences* – the UK is a multicultural country with a mix of different ethnic groups and language

Key terms

Jargon: technical language that is understood by people in particular industry or area of work

Slang: an informal type of language that is used by a particular group of people

Acronym: an abbreviation that stands for a longer phrase, such as 'NHS' for National Health Service

Dialect: a localised version of a language

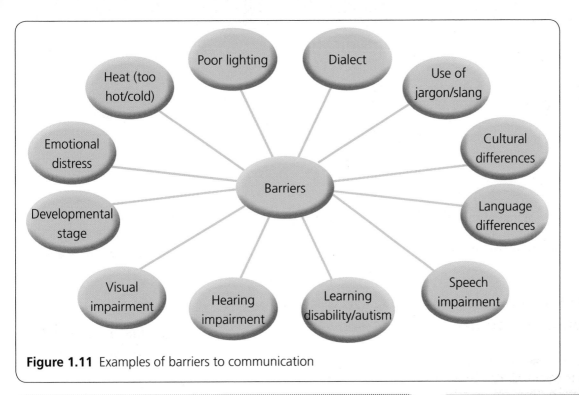

Figure 1.11 Examples of barriers to communication

communities. English may be a second or even third language for some children and adults, and may not be spoken or understood at all by others. Communication in written and spoken English may not be easy or even possible for people in this situation. Similarly, people from different cultural groups may interpret non-verbal behaviour in different ways, misunderstanding messages.

▶ *jargon, slang and use of acronyms* – these forms of language only make sense to people with specialist knowledge. A person who doesn't have this specialist knowledge won't understand the message. Practitioners working in children and young people settings sometimes use jargon and acronyms to communicate quickly with each other. Teenagers sometimes use forms of slang to communicate with each other in ways their parents and teachers don't understand.

▶ *dialect* – people who speak English using a regional dialect (for example Glagwegian or Liverpudlian) pronounce words in different ways. They may also use some words that are specific to the local area. A child or adult who isn't from the same area may not understand a local dialect.

▶ *distress, emotional difficulties and health problems* – some conditions, depression and stroke for example, may affect an individual's ability to send and receive messages effectively. Illness and injuries can also cause people to withdraw from communication situations. Similarly, when a person is angry, aggressive or upset they may find it difficult to communicate; their own communication may be misunderstood by others.

Reflect

Can you think of any slang terms that are used by people in your local area or jargon used in your workplace? Do you think that adults or other young people from a different area would know what these terms mean?

Reflect

Can you think of any times or circumstances where your ability to communicate has been affected because you were upset or unwell? Did other people recognise this and adapt their communication approach in any way?

How can you overcome communication barriers?

Your assessment criteria:

3.2 Demonstrate how to reduce barriers to communication in different ways

Barriers to communication can often be overcome, or at least reduced, by making changes to the environment, adapting your approach or by using support services that help people to overcome communication difficulties.

Adapting the environment

Environmental changes might include:

► replacing poor lighting with brighter lighting

► reducing background noise or creating some quiet areas away from noisy activity

► putting up multilingual posters and displaying signs clearly

► fitting electronic devices such as **induction loop** systems for hearing impaired people.

Adapting your approach to communication

In order to improve communication, health and social care practitioners can adapt their approach by:

► making sure they can be seen clearly, facing both the light and the person to whom they are talking

► making sure their mouth is visible when speaking

► minimising background noise

► using eyes, facial expressions and gestures to communicate where necessary and appropriate.

Timing

Speaking clearly and slowly and repeating and, if necessary, rephrasing what you say can make communication more effective with some service users, their relatives and colleagues. Speaking a little more slowly can help where a person has a hearing or visual impairment, a learning disability, or is anxious or confused. The pace of communication may need to be slower to give the person time to understand what is being said to them. It is also important to allow time for the person to respond. This can mean tolerating silences whilst the person thinks and works out how to reply.

Using support services and specialist devices

Health and social care practitioners should understand the language needs and communication preferences of the children and adults with whom they work. If a child or adult has difficulty communicating in English, or has sensory impairments or disabilities that affect their communication skills, specialist communication

Key terms

Induction loop: a system that boosts sound for hearing aid users

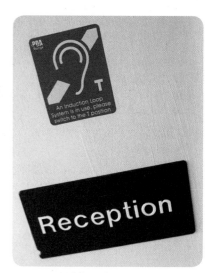

This symbol indicates a communication loop is available for hearing aid users

support may be needed. Learning a few words of another person's language or developing some basic sign language skills can really help a practitioner to establish a positive, supportive relationship with a service user, their relatives or with colleagues.

A range of electronic devices exist to help people overcome communication difficulties. These include hearing aids, text phones, telephone amplifiers and hearing loops. Electronic devices can be used both to send and receive messages.

Investigate

Visit the websites of the Royal National Institute for the Deaf (www.RNID.org.uk) and the Royal National Institute for the Blind (www.RNIB.org.uk).
Find out about the range of services that these groups provide for people who have sensory impairments. Produce a summary of the different forms of communication support that are available to people with visual or hearing impairments.

Case study

Mrs O'Sullivan, aged 78, is being admitted to a residential care home for a three-week respite period for the first time. Alex, a support worker, has been given the job of meeting and showing Mrs O'Sullivan around. Alex knows that Mrs O'Sullivan has become deaf because of injuries she received in a car accident.

On arrival Mrs O'Sullivan is accompanied by her daughter and by a social worker. When Alex introduces herself to Mrs O'Sullivan, her daughter answers by saying, 'You are wasting your time. She doesn't communicate any more.'

1. Suggest reasons why Mrs O'Sullivan may communicate less than she used to.
2. What could Alex do to maximise communication with Mrs O'Sullivan during her brief visit?
3. What kinds of extra help and support might improve Mrs O'Sullivan's ability to communicate effectively during her three-week respite break?

Practical Assessment Task   3.1   3.2

What kinds of barriers to effective communication occur in the health or social care setting where you work or are on placement? Complete the table below by identifying three examples of barriers to effective communication that you are aware of, and then demonstrate ways of overcoming each barrier.

Barrier to communication	How does this make communication less effective?	How have you tried to overcome this barrier?
Example 1		
Example 2		
Example 3		

Your evidence for this task must be based on your practice in a real work environment and must be witnessed by, or be in a format acceptable to, your assessor.

How can you check communication is effective?

Effective communication in health and social care settings helps practitioners, service users and others who visit the setting to form good relationships and to work well together. People communicate most effectively when they:

- ▶ feel relaxed
- ▶ are able to empathise with others
- ▶ experience warmth and genuineness in the relationship.

There are a number of ways of checking that your communication is effective. What you need to know is that the 'messages' you send are received and understood correctly by the person with whom you are communicating. You can do this by using active listening and clarifying or repeating techniques.

Active listening

Active listening involves paying close attention to what the other person is saying whilst also noticing the non-verbal messages they are communicating. People who are good at active listening also tend to be skilled at using minimal prompts. These are things like nods of the head, 'Mm' sounds, and encouraging phrases like 'Yes, I see' or 'Go on'. Skilful use of minimal prompts encourages the person you are communicating with to keep speaking or to say a little more.

Clarifying or repeating

You can ensure that your communication has been understood by clarifying (repeating back, summarising or rephrasing) aspects of what the person has said during the conversation. You could say something like, 'Can I just check that you meant …?' or, 'Do you mean …?' You should try not to clarify too often in a conversation as this will interrupt the speaker's flow; it might also make them think you are 'parroting', which may appear insincere.

Key terms

Empathise: understand another's feelings

Minimal prompts: unobtrusive sounds and behaviours that encourage the other person to talk

Reflect

Think about your own approach to listening. Are you an active listener or this is something you need to work at?

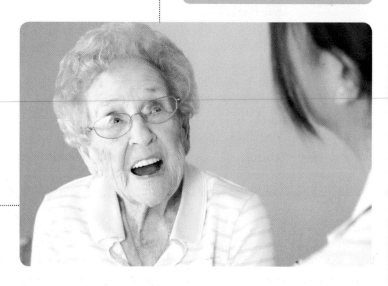

How can you obtain communication support and assistance?

You should always seek support and assistance if you encounter communication problems with any service users, visitors or colleagues. You may be able to obtain help from:

- ▶ your supervisor, line manager or mentor
- ▶ senior and experienced colleagues
- ▶ a service user's relatives
- ▶ specialist practitioners, such as speech and language therapists, psychologists or special needs teachers
- ▶ interpreting services and organisations which work with recent immigrants and asylum-seeking families where use of English is a barrier to effective communication
- ▶ specialist organisations which provide support for people who have sensory impairments, disabilities and language problems.

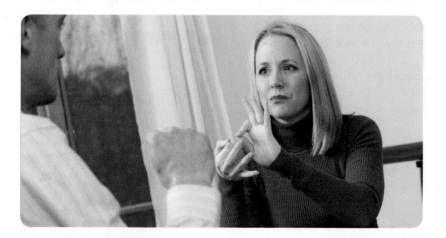

Practical Assessment Task   3.3   3.4

How do you ensure that your communication with people has been understood? Are you able to use the checking techniques described above?

1. Working with a service user or an adult who attends your workplace, demonstrate that you are able to find ways of checking that your communication with them has been understood.

2. Make notes on the sources of information and support or services that you could use to enable more effective communication with this or another person if the need arose.

Your evidence for this task must be based on your practice in a real work environment and must be witnessed by, or be in a format acceptable to, your assessor.

Confidentiality

What is confidentiality?

Confidentiality is not about keeping secrets; it is about protecting an individual's right to *privacy*. You may obtain private, personal information from service users, their relatives or from other practitioners as part of your work role. As a health and social care practitioner you have a duty to:

▶ keep personal information about service users private

▶ only share information about service users with those who have a right to know or when a person has given their permission to disclose information about them.

Your workplace will have a confidentiality policy that sets out the rules and procedures on sharing confidential information. You should read this and make sure that you follow it in your practice. You may be asked to sign a confidentiality agreement as part of your employment contract. Again, you should have a clear understanding of what this means in practice.

Your assessment criteria:

4.1 Explain the term confidentiality

4.2 Demonstrate confidentiality in day-to-day communication, in line with agreed ways of working

Key terms

Confidentiality: ensuring information is only accessible to people who are authorised to know about it

Investigate

Obtain a copy of the confidentiality policy of your workplace. Identify the main points and how they affect your work role. What are you expected to do to protect confidentiality in your workplace?

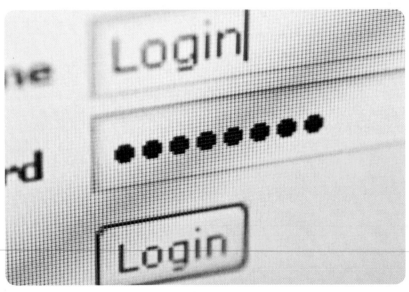

Passwords to gain access to computerised records are an important way of protecting confidentiality

How can you demonstrate confidentiality?

There will be many occasions in your day-to-day work when you will need to share information about service users. This information can be shared with your work colleagues without breaching confidentiality because everybody in the team needs to know about each service user. However, you can promote and demonstrate confidentiality by:

▶ only talking about service users in areas of the setting where you cannot be overheard by non-staff members

▶ not revealing confidential information about one service user to another who may remember and pass it on

▶ using service users' first names or initials only when discussing or writing up your observations about them

▶ storing written records about service users in locked cupboards or cabinets and making sure you put them back in the correct place after using them

▶ using a secure password to access computers that contain information about service users

▶ making sure service users only have access to their own records

▶ referring service users' relatives to the service users' key worker when they request information relating to their relative.

Maintaining confidentiality outside work

You should not talk, gossip or complain about the people you work with when you are at home or when you are socialising with your friends. This is a serious breach of confidentiality and might lead to disciplinary action by your employer.

Reflect

Think about the ways in which you demonstrate confidentiality through your care practice. What do you do, or not do, to promote confidentiality at work?

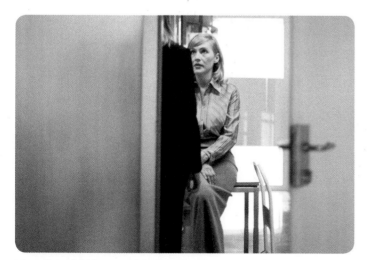

You should always ensure that you can't be overheard when discussing confidential issues with your colleagues

When should confidential information be passed on?

Disclosure of information to people other than your immediate work colleagues about a service user's background, personal problems, care needs or health issues, normally only happens with the consent of the service user or their next of kin. However, there are exceptions to this rule. For example, confidential information can be passed on if a person requires an assessment or specialist support from a practitioner who is not a member of your work team.

There may also be times when you have to reveal what you have been told, or have seen, to a more senior person at work or to an external organisation. A service user's, family member's or colleague's request that you maintain confidentiality can be overridden if:

▶ what they say suggests an individual may be at risk of harm

▶ they reveal information that can be used to protect another person from harm

▶ a court or a statutory organisation, such as a Mental Health Act tribunal, asks for specific information about a person.

Your assessment criteria:

4.3 Describe situations where information normally considered to be confidential might need to be passed on

4.4 Explain how and when to seek advice about confidentiality

Case study

Kwame Adams is a social worker in the Care of Older People team. Peter McVey, aged 84, is one of Kwame's clients. Peter lives in the downstairs part of a terraced house on his own. He has lived in the same house for the past 52 years and is very reluctant to move. Peter has Parkinson's disease, and has difficulty moving around and meeting his own physical needs. Beatrice, aged 23, is Peter's niece. She has a key to his home and comes around twice a day to help him get dressed and to prepare food for him. Peter and Beatrice get on very well.

Kwame recently became concerned about the way Beatrice is looking after Peter. He noticed that Peter seems a little anxious when Beatrice comes to the house. He has also noticed that Beatrice is dressing Pete in the same clothes every day. The last time Kwame came to the house Peter complained about being hungry. He said that Beatrice now collects his pension and does his shopping, but that the fridge is always empty. When Kwame asked Peter whether he would like him to speak with Beatrice about the way she is looking after him and the lack of food, Peter said, 'No, you mustn't. She might get angry and go away for good'.

1. What is the confidentiality dilemma in this situation?

2. What might be the advantages and disadvantages of Kwame speaking to Beatrice about his situation?

3. What do you think Kwame should do to meet his responsibilities as a social worker?

When should you seek advice about confidentiality?

It is best to treat everything you learn about children and their families in your workplace as confidential information; it is advisable to check with your supervisor before you pass on confidential information. Similarly, it is always best to tell your supervisor if you receive any information that concerns you. If someone says they want to tell you something 'in confidence', you should say that you may not be able to keep the information to yourself because part of your job involves safeguarding children's welfare. It is then up to the person to decide whether to tell you.

Practical Assessment Task | 4.1 | 4.2 | 4.3 | 4.4

Practitioners in health and social care settings should communicate with others (service users, their families, colleagues) in ways that apply and protect the principle of confidentiality. Using your knowledge of confidentiality and what you have learnt from the confidentiality policy of your workplace, carry out the following tasks:

1. Explain the term *confidentiality*, illustrating your explanation with two examples of situations when it is important to keep information confidential in your workplace.

2. Demonstrate how you protect confidentiality and follow the confidentiality procedures of your work setting in your day-to-day communication with others.

3. Describe two situations that could occur, or which have occurred, in your workplace, when information normally considered confidential needs to be passed on.

4. Explain how and when you would seek advice about the confidentiality issues involved in question 3 above.

Your evidence for this task must be based on your practice in a real work environment and must be witnessed by, or be in a format acceptable to, your assessor.

Are you ready for assessment?

AC	What do you know now?	Assessment task	✓
1.1	Identify the different reasons people communicate	Page 7	
1.2	Explain how effective communication affects all aspects of your work	Page 11	
1.3	Explain why it is important to observe an individual's reactions when communicating with them	Page 13	

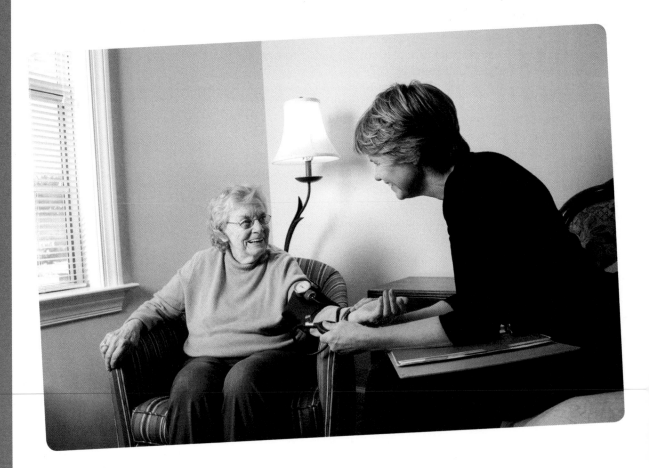

AC	What can you do now?	Assessment task	✓
2.1	Show how to find out an individual's communication and language needs, wishes and preferences	Page 21	
2.2	Demonstrate communication methods that meet an individual's communication needs, wishes and preferences	Page 21	
2.3	Show how and when to seek advice about communication	Page 21	
3.1	Identify different barriers to effective communication	Page 25	
3.2	Demonstrate ways to reduce barriers to effective communication	Page 25	
3.3	Demonstrate ways to check that communication has been understood	Page 27	
3.4	Identify sources of information and support or services to enable more effective communication	Page 27	
4.1	Explain the term 'confidentiality'	Page 31	
4.2	Demonstrate confidentiality in day-to-day communication in line with agreed ways of working	Page 31	
4.3	Describe situations where information normally considered to be confidential may need to be passed on	Page 31	
4.4	Explain how and when to seek advice about confidentiality	Page 31	

2 | Introduction to personal development in health, social care or children and young people's settings (SHC 22)

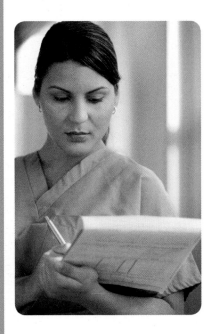

Assessment of this unit

This unit introduces you to the concepts of personal development and reflective practice, and the key part they play in work roles with people in health and social care settings.

You will be assessed on both your knowledge of personal development and reflection, and on your ability to apply this in relation to your own development as a practitioner. The 'What you need to know' chart below identifies the knowledge-based criteria you must cover in your assessment evidence. You also need to produce evidence of your practical ability to assess and plan for your own learning and development as a practitioner. The 'What you need to do' criteria listed opposite must be assessed in a real work environment by a vocationally competent assessor.

Your tutor or assessor will help you to prepare for your assessment and the tasks suggested in the chapter will help you to create the evidence that you need.

AC	What you need to know
1.1	Describe the duties and responsibilities of own work role
1.2	Identify the standards that influence the way the role is carried out
1.3	Describe ways to ensure that personal attitudes or beliefs do not obstruct the quality of work

AC	What you need to do
2.1	Explain why reflecting on practice is an important way to develop knowledge, skills and practice
2.2	Assess how well your own knowledge, skills and understanding meet standards
2.3	Demonstrate the ability to reflect on work activities
3.1	Identify sources of support for own learning and development
3.2	Describe the process for agreeing a personal development plan and who should be involved
3.3	Contribute to drawing up own personal development plan
4.1	Show how a learning activity has improved own knowledge, skills and understanding
4.2	Show how reflecting on a situation has improved own knowledge, skills and understanding
4.3	Show how feedback from others has developed own knowledge, skills and understanding
4.4	Show how to record progress in relation to personal development

Assessment criteria 2.1–4.4 must be assessed in a real work environment.

This unit also links to some other mandatory units:

SHC 21	Introduction to communication in health and social care settings
SHC 24	Introduction to duty of care in health and social care
HSC 025	The role of the health and social care worker

Some of your learning will be repeated in these units and will give you the chance to review your knowledge and understanding.

Do you understand your work role?

Here we focus on ways in which you can develop the knowledge, skills and values needed to perform your work role effectively. A clear understanding of the requirements of your work role is needed for this. You should understand:

▶ what you need to do as part of your work role

▶ the aspects of your work role you do well or carry out competently at the moment

▶ the areas of practice you need to improve on through further training or by gaining more experience.

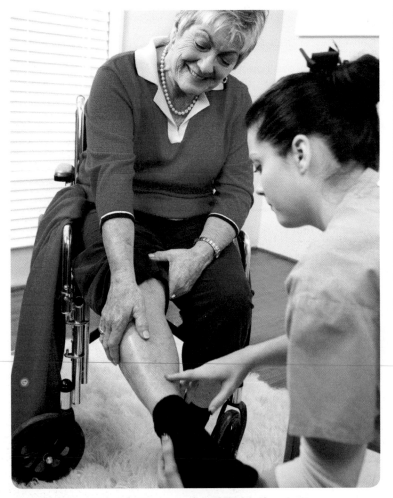

Competence in a health or social care work role is achieved through training and experience

Key terms

Job description: a written outline of the duties and responsibilities of a work role

Duties: things a person is expected or required to do

Responsibilities: what a person is expected to do

Person specification: a written outline of the qualifications, experience and qualities needed to perform a particular work role

Collaborate: work together with others to achieve a shared goal

Investigate

What does your job description say about the duties and responsibilities associated with your work role? Ask your employer for a copy of your job description if you don't have one. If you are a student on placement, check your placement guidelines to identify the duties and responsibilities associated with your work role.

Understanding your duties and responsibilities

Everybody who is employed or working voluntarily in health and social care settings should have a job description. Your job description should be written for your particular work role and should clearly outline your work-related duties and responsibilities. Typically, during the recruitment process, employers also produce a person specification that identifies the qualifications, experience and qualities or abilities that a person requires for a particular job. If you are a student on placement, your school or college and the placement organisation should collaborate to produce guidelines relating to your role.

The duties and responsibilities associated with your work role will depend on the kind of setting you work in, and the priorities and focus of the organisation that employs you. For example, if you work as a support worker in a day centre for older people, your practical duties and responsibilities are likely to be different to those of a person who works as a health care support worker with adults in a hospital setting.

Reflect

In what ways do you think the duties and responsibilities of a practitioner working with older people in a residential care setting and older people in a hospital setting would be similar and different?

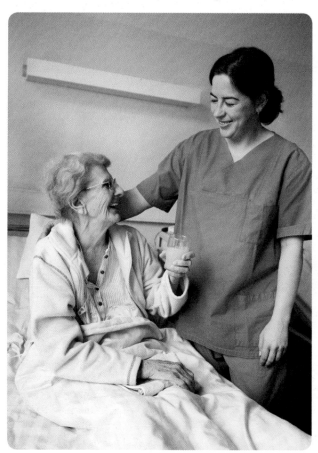
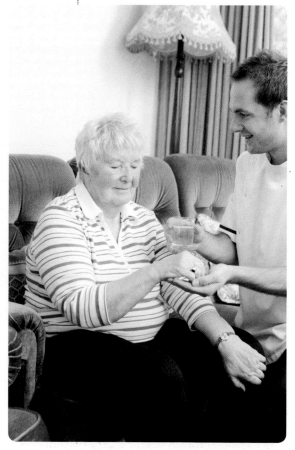

Positive relationships with service users are based on trust and the belief that individuals have in your competence as a care practitioner

Aptitude and skills

Work with adults in health and social care settings is varied. It can be physically and mentally demanding. You may have fantastic, enjoyable days filled with positive experiences. You may also have very challenging, tiring and distressing days when your patience is really tested. Whatever kind of day you are having, you must always work to meet the needs of the people who use your care setting. These needs will be diverse, so you will need to be flexible and adaptable in your approach.

At interview, you will need to demonstrate that you have the aptitude for the kind of day-to-day work that a particular role involves. You will also need to show that you have the skills needed for a particular role or that, because of your aptitude and willingness to learn, you have the potential to develop the necessary skills.

Teamworking skills are central to any health or social care worker's practice; in this sector people don't usually work as individual practitioners, they work in teams. You must be able to co-operate and collaborate in order to provide safe, supportive care and assistance for the people who use your care setting.

Reflect

What would you say are the strengths and abilities that you bring to your health or social care role? How would you explain this to a prospective employer?

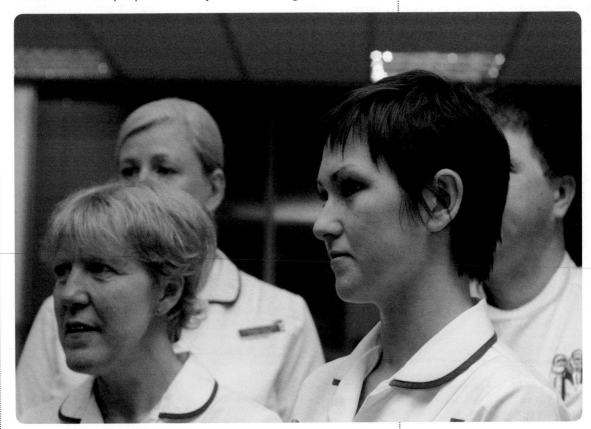

Care teams can consist of practitioners from all kinds of backgrounds and age groups

Starting a new job

When anyone starts a new job, they need clear guidance on what is expected of them. When you start at a new setting, your manager should ensure that you have an **induction** covering:

▶ practical issues such as the layout of the work setting and the normal routines

▶ any special ideas and values that underpin the work of the setting

▶ the **policies** and **procedures** used in the setting, especially in relation to health and safety

▶ an introduction to your colleagues and other support workers

▶ an introduction to the service users and their relatives who use the setting.

The induction phase of a new job can feel overwhelming – there is so much new information to take on board. It is okay to ask questions about things you don't understand, can't remember or are not sure about. Not asking questions can result in mistakes being made. Don't worry about looking silly: it shows professionalism and maturity to clarify issues.

Your supervisor and work colleagues will expect you to ask questions and to seek their help when you start your job or placement. It is a good idea to make use of their greater experience and the assistance they are able to offer.

Your assessment criteria:

1.1 Describe the duties and responsibilities of own role

Key terms

Induction: a period of basic training

Policies: written documents that set out an organisation's approach to a particular issue

Procedures: documents that set out in detail how a particular issue should be dealt with or how particular tasks should be carried out

Case study

Rachel, aged 29, has three children. They are aged 12, 11 and 5. Rachel has been a full-time housewife and mother since her first child was born. She enjoys caring for her children and feels that she is good at meeting their needs and managing their behaviour. She says that the key is to be strict with them about their behaviour. Rachel would like to apply for a job at a day centre for young people with learning disabilities. She thinks that her experience of looking after her children and her caring personality, together with the fact that she 'loves playing with children', should be enough to get her an interview and hopefully the job.

1. Identify one way that your work role and responsibilities are similar to and one way in which they are different from those Rachel describes in relation to caring for her children.

2. Do you think that Rachel has the right kind of aptitude for working with young people with learning disabilities in a day centre?

3. Describe the kind of skills that Rachel would need to develop or demonstrate in order to get a job like the one that you do at the moment.

What are the standards that influence your role?

All health and social care settings have to operate within a legal framework, and to follow the guidance and rules of **regulatory bodies**. Health and safety laws and childcare practice standards are very important elements of this framework. Examples of standards that affect your role can be found in:

- ▶ codes of practice
- ▶ internal policies and procedures
- ▶ legislation (such as the Health and Safety at Work Act, 1974)
- ▶ National Minimum Standards
- ▶ National Occupational Standards.

Internal policies and procedures

Your employer should have produced and made you aware of a range of policies and procedures that cover the standards of practice you need to achieve. Policies and procedures are usually explained during induction training and many settings have additional training sessions or staff meetings where practitioners have the opportunity to learn more.

You need to know how the different policies and procedures used in your work setting impact on your work role. Following them carefully should ensure that you are working to the expected legal and regulatory standards. Your senior colleagues and the manager of your workplace should be able to explain any of the workplace's policies and procedures so it is worth asking about any that you are unsure of or which you don't understand.

The Health and Safety at Work Act (1974)

The Health and Safety at Work Act (1974) is the key law affecting the health and safety rights and responsibilities of employers and employees in your workplace. Employers are responsible for providing:

- ▶ a safe and secure work environment
- ▶ safe equipment
- ▶ information and training about health, safety and security.

Employees (practitioners and students) have a responsibility to:

- ▶ work safely within the care setting
- ▶ monitor their work environment for health and safety problems that may develop
- ▶ report and respond appropriately to any health and safety risks.

Your assessment criteria:

1.2 Identify standards that influence the way the role is carried out

Key terms

Regulatory bodies: organisations that set standards and rules for care practitioners to follow

Reflect

Did you have an opportunity to find out about and discuss the policies and procedures of your work setting when you started your job or placement? Where would you find a copy of the policies and procedures if you wanted to check something today?

Practitioners and students carry out their legal responsibilities by:

▶ developing an awareness of health and safety law

▶ working in ways that follow health and safety guidelines, policies and procedures

▶ monitoring the work environment for health and safety hazards

▶ where it is safe to do so, dealing directly with hazards that present a health and safety risk

▶ reporting health and safety hazards or the failure of safety systems or procedures to a supervisor or manager.

Your employer's health and safety policy should cover the key points of this legislation. You should have a good understanding of what it says and how this affects your work role.

Your assessment criteria:

1.2 Identify standards that influence the way the role is carried out

Case study

Hannah Kinnaird is a student taking a Diploma in Adult Health and Social Care course at a local college as part of her apprenticeship in social care. She will work on placement at Chillerton Grange residential care home three days each week and attend college on the other two days. Hannah has never worked in a residential care home before and is very excited to be starting a placement at Chillerton Grange. Hannah has just visited the care home to meet Mrs Lloyd, the home manager and her supervisor. She is feeling a bit frustrated and grumpy because Mrs Lloyd gave her a folder containing information about Chillerton Grange and about the policies and procedures that apply in the setting. Hannah doesn't really want to read these but has been told that she will need to show she understands the health and safety policy and procedures before she can spend time with the residents.

1. Identify the main piece of health and safety legislation that is likely to be covered by the policies and procedures of Chillerton Grange residential home.

2. Describe the health and safety responsibilities Hannah will have when she starts working at Chillerton Grange.

3. Give two reasons why Hannah needs to understand what the policies and procedures say about health and safety.

Investigate

The website of the sector skills councils responsible for health and social care (www.skillsforcare.org.uk and www.skillsforhealth.org.uk) of information on standards that apply to work with adults in health and social care settings. You can also find copies of the National Occupational Standards on this website.

National Occupational Standards

The aim of the National Occupational Standards (NOS) relating to adult health and social care practice is to:

▶ raise the quality of care provision in adult health and social care settings

▶ identify the knowledge, skills and understanding needed by competent practitioners for work with adults in health and social care settings.

▶ The National Occupational Standards are also used to develop care qualifications (such as this one!) and courses that seek to improve practice in the sector. Employees and students are responsible for working to the NOS. Your employer or placement provider should provide you with ongoing support and suitable training opportunities to enable you to achieve and maintain acceptable standards of practice. You have a duty to make the most of these opportunities.

How can you keep personal views and work separate?

Everyone has attitudes and beliefs that are developed in childhood, through experience and in the course of our relationships with others. In many ways, our attitudes and beliefs reflect who we are – they inform our views and opinions. However, practitioners in children and young people's settings must avoid judging others and should not express their personal attitudes and beliefs too forthrightly. In particular, it is important not to discuss or put down the attitudes and beliefs of others (service users, colleagues, visitors). There must be some separation between your own personal views and the way you relate to others in the workplace. You need to accept difference, avoid challenging the beliefs of others and should not get into conflict over attitudes and beliefs in general. You can do this by:

▶ discussing issues openly and by contributing your thoughts and ideas to meetings and discussions

▶ listening to the ideas, views and opinions of others in an open-minded way

▶ allowing people to work in ways that suit them if the outcome is acceptable – people don't always have to do things your way!

▶ avoiding confrontation, as this creates hostility and may damage the confidence of individual colleagues and the morale of the team in general.

Your assessment criteria:

1.3 Describe ways to ensure that personal attitudes or beliefs do not obstruct the quality of work

Reflect

Have you ever expressed your personal views about service users or issues affecting them at work or heard other people doing so? What impact did this have on yourself and others? What benefits are there in remaining neutral on contentious or sensitive subjects?

Case study

Carrie is the main carer for her physically disabled son Paulo, aged 23. Carrie's partner works long hours and often leaves home early in the morning to travel to work. This means that Carrie has to get Paulo up, washed and dressed on her own. This morning Carrie and Paulo arrived half an hour late for a regular appointment with the practice nurse at the local health centre. Carrie doesn't like taking Paulo to see the practice nurse as Celia, the nurse, often makes comments she feels are critical. Celia clearly isn't impressed when Carrie and Paulo arrive late for appointments and has also made comments about them 'looking half-dressed today'. Carrie feels criticised by this and is going to make a complaint if Celia says anything else or looks irritated again when she brings Paulo for his next appointment.

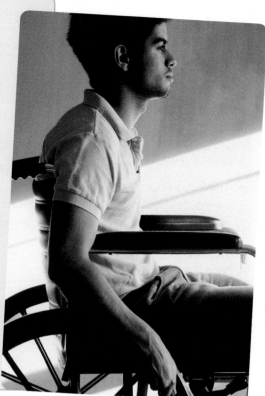

1. What mistake is Celia making in relation to Carrie and her son?

2. What does Celia say or do that suggests she is being judgemental towards Carrie?

3. What do you think Celia could do to deal with this situation in a more constructive way?

Knowledge Assessment Task   1.1   1.2   1.3

You have been asked to take part in a vocational studies day at a nearby secondary school. The pupils at the school are interested in the 'world of work' and have been told that there will be a poster display with information about a range of local jobs. You should produce a poster that could be used on the day. Carry out the following tasks:

1. Describe the duties and responsibilities of your own role.

2. Identify standards that influence the way your work role is carried out.

3. Describe how you ensure that your personal attitudes and beliefs do not obstruct the quality of your work.

Keep your written work as evidence towards your assessment.

Reflecting on own work activities

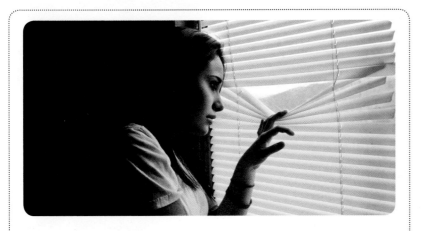

Why use reflection?

Reflection is an important skill for health and social care practitioners. Reflection involves:

- looking inward (contemplating)
- examining your own practice
- thinking about what you have done and the reasons why.

Reflection can lead you to consider your actions and practice from new angles. Being able to look critically at particular experiences or areas of your own practice is now accepted as an important way of learning and developing. You should be able to reflect on both positive and negative aspects of your practice as a care worker. If things are not going so well, or you feel you need support in a particular area, you could follow up your reflections by talking through issues with your colleagues or supervisor. It is this kind of action that helps us to learn from our mistakes and from difficult experiences. Similarly, if a situation has gone extremely well, you can learn from it by reflecting on just how and why it went right. Learning the lessons of success is as important as learning lessons from failure.

Reflection will help to make you more self-aware and your practice more effective. It ensures you consider:

- how best to meet service users' needs
- what your own skills and knowledge are
- how to adapt in different circumstances.

There are lots of opportunities for reflection during the working day, as well as afterwards. For example, opportunities for reflection arise:

- in appraisals or supervision sessions
- during team meetings

Your assessment criteria:

2.1 Explain why reflecting on work activities is an important way to develop knowledge, skills and practice

2.2 Assess how well own knowledge, skills and understanding meet standards

Key terms

Reflection: thinking carefully about something in an open-minded way

Reflect

Do you currently use reflection to improve your care practice? What might be the benefits of using a reflective journal to record your thoughts about practice-related issues?

- ▶ on training courses
- ▶ when talking to colleagues, service users or visitors
- ▶ when thinking about work incidents or events that have happened.

In addition to clarifying your own thoughts, these opportunities may give you the chance to receive feedback, to hear others' perspectives and to see how they deal with issues, problems and challenges.

How can you meet the standard?

Reflection will help you to assess your own development and the extent to which you meet expected standards of performance for your work role. Your work setting may provide guidance on reflection and self-evaluation. Supervision and performance review sessions with your manager, supervisor or tutor may also give you an insight into areas where you need guidance and support and areas where you may benefit from further development.

The process of appraisal

Your regular supervision sessions and annual appraisals provide ideal opportunities to assess the extent to which you meet expected standards of practice. You should be able to discuss the strengths and weaknesses of your performance and skills with your supervisor or manager. To benefit from appraisal, you will need to be totally honest with yourself, without being overly self-critical. The aim of your appraisal is to discuss your past and present performance in your work role and to plan for your future development.

Figure 2.1 What is appraisal?

Appraisal is time to:	Appraisal is *not* time to:
• listen	• be disciplined or told off
• discuss	• moan or complain
• plan.	• be surprised or shocked by what is said.

Key terms

Self-evaluation: assessing your own skills, abilities, achievements and professional development needs

Appraisal: an assessment of an individual's skills, achievements, learning and professional development needs

Reflect

Obtain a copy of the appraisal or performance review forms used in your work setting. Find out what questions are asked and what you are required to reflect upon as part of the appraisal or performance review process. Think about how you achieve expected standards in the way you approach your own work role.

How do you reflect on your work?

Reflection involves being able to stand back and think objectively about:

Your assessment criteria:

2.3 Demonstrate the ability to reflect on work activities

▶ your past and current work performance

▶ whether you are meeting your goals

▶ whether you are achieving the standards of practice expected of someone in your work role.

Reflection is not always easy as you must be totally honest with yourself, and a little bit self-critical. As well as reflecting on your own views, you should also take into account feedback from other people about your work performance. As part of your reflective approach, you will need to be able to think about alternative approaches, activities, strategies and solutions to the opportunities, problems and challenges that exist in your work setting. Figure 2.2 illustrates the reflective process and identifies the kinds of questions that you may ask in order to reflect on an issue, incident or experience.

Description (What happened?)

Feelings (What were you thinking and feeling?)

Action plan (If it happened again what would you do?)

A reflective cycle

Evaluation (What was good and bad about the experience?)

Conclusion (What else could you have done?)

Analysis (What sense can you make of the situation?)

Figure 2.2 Reflective questions

Using a reflective journal

It is a good idea to record your reflections, perhaps in a diary or journal, so that you can look back and consider how things have changed over time. This can also help to focus your attention on areas where you need to develop your knowledge, skills or practice.

It is best to see reflection as an ongoing process of learning and development. You can learn both from your successes and from the situations that haven't gone quite so well. It is important to take a variety of perspectives, including peer observations and service user feedback, into account when reflecting on your performance and practice development.

Case study

Kelly is an experienced care assistant; she has worked on a hospital surgical ward for three years, mainly with adults and older people recovering from back, hip and knee surgery. At the start of the new year, Kelly was transferred to work in the maternity unit outpatients department. Kelly struggled to adapt to the different ways of working, especially the lack of physical care-giving, in the outpatients department. At first she felt overwhelmed by the amount of administrative work and the level of emotional support that many of the women outpatients (and their partners) needed. She wasn't used to listening to people's concerns or to assisting nursing and medical staff with their work. Kelly became unmotivated at times and was seen to be impatient with some of the people who arrived late for appointments. Jane, the unit midwifery manager, asked Kelly to reflect a bit more on her approach to her new role. Kelly wrote down her thoughts and feelings a couple of times a week. This really seemed to help as Kelly became more aware of the needs the pregnant women and their partners have and realised that her role should involve providing more background support, reassurance and information for people. As a result, Kelly felt much happier in her new job and became a more effective team member.

1. What did Kelly need to do in order to reflect on her work role and practice?

2. What do you think were the benefits for Kelly of becoming a more reflective practitioner?

3. How do you think others may have benefited from Kelly's ability to reflect on her practice?

Practical Assessment Task   2.1   2.2   2.3

Reflection is an important part of health and social care practice. Using an appropriate method to record your reflections (such as a written or audio diary or journal), spend some time thinking about aspects of your practice with service users and their relatives. Your assessor will ask you some questions about your reflections in order to assess whether you are able to reflect effectively on your own work activities. You should be able to:

► explain why reflecting on practice is an important way of developing knowledge, skills and practice

► assess how well your own knowledge, skills and understanding meet the standards associated with your job and work setting

► demonstrate the ability to reflect on your work activities.

Your evidence for this assessment activity must be based on your practice in a real work environment.

Agreeing a personal development plan

Your personal development plan

A personal development plan is a document where you record:

▸ **objectives** for your development

▸ activities to meet these objectives

▸ timescales for achieving objectives

▸ timescales for reviewing progress.

A personal development plan should help you to focus your efforts on developing your professional knowledge, skills and practice. You will benefit from the help and support of others when you are completing your personal development plan.

Learners can be supported in a number of different ways (see Figure 2.3) to achieve their learning and development goals. The relevance of each form of support will depend on an individual's particular development needs.

You will probably benefit from several forms of support during your course; you should use all the sources of support that are available to help you address any weaknesses and develop your practice. It is important to know how you can access different sources of support, and to seek help when you need it. Tutors and workplace supervisors see asking for support as a sign of maturity rather than as an indication of incompetence or lack of ability.

Your assessment criteria:

3.1 Identify sources of support for own learning and development

Key terms

Objectives: aims or goals that a person seeks to achieve

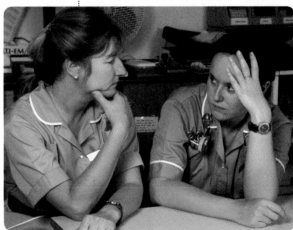

Your supervisor should be able to help you to create a personal development plan

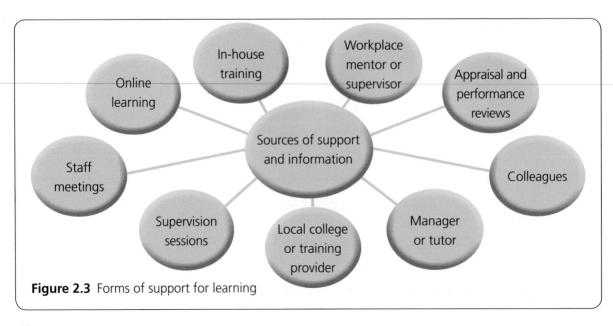

Figure 2.3 Forms of support for learning

Using training opportunities

You may be able to meet your development goals by attending a formal training course or a less formal information study day held at your work setting, at a local college or in a setting managed by external training providers. If you are thinking about taking this approach, you need to ensure that the training opportunities you choose are:

▶ accessible

▶ suitable for your development needs

▶ affordable

▶ achievable within your time constraints.

Larger employers in health and social care sector may offer in-house training during or after work hours. You should try to make the most of these opportunities as they have the added benefit of being based in your workplace around the specific needs of staff in your setting. In addition to any training benefits, participation also contributes to teamwork effectiveness.

Staff meetings

Team members usually meet regularly at staff meetings. Practitioners can discuss practice issues, sharing information about policies and procedures, and good practice solutions. Managers and senior colleagues may also impart information about future developments in the setting. Some settings use staff meetings to allow practitioners to report on training events and courses they have attended. This enables other staff members to share the key learning points, to consider how they may incorporate them into their practice, and to assess whether they too would benefit from attending the course.

Reflect

How do you contribute to staff meetings in your work setting? Do you use them as learning and development opportunities? Think about ways in which you could increase your participation to get more out of the meetings you attend.

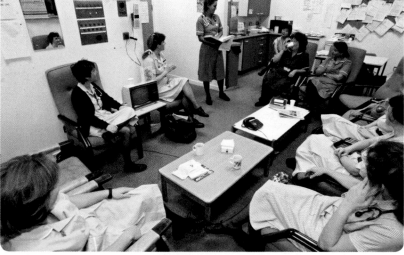

Staff meetings are ideal opportunities to share information and discuss teamwork issues

How do you create your personal development plan?

Agreeing a personal development plan

To create a personal development plan you need to:

▶ assess your skills and abilities at a **baseline** point

▶ develop your understanding of the knowledge, skills and standards of practice that are expected for your work role

▶ construct a plan that will enable you to progress from where you are now to the point you would like to be.

Personal development planning involves collaboration between you and your supervisor. You will need time and support to create your personal development plan. You will certainly have to discuss your training and development needs over the next year or so with your supervisor before you begin writing your plan.

Contributing to your personal development plan

Remember that your personal development plan is a way of addressing your development needs and of achieving progress towards being a more effective care practitioner. So, your personal development plan should specify a range of objectives, being quite specific about how you intend to achieve them.

Identifying development objectives and creating a plan to achieve them is a valuable exercise in breaking down your goals into achievable chunks. Establishing achievable objectives is very important. When people do not achieve their objectives or feel stressed by them, it is often because they are overwhelmed by the size of the task.

The objectives that you set are the destination point in a development journey. They should fill in the knowledge and skills gaps, or address the development needs you identified during the initial self-assessment process. Using the SMART approach is a good way of ensuring you set development goals that you can achieve. That is, each objective should be:

▶ **S**pecific (clear and detailed)

▶ **M**easurable (so you'll know when you've done it)

▶ **A**chievable (realistic)

▶ **R**elevant (addresses a need that you've already identified)

▶ **T**ime-limited (you'll do it by a set time, a deadline).

It is important to set dates for achieving goals and to undertake activities that produce evidence, so you can prove that you are developing.

Key terms

Baseline: the starting point or point at which something is first measured

Reflect

Can you think of any particular development goals that you would like to achieve in the next six months? Consider goals in relation to your knowledge, skills, practice, values, beliefs and career aspirations, for example.

Figure 2.4 A personal development plan

Goals	Actions	Deadline for completion
I want to become a more effective communicator	• Review learning from Diploma unit on communication and induction training • Talk more in meetings – don't be so shy • Volunteer to meet relatives and visitors to the workplace • Concentrate on being an active listener	End Nov (6 months)
I want to develop the skills needed to be a key worker for an individual	• Discuss opportunities to extend skills and responsibilities with manager and supervisor • Seek and take additional training on key worker role and responsibilities. • Arrange to shadow key worker for an individual in the workplace. • Take on key worker role for an individual with supervision from manager/supervisor.	End Nov (6 months)
I want to gain experience of caring for individuals with dementia	• Discuss learning and practice development needs with manager. • Identify opportunities to work with individuals with dementia each week. • Attend in-house dementia workshop and complete dementia awareness module of Diploma course. • Shadow and support colleagues experienced in providing dementia care • Begin working with individuals with dementia on a regular basis	End of August (2 months)
I want to learn to use the computer system to make entries into individual's records	• Attend in-house training workshop and complete online skills course • Begin writing feedback report on individual's using the computer rather than by hand. • Complete Handling Information unit of Diploma course, demonstrating competent skills in computer use.	End of Sept (3 months)
I want to complete my Adult Health and Social Care Diploma	• Plan study time each week and organise course study plan. • Identify learning and assessment opportunities at work every week. • Complete one unit each month, arranging regular assessment of competence	End of July (12 months)

Monitoring and evaluating your plan

To show you are building up skills and knowledge, you will need to monitor your development and progress; your personal development plan is a good tool for this. It should contain information on your current skills, abilities and achievements (the baseline) and your development objectives (where you want to be). Reviewing your progress towards these objectives is a good way of checking whether you have acquired new skills and knowledge.

Being flexible

It is very important to remember that a personal development plan is only a *plan*. In other words, it is about things that you would like to happen but it is also *flexible*. You should see it as a tool to help you achieve your development objectives, giving direction and guidance. You are advised to look at it regularly and to use it as a central part of your ongoing development as a practitioner. You should arrange to discuss and update your plan on a regular basis, so that it always reflects your needs, achievements and objectives in an up-to-date way. Informally, you can ask yourself a number of review questions to assess your development:

▶ Are you making progress towards your objectives?

▶ Are the actions that you have identified to achieve your objectives working?

▶ Have you got the skills and knowledge you need and are you starting to use them in the workplace?

You should remember that if your work or personal circumstances change, it may not be possible for you to meet all of the objectives in your personal development plan within the original time scale. Some or all of your objectives may need to be modified or rescheduled to reflect your new situation. So, it is essential to review your personal development plan and to check your own progress at regular intervals. Do not wait for your six-monthly appraisal or annual performance review meeting when it may be too late to alter things.

Your assessment criteria:

3.1 Identify sources of support for own learning and development

3.2 Describe the process for agreeing a personal development plan and who should be involved

3.3 Contribute to drawing up own personal development plan

Discuss

In a small group or with a work colleague, share your thoughts or ideas in relation to the three questions on the left. Consider whether you have reached a point where you need to change or adapt your personal development plan.

Practical Assessment Task   3.1 3.2 3.3

Personal development planning is an efficient and effective way of ensuring that you identify and focus on your learning and development needs. You should be able to demonstrate that you know how the personal development planning process works in your workplace. Your assessor will ask you to provide evidence showing that you are able to:

▶ identify sources of support that will promote your own learning and development

▶ describe the process used in your workplace for agreeing a personal development plan, identifying the people who are involved in this

▶ contribute to drawing up your own personal development plan.

You may want to make notes to help you to prepare for your assessment. The evidence that you produce for this assessment task must be based on your practice in a real work environment.

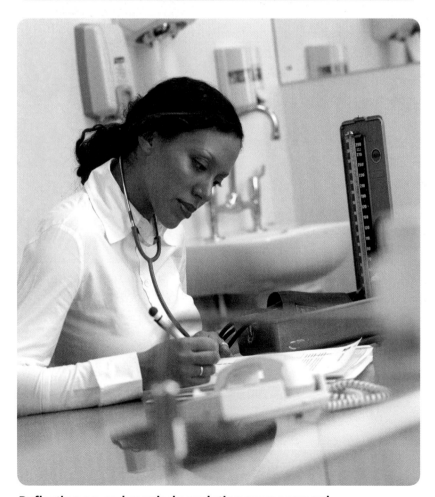

Reflecting on and regularly updating your personal development plan is an important way of ensuring that you keep making progress

How can you improve your knowledge, skills and understanding?

Having worked through this chapter, you should now understand your own work role, know how to reflect on this, and find out about the standards of practice expected of you. You should also have agreed a personal development plan. Here we will look at ways of developing your own knowledge, skills and understanding in order to become a better practitioner.

Improvement through learning activities

When you have agreed a personal development plan, the next step is to develop your knowledge, skills and understanding in ways that meet your development needs. As well as increasing your confidence, training and other development activity should:

▶ broaden and deepen your knowledge

▶ improve and extend your range of skills.

Although learning and development can happen without planning, having a personal development plan to reflect on will enable you to achieve your development goals more effectively. However, you should remember that going on courses and attending training events will not automatically result in your development. You need to think and do things differently before you can claim that you have learnt something new.

Your assessment criteria:

4.1 Show how a learning activity has improved own knowledge, skills and understanding

4.2 Show how reflecting on a situation has improved own knowledge, skills and understanding

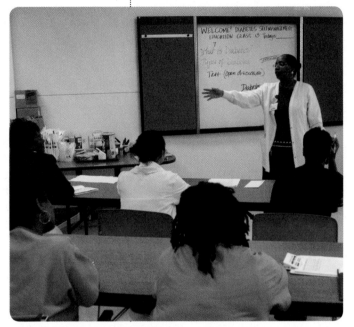

Short courses and organised training sessions are effective ways of extending knowledge

---

Practical Assessment Task   4.1

Identify some examples of learning activities (either formal or informal) that you have participated in and which you believe you have learnt from. Your assessor will need to know:

▶ what the learning activities involved

▶ how you participated in the learning activities

▶ how the learning activities improved your knowledge, skills and understanding.

Keep any notes you write as evidence towards your assessment. Your evidence for this assessment activity must be based on your practice and experience in a real work environment.

Improvement through reflection

Reflection should enable you to improve the knowledge, skills and understanding you have in relation to:

- ▶ interactions with service users and their relatives
- ▶ interventions and activities you provide for service users
- ▶ relationships with colleagues and visitors to the setting
- ▶ your input into team activities and meetings
- ▶ your relationships with service users.

Reflection will enable you to build on your achievements and address weaknesses in your performance, always aiming to become a better practitioner. To achieve this you need to be able to:

- ▶ reflect in action – that is, to think on your feet to deal with issues that arise unexpectedly (a resident or service user's aggression, for example)
- ▶ reflect on action – that is, to think through issues after the event (perhaps, how an activity or intervention could have been managed differently).

Your ability to use reflection will help in your relationships with service users and colleagues. Service users and their families will expect you to be able to sum up their progress and response to care and treatment in a courteous, respectful and constructive way. Reflecting on your practice, on your observations of service users and on your relationships with them and their relatives or visitors will help you to become a more professional and effective practitioner.

Reflect

Can you think of an instance where you have either reflected in action or reflected on your past actions and been able to improve your practice as a result?

Practical Assessment Task   4.2

How has the use of reflection helped to improve your practice or promote your learning and development? Your assessor will ask you about your use of reflection in the workplace. He or she will require evidence that shows how reflecting on a situation has improved your own knowledge, skills and understanding. You can produce this evidence by carrying out the following task:

1. Identify and describe a practice situation that you have reflected on.
2. Describe how the process of reflection helped you to learn from the situation or develop some aspect of your knowledge, skills or understanding.

Keep any notes you write as evidence towards your assessment. Your evidence for this assessment activity must be based on your practice and experience in a real work environment.

How can you use feedback to improve your performance?

Being open to feedback is one of the hardest aspects of working and studying, especially if you receive critical comments. When this happens you may be defensive or dismissive as a way of protecting yourself. Instead, you should listen carefully, keep any feedback in perspective and try to respond constructively. Ask for clear examples of any areas of weakness or underperformance, for ideas about how you could improve in these areas and for suggestions about who could help you to improve.

Your assessment criteria:

4.3 Show how feedback from others has developed own knowledge, skills and understanding

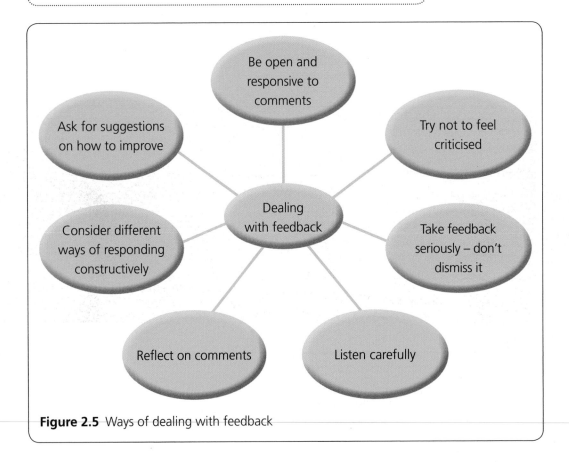

Figure 2.5 Ways of dealing with feedback

Feedback from professional practitioners can help you to develop your knowledge and skills quickly, which can be especially helpful when you are settling into a new role. However, be wary of reading too much into comments from your friends at work and take no notice of anyone who encourages you to take short cuts to save on time and effort. Possible sources of feedback from colleagues include team meetings, communication books or diaries and informal conversations. Good team spirit, approaches for help or advice, and people wanting to work with you are good indications that you are making a positive contribution to practice.

You may receive feedback formally and informally through, for example:

▶ appraisals

▶ mentoring

▶ team meetings

▶ training opportunities

▶ peer observations

▶ service users' questionnaires or feedback

▶ conversations with colleagues and visitors.

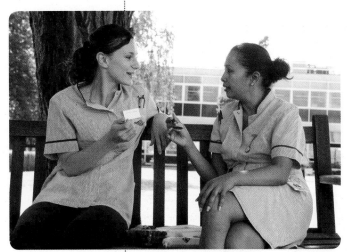

Colleagues can give you constructive feedback on both the positive and less effective aspects of your care practice

Formal appraisals provide feedback on performance, specifically whether you are meeting expected standards of practice. The aim is to acknowledge competence and identify areas for improvement, not to criticise you.

Mentors are a good source of feedback: they may be models of good practice, or may offer you advice and guidance. Colleague feedback from people who often observe you can be constructive. Questionnaire responses from service users and their relatives provide a very important source of feedback. You need to take on board their feelings, observations and comments, even though they may see things very differently from you. Feedback from service users can really help you to improve your practice – you will get a better view of how they see you and experience your practice.

You need to be honest when giving feedback to people and open-minded when receiving it.

How can you record your personal progress?

Your assessment criteria:

4.3 Show how feedback from others has developed own knowledge, skills and understanding

4.4 Show how to record progress in relation to personal development

You need to collect evidence of your personal development for performance review and appraisal purposes. However, it is also important for you to be able to see what you have achieved compared to your development plan. A portfolio of evidence containing your curriculum vitae (CV), certificates, personal development plan and other evidence of your progress can be a boost to your confidence and professional self-image too. You can record evidence of your progress, development and achievements in:

▶ your CV

▶ your portfolio of achievement

▶ a training folder or file kept at work

▶ other workplace records.

Your records

Use your CV to demonstrate your knowledge and experience. You should record your school and college qualifications, as well as any other professional development courses that you have undertaken. It is useful to keep your CV on a computer as this makes updating and sending the document easy. Having an up-to-date CV means you can apply for posts that come up unexpectedly.

A portfolio of achievement is typically a file containing your certificates and records of training and development. It can be given to prospective employers to demonstrate what you have done. A training folder or file may contain your personal development plan and appraisal documents, as well as records about training events you have attended.

Keep your records in a file or portfolio that is easy to access and update

Practical Assessment Task

4.3 **4.4**

Feedback from others is an important source of information that can be used to help you to learn and develop your practice. In this final activity, you will need to demonstrate to your assessor:

▶ how feedback from others (colleagues, service users or your manager, for example) has enabled you to develop your own knowledge, skills and understanding of your work role and practice

▶ that you are able to record progress in relation to your learning and development in an appropriate and effective way.

Keep any notes you write as evidence towards your assessment. Your evidence for this assessment activity must be based on your practice and experience in a real work environment.

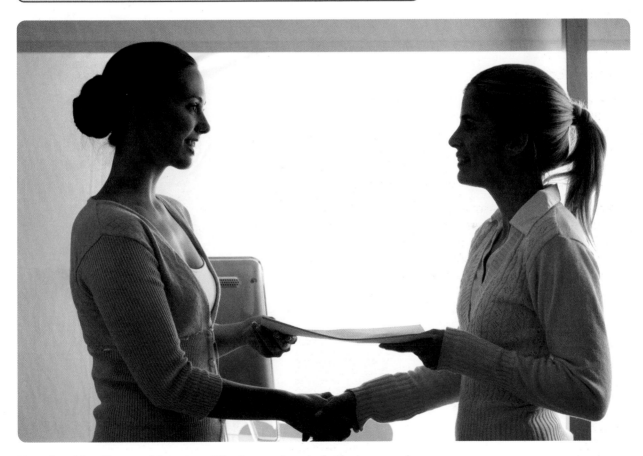

You should collect and keep certificates and awards that you gain as they provide evidence of your achievements and ability

Are you ready for assessment?

AC	What do you know now?	Assessment task	✓
1.1	Describe the duties and responsibilities of own work role	Page 43	
1.2	Identify the standards that influence the way the role is carried out	Page 43	
1.3	Describe ways to ensure that personal attitudes or beliefs do not obstruct the quality of work	Page 43	

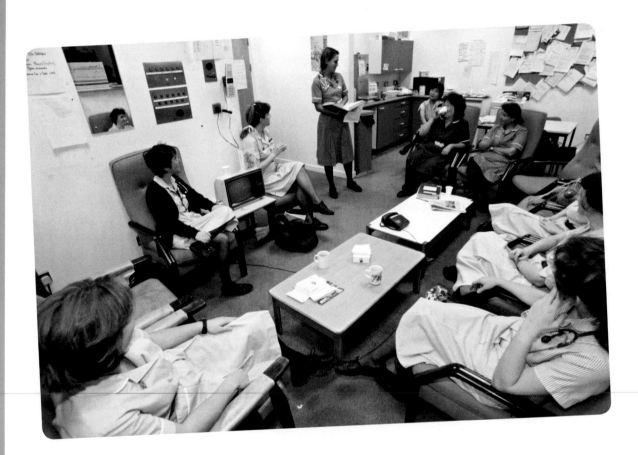

AC	What can you do now?	Assessment task	✓
2.1	Explain why reflecting on practice is an important way to develop knowledge, skills and practice	Page 47	
2.2	Assess how well your own knowledge, skills and understanding meet standards	Page 47	
2.3	Demonstrate the ability to reflect on work activities	Page 47	
3.1	Identify sources of support for own learning and development	Page 53	
3.2	Describe the process for agreeing a personal development plan and who should be involved	Page 53	
3.3	Contribute to drawing up own personal development plan	Page 53	
4.1	Show how a learning activity has improved own knowledge, skills and understanding	Page 54	
4.2	Show how reflecting on a situation has improved own knowledge, skills and understanding	Page 55	
4.3	Show how feedback from others has developed own knowledge, skills and understanding	Page 59	
4.4	Explain how and when to seek advice about confidentiality	Page 59	

3 | Introduction to equality and inclusion in health and social care settings (SHC 23)

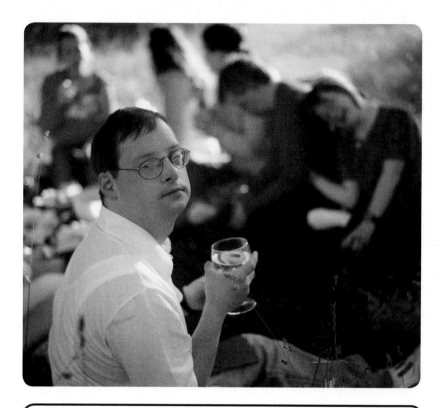

Assessment of this unit

This unit introduces you to the concepts of equality and inclusion and their importance in work with people in health and social care settings. It focuses on the meaning of key words and ideas relating to equality and inclusion, forms of discrimination that can occur in care settings and legal aspects of health and social care work. You will also develop your knowledge of ways of working with people in an inclusive, anti-discriminatory way and the sources of information, advice and support that you could use to develop your practice in this area.

To successfully complete this unit you will need to produce evidence of your knowledge of concepts, practices and the law relating to equality and inclusion as shown in the 'What you need to know' chart opposite. You also need to produce evidence of your practical ability to promote equality and work in an inclusive way in your workplace, as shown in the 'What you need to do' chart.

Your tutor or assessor will help you to prepare for your assessment and the tasks suggested in the chapter will help you to create the evidence that you need.

CHAPTER 3

AC   What you need to know

1.1	The meaning of diversity, equality, inclusion and discrimination
1.2	The ways in which discrimination may deliberately or inadvertently occur in the work setting
1.3	How practices that support equality and inclusion reduce the likelihood of discrimination
3.1	A range of sources of information, advice and support about diversity, equality and inclusion
3.2	How and when to access information, advice and support about diversity, equality and inclusion

AC   What you need to do

2.1	Identify which legislation and codes of practice relating to equality, diversity and discrimination apply to your own work role
2.2	Show you can interact with individuals in ways that respect their beliefs, culture, values and preferences
2.3	Describe how to challenge discrimination in a way that encourages change

Assessment criteria 2.1–2.3 must be assessed in a real work environment.

This unit also links to some of the other units:

HSC 026	Implement person-centred approaches in health and social care
CMH 02	Understand mental health problems
SSMU 2.1	Introductory awareness of sensory loss

Some of your learning will be repeated in these units and will give you the chance to review your knowledge and understanding.

Understanding the importance of equality and inclusion

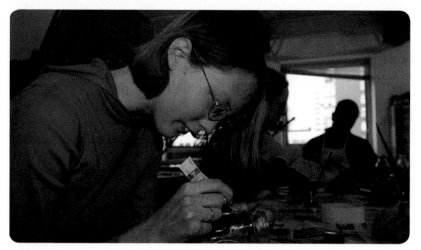

Creative activities are a practical way of promoting inclusion and interaction in care settings

Key terms

Diversity: the range of differences (social, cultural, language, ethnic, ability and disability) within a population

What are diversity, equality and inclusion?

Diversity

As a care practitioner you will work with colleagues, service users and other adults from a wide range of social, cultural, language and ethnic backgrounds. You will work with men and women, people with different types of ability and disability, individuals who speak different languages and who have different cultural traditions, as well as people who could be described as middle class, working class, as 'black', 'white' or of mixed heritage. You should value and treat each person fairly and equally.

The **diversity** of the United Kingdom population is vast; if you think about the local area where you live, you can probably identify a number of different sub-groups within the community. This means that the population consists of individuals with a huge range of different characteristics. These differences impact on people's needs. As a result, you have a responsibility to value difference as a way of meeting people's individual needs.

Figure 3.1 Religious diversity in the UK

Ethnic group	Population	Proportion of total UK population
White	54,153,898	92.1%
Mixed race	677,177	1.2%
Indian	1,053,144	1.8%
Pakistani	747,285	1.3%
Bangaldeshi	283,063	0.5%
Other Asian (non-Chinese)	247,644	0.4%
Black Caribbean	565,876	1.0%
Black African	485,277	0.8%
Black (others)	97,585	0.2%
Chinese	247,403	0.4%
Others	230,615	0.4%

Equality

You will probably know from your own experience of service users, and perhaps from being a service user yourself, that people who need care want to be treated equally and fairly. This doesn't always mean that all service users should be treated *the same*. Equality in health and social care settings is about making sure each person has the appropriate opportunities to receive care and treatment, and to make decisions to the best of their ability and in line with their own interests. Your role as a care practitioner will involve informing and supporting each individual so that they benefit from forms of care, services and facilities that are best suited to their particular needs. Valuing service users as individuals is a very important first step in promoting this kind of equality of opportunity.

Inclusion

A health or social care service must promote social inclusion in order to offer equality of opportunity to those who use it. An inclusive health or social care service works hard at:

▸ identifying and removing barriers to access and participation

▸ enabling people to use the full range of services and facilities

▸ welcoming, valuing and supporting everyone who uses the care setting.

Inclusion doesn't happen by chance. The people who work in health and social care settings have to:

▸ be honest and reflective about how their workplace operates

▸ be critical in a constructive way, so that positive changes can be made

▸ work at identifying *actual* barriers to access and participation

▸ remain alert to *potential* barriers that may exclude some people

▸ act in practical ways to remove actual and potential barriers

▸ place the individuals who need care at the centre of planning and support-giving processes.

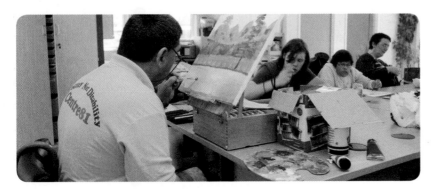

Inclusion is about providing opportunities for all

Investigate

How is the individuality of each service user acknowledged and celebrated in the care setting where you work or where you are on placement? Find out about the way in which a person's background, abilities and achievements are assessed and documented, for example. You might also think about the ways in which practitioners talk to service users, and talk about them to others, providing feedback on their particular abilities, achievements or needs.

Key terms

Equality: treating a person fairly or in a way that ensures they are not disadvantaged

Equality of opportunity: a situation in which everyone has an equal chance

Social inclusion: the process of ensuring that all members of society have access to available services and activities

Reflect

How diverse is your work setting? Do people from a diverse range of social and cultural backgrounds use the services? Are members of some social or cultural groups noticeably less well represented or absent altogether?

What is discrimination?

Diversity is not welcomed or celebrated by everyone, despite the fact that the UK has been a multicultural society for many years. Diversity and difference frightens some people, leading to a view of people as either 'them' or 'us'. This can result in unfair treatment or **discrimination** against those who are different from the majority. People who use or work in health and social care services can suffer discrimination due to:

▶ skin colour and other physical characteristics

▶ disability or health status

▶ gender (as a man or a woman)

▶ social background and family circumstances

▶ culture, traditions and way of life.

Unfair discrimination that is obvious and deliberate is known as **direct discrimination**. Unfair discrimination that happens inadvertently or which is carried out in a secretive, hidden way is known as **indirect discrimination**.

Prejudice is at the root of discrimination. A prejudice is an opinion, feeling or attitude of dislike concerning another individual or group of people. Prejudices are typically based on inaccurate information or unreasonable judgements. When a person acts on a prejudice, they become involved in discrimination. People are not born with prejudices – these have to be learnt (see Figure 3.3). However, children can be quick to pick up these views if they hear others talking in a prejudiced way. Acknowledging diversity, challenging prejudices and tackling all forms of discrimination are important elements of anti-discriminatory practice in health and social care work.

Your assessment criteria:

1.1 Explain what is meant by diversity, equality, inclusion and discrimination

Key terms

Discrimination: unfair or less favourable treatment of a person or group of people in comparison to others

Direct discrimination: obvious and deliberate unfair treatment

Indirect discrimination: unfair treatment that occurs inadvertently

Prejudice: an unreasonable or unfair dislike or preference towards a person or a group of people

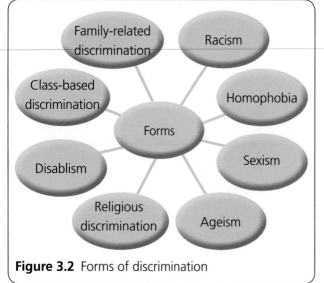

Figure 3.2 Forms of discrimination

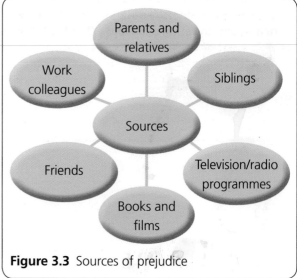

Figure 3.3 Sources of prejudice

Case study

In 1963 Jane Elliot, a teacher in a small primary school in the USA, carried out an experiment. She divided the children in her class into two groups based on their eye colour. On the first day of the experiment the blue-eyed children were told that they were the better group and were treated more favourably. They had more privileges such as second helpings at lunchtime and extra playtime. Jane Elliot also ridiculed the brown-eyed children and continually put them down. On the second day, she made the brown-eyed children the favoured group. This time they had all of the advantages and the blue-eyed children were told they were the bottom group.

Imagine that you were one of the children in Jane Elliott's class.

1. How would you have felt on the day you were in the less favoured group?

2. How do you think you would have felt when you were told you weren't as good as other children because of the colour of your eyes?

3. How do you think you would have reacted towards your friends when they were in the favoured group?

4. How do you think you would have felt when you were in the favoured group?

The results of Jane Elliot's experiment were startling. Children of different eye-colour who had previously been friends fought and put each other down. When children were in the favoured group, they did better in maths and word tests than the children who were not. The same children performed badly when they were in the other group. Jane Elliot concluded that self-esteem and self-image were adversely affected when children experienced discrimination.

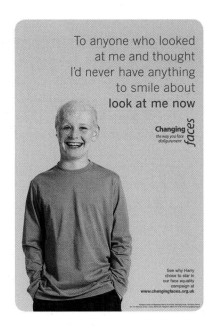

To anyone who looked at me and thought I'd never have anything to smile about look at me now

Changing faces
the way you face disfigurement

See why Harry chose to star in our face equality campaign at www.changingfaces.org.uk

Knowledge Assessment Task   1.1

You have been asked by your workplace manager to produce a leaflet or a poster as part of an inclusion campaign. The aim is to raise care practitioners' awareness of equality and inclusion issues in health and social care settings. Your leaflet or poster should explain what *diversity*, *equality*, *inclusion* and *discrimination* mean in relation to practice in your setting; use words and images to communicate the meaning of each term as clearly as possible. Keep the work you produce as evidence towards your assessment.

Why does discrimination happen in health and social care settings?

Your assessment criteria:

1.2 Describe ways in which discrimination may deliberately or inadvertently occur in the work setting

As Jane Elliot's experiment showed, discrimination can damage a person's self-esteem and self-confidence, and is a barrier to equality of opportunity. So, discrimination should always be avoided in health and social care settings. Where discrimination does occur, health or social care practitioners should be able to recognise and challenge it.

Health and social care practitioners and organisations generally aim to be inclusive and welcoming to everybody who wishes to use their services. Despite this, overt discrimination does sometimes occur in health and social care settings. This can be the result of:

▶ individual staff members favouring some service users or treating others in a less favourable way because of prejudices that they hold

▶ health and social care organisations deliberately setting out to attract or admit service users from particular backgrounds or areas, while making it difficult for others to obtain places

▶ members of staff expressing their prejudices, values and beliefs in the way they talk to service users, relatives or their colleagues

▶ employment policies that result in staff being recruited from a narrow range of backgrounds and age groups

▶ a gender-biased approach to providing care, treatment or leisure activities for men and women

▶ not adapting or providing facilities and services for people who have disabilities, language or communication needs or mental health problems, for example.

Key terms

Stereotypes: set and often ill-informed generalised ideas, for example, about the way people from certain backgrounds behave or feel

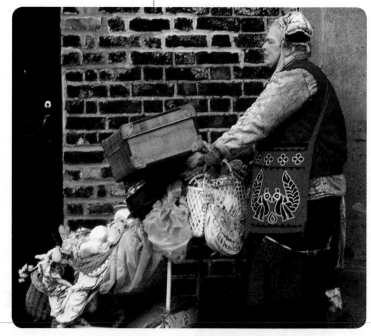

Prejudices about homelessness, mental illness and substance misuse can lead to discrimination in health and social care settings

Deliberate discrimination within health and social care settings is relatively unusual. Where discrimination does occur it usually happens inadvertently or by accident. Health or social care practitioners may not be aware that the way they practise, talk or operate the service favours some people but disadvantages others. This can happen because:

▶ some practitioners lack cultural awareness and knowledge about the lifestyles of different groups

▶ health or social care practitioners may promote gender or cultural **stereotypes** by encouraging people to adopt particular work or domestic roles or by responding to people's behaviour in stereotypical ways

▶ information leaflets and other resources are outdated, gender- or culture-specific

▶ admissions policies and practices in the setting impose conditions that some people are unable to meet

▶ diversity and difference is not celebrated (for example, by celebrating different cultural festivals or telling of stories from a wide range of cultural traditions)

▶ the recruitment process results in the selection of applicants who will 'fit in' because they are 'people like us'.

Reflect

How socially and culturally diverse is the staff group in the health or social care setting where you work or are on placement? Is the staff group representative of the local community?

Investigate

Look at and review the range of leisure and recreational resources available for people in the care setting where you work or are on placement. Do the books, games, equipment and visual images Reflect a diversity of lifestyles, traditions and social backgrounds?

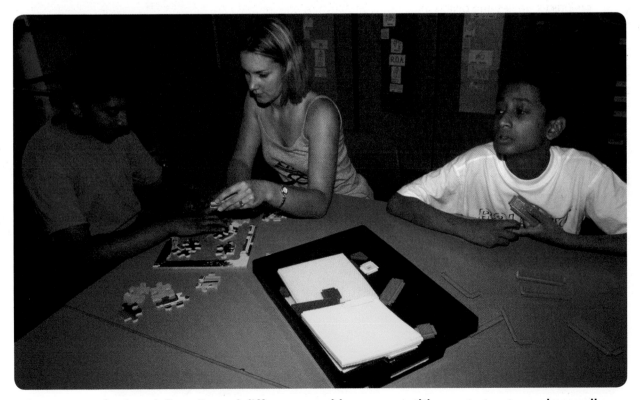

Awareness of cultural diversity and difference enables care practitioners to treat people equally and with respect

How can you promote equality and inclusion?

Seeing each service user or colleague with whom you work as an individual with unique qualities and particular needs is an important way of avoiding the stereotyping that sometimes leads to inadvertent discrimination. As a health or social care practitioner, you should be able to provide support, assistance and care for each person in ways that are appropriate to their abilities, interests and needs. Strategies for promoting equality and inclusion include:

▶ valuing individuals equally whilst acknowledging their individuality and differences

▶ using effective communication skills to develop strong and trusting relationships with all service users and their families

▶ adapting your approach to each individual's particular needs so that they obtain the support and assistance required to enjoy equality of opportunity

▶ ensuring that people from diverse backgrounds are represented in the range of images and resources (posters, books, displays, leaflets, DVDs, photographs) that service users and visitors see in the setting

▶ using resources that challenge stereotypes by showing both men and women in caring, employment and leadership roles, disabled people undertaking a full range of activities and people from a variety of cultural backgrounds in everyday life situations.

Your assessment criteria:

1.2 Describe ways in which discrimination may deliberately or inadvertently occur in the work setting

1.3 Explain how practices that support equality and inclusion reduce the likelihood of discrimination

Reflect

What do you do within your care practice to promote equality and inclusion? Try to identify two or three ways in which you do, or could do, this.

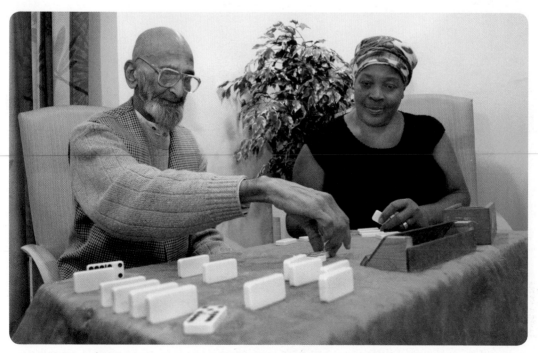

Giving people choices and providing opportunities for them to pursue their interests is a way of respecting individuals' rights and identity

The ways in which gender, ethnicity, culture and social background are portrayed in a person's early years have an impact on the expectations they develop about their future. Everyone should be encouraged and supported to believe that they can:

▶ take an active role in society

▶ achieve success in a variety of ways

▶ aspire to valued, responsible and influential positions in life.

Reflect

How are service users who use English as an additional language included and supported in the setting where you work or are on placement? Do you think anything else could be done to improve the inclusion of people with language support needs?

Knowledge Assessment Task 1.2 1.3

You have been asked to produce an information leaflet that could be included in the induction training materials given to new employees at your workplace. Your manager has asked you to produce an informative leaflet that:

▶ describes ways in which discrimination may deliberately or inadvertently occur in the work setting

▶ explains how promoting equality and inclusion reduces the likelihood of discrimination occurring.

Your leaflet should include practical examples and suggestions relevant to the people who use your setting. It can include images, words, diagrams and tables but should focus on how discrimination occurs and how it can be prevented through equality and inclusion strategies. Keep your written work as evidence towards your assessment.

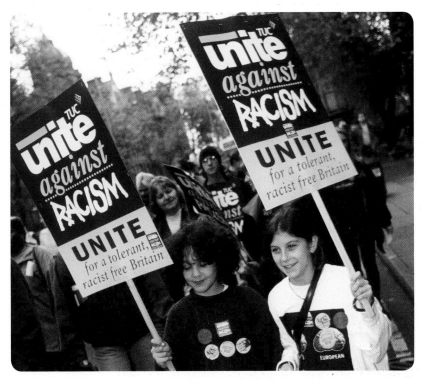

Anti-discriminatory practice challenges prejudices such as racism

Working in an inclusive way

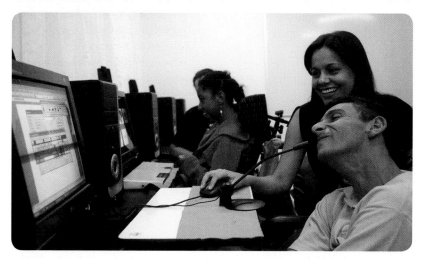

With adapted equipment and aids, many people can overcome their disabilities to participate more fully in work and education

Your assessment criteria:

2.1 Identify which legislation and codes of practice relating to equality, diversity and discrimination apply to own role

Key terms

Legislation: another term for written laws, such as Acts of Parliament

Code of practice: a document setting out standards for practice

Policies: plans of action

Procedures: documents that specify ways of doing something or dealing with a specific issue or problem

What is the legal framework for health and social care practice?

Health and social care practitioners have to work within a framework of legislation, codes of practice, policies and procedures that are designed to promote equality and inclusion and prevent discrimination.

The health and social care legal framework promotes diversity and protects the rights of individuals (service users, families and practitioners) in care settings. You need to be able to identify examples of legislation, codes of practice and policies and procedures relating to equality, diversity, discrimination that affect your role. You should also know about the legal responsibilities health and social care employers and employees have for promoting diversity and rights.

In health and social care settings, the main statutes promoting diversity and equality and protecting people from discrimination are:

▶ The Human Rights Act (1998)

▶ The Race Relations Act (1976) and the Race Relations (Amendment) Act (2000)

▶ The Disability Discrimination Act (1995) and (2005)

▶ The Special Educational Needs and Disability Act (2001)

▶ The Public Order and Racial and Religious Hatred Act (2006).

These laws influence the rights of individuals and standards of quality in care provision. Every health and social care organisation needs to have policies and practices that put these laws into action.

The Equality and Human Rights Commission is an independent public body responsible for:

▶ providing information and advice on equalities issues

▶ working with employers, service providers and organisations to help them develop best practice on equalities issues

▶ working with policymakers, lawyers and the government to make sure that social policy and the law promote equality

▶ enforcing anti-discrimination laws to tackle unfair treatment and discrimination.

The Human Rights Act (1998) (updated 2000)

This piece of legislation is an important equality law that gives people who live in the UK a range of basic human rights. The right to life and the right to freedom from unfair discrimination can be used to gain access to health and social care services. The Act helps people who have disabilities or who feel they are being discriminated against to assert their rights to care. This now includes the right not to be evicted from a care home if the owners believe that an individual's needs have become too expensive for them to meet.

Investigate

Use the Equality and Human Rights Commission website (www.equalityhumanrights.com) to find out about the rights of disabled people and those with mental health problems.

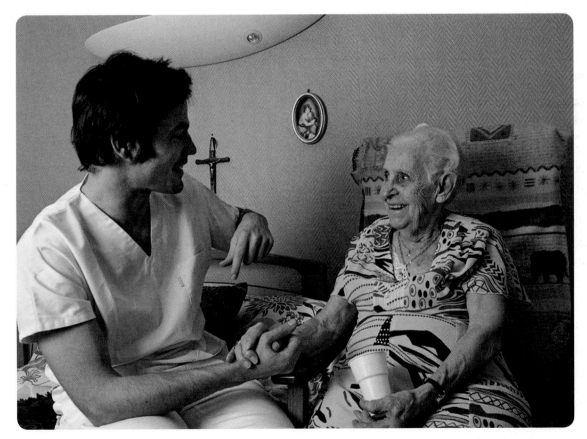

Acknowledging and accepting an individual's beliefs and identity is an important part of care practice

The Race Relations Act (1976) and Race Relations (Amendment) Act (2000)

The Race Relations Act (1976) made racial discrimination unlawful. The Act defined racial discrimination as 'less favourable treatment on racial grounds'. The Race Relations (Amendment) Act (2000) extended and strengthened the 1976 law by making racial discrimination by public authorities, such as the Police, NHS and local authorities, unlawful. These Race Relations Acts aim to eradicate racial discrimination and to promote equal opportunities for members of all ethnic groups.

The Public Order Act (1986) and the Racial and Religious Hatred Act (2006)

The Public Order Act (1986) made it an offence to use words or behaviour, or to display written material, that is intended to stir up racial hatred. The Racial and Religious Hatred Act 2006 also made it an offence to engage in acts intended to stir up religious hatred.

The Disability Discrimination Act (1995) and (2005)

This Act safeguards the rights of disabled people; 'less favourable treatment' of disabled people in employment, the provision of goods and services, education and transport is unlawful. The aim of the Act is to ensure that disabled people receive equal opportunities and that employers, traders, transport and education providers make 'reasonable adjustments' to their premises and services to allow access.

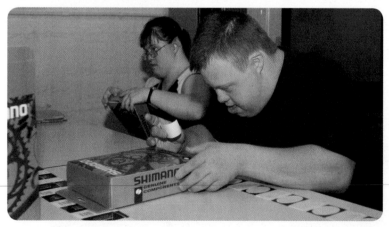

It is illegal to treat people with disabilities less favourably simply because they have some form of disability

The Special Educational Needs and Disability Act (2001)

This Act was created to help establish legal rights for disabled children and those with special educational needs in compulsory and post-16 education, training and other student services. It extended the Disability Discrimination Act (1995) and sought to prevent unjustified discrimination against disabled learners of all ages.

Reflect

Which of these pieces of legislation have you heard of, if any? What impact do you think each may have on your own work role and the way that you practice and provide care or support?

Case study

Alex, aged 42, signed on with a recruitment agency to do temporary care work. When he applied, Alex made it clear to the agency that he has a hearing impairment and uses a hearing aid and lip reading to communicate in face-to-face situations. Alex's previous experience as a health care support worker seemed to make him suitable for the type of work the agency was advertising. After he had completed an application form and sent in various documents, the agency asked Alex to take part in a telephone interview using *TypeTalk* (a telephone service for hearing-impaired people). Despite a good interview performance, the recruitment agency said that Alex was unsuitable for the work they had because of his hearing impairment. Alex reported the agency to the Equality and Human Rights Commission and is intending to take them to court on the grounds of 'disability discrimination'.

1. What kind of disability does Alex have?
2. How has Alex experienced disability discrimination in this situation?
3. What rights does Alex have under the Disability Discrimination Acts?

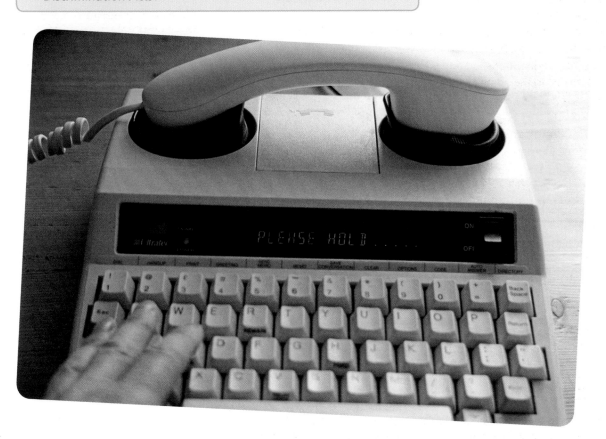

The Equality Act 2006 and 2010

The 2006 Act created the Equality and Human Rights Commission, outlawed discrimination relating to religion, belief and sexual orientation and placed a duty on public bodies to promote gender equality. The main aim of the 2010 Act was to bring together and simplify a range of complicated anti-discrimination laws in Great Britain. The Equality Act 2010 requires equal treatment in access to employment as well as private and public services for all people regardless of their age, disability, marital status, race, religion or belief, gender/sex, or sexual orientation. Employers and service providers are under a duty to make reasonable adjustments to their workplaces to overcome barriers experienced by disabled people.

Codes of practice

Codes of practice provide guidelines on implementing the often complicated legislation that affects health and social care practice. Examples of codes of practice relevant to your work in health and social care settings include:

▶ the codes of practice on equalities issues produced by the Equalities and Human Rights Commission

▶ the codes of practice for social care workers and employers of social care workers produced by the General Social Care Council (www.gscc.org.uk)

▶ the standards of proficiency for registered health professionals produced by the Health Professions Council (www.hpc-uk.org)

▶ the code of conduct for registered nurses and midwives produced by the Nursing and Midwifery Council (www.nmc.org.uk).

Codes of practice provide guidance and rules on ways of implementing legislation and policy, as well as guidance on professional standards of behaviour and standards of practice. They identify what health and social care practitioners should do in specific situations.

Government charters identify entitlement to services and define national standards of care that people can expect to receive; the policies produced by individual care organisations also incorporate the legal framework of health and social care and should be used in practice by all employees.

Your assessment criteria:

2.1 Identify which legislation and codes of practice relating to equality, diversity and discrimination apply to own role

Investigate

Use the Equality and Human Rights Commission website (www.equalityhumanrights.com) to find out about the rights of disabled children and adults.

Investigate

What does the inclusion policy in the setting where you work or are on placement say about treatment and integration of disabled people? Find out and make some notes on how this affects your role as a health or social care practitioner.

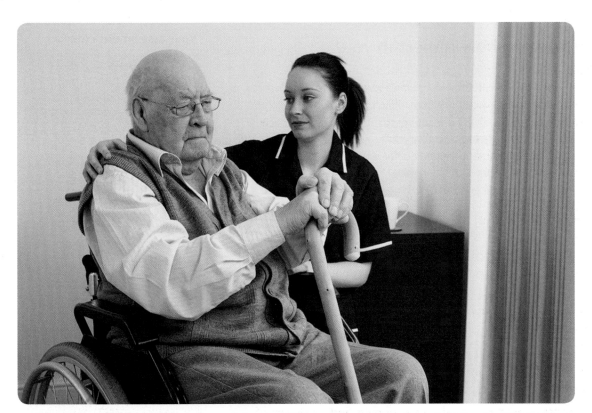

Codes of practice provide care practitioners with guidance on ways of delivering inclusive and non-discriminatory care and support for service users

Practical Assessment Task   2.1

How do legislation and codes of practice influence the ways in which you practise in your work setting? Create a table identifying the ways in which the legal framework affecting work with health and social care provision influences the way you promote equality and diversity and challenge discrimination through your work role.

Your evidence for this task must be based on your practice in a real work environment and must be presented in a format acceptable to your assessor.

Example of legislation	How does this affect your practice?

How can you show respect in your interactions?

Interacting with service users and their families in ways that clearly demonstrate respect is a very important part of inclusive practice in health and social care settings. Everybody who uses your care setting should be valued and respected for who they are, whatever their physical characteristics or their social or cultural background. People feel respected when you:

▶ treat them as an equal while recognising their individual needs, wishes and preferences

▶ acknowledge and recognise that their beliefs, culture and traditions are an important part of who they are

▶ use inclusive, non-discriminatory language that avoids stereotypes, prejudices and **stigmatised** terms

▶ are open-minded and prepared to discuss their needs, issues and concerns in a way that recognises the unique qualities of each person, as well as the characteristics they share with others

▶ show interest in their cultural and religious traditions and take part in an appropriate way in celebrating festivals and events that are significant for them and their community.

Your assessment criteria:

2.2 Show interaction with individuals that respects their beliefs, culture, values and preferences

Key terms

Stigmatised: socially disapproved of

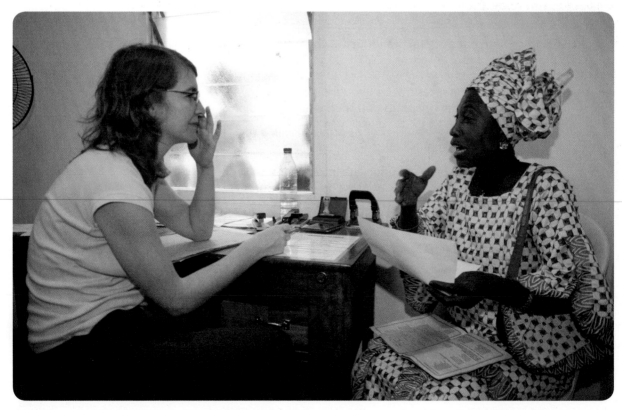

Careful, active listening is an important part of showing respect in care-related interactions

Case study

Edith Goldman, aged 83, is no longer able to live independently. Her son has reluctantly decided that Edith needs to move to a care home. He has tried to talk to Edith about her needs and what she would like but is unsure how much Edith is able to understand. Edith has a diagnosis of dementia and has been supported at home by two home care workers for the past year. Both of the home care workers were Jewish and understood Edith's religious and cultural needs. Edith had very strong connections with the Jewish community in her local area and was a regular visitor to her local synagogue before she became too unwell to attend. Edith's son is now looking for a Jewish nursing home, as he knows that Edith's faith and Jewish customs and traditions have been important to her throughout her life.

1. Identify two aspects of care provision that would need to take Edith's religious beliefs into account.

2. How might the care staff at a Jewish care home help Edith to express her religious faith?

3. Explain why it would be better for Edith to live in a Jewish care home rather than a secular (non-religious) home.

Practical Assessment Task   2.2

How do you use your interactions with service users and their families to show respect for their culture, beliefs, values and preferences? Complete an interaction diary over the next week, recording when your approach and behaviour showed respect for individuals':

▶ beliefs and culture

▶ values

▶ preferences.

You should use examples that were witnessed by a senior colleague, your workplace assessor or manager; ask that person to confirm that you did show respect during the interactions you describe. Your evidence for this task must be based on your practice in a real work environment and must be witnessed by, or be in a format acceptable to, your assessor.

How can you challenge discrimination and encourage change?

Your assessment criteria:

2.3 Describe how to challenge discrimination in a way that encourages change

Equality and inclusion for all service users requires that everyone in a health or social care setting is committed to anti-discriminatory practice. You can ensure that your own practice is inclusive and non-discriminatory by:

▶ showing equal concern for all service users

▶ valuing difference and individuality

▶ valuing the personal beliefs of everyone you work with

▶ developing your knowledge and awareness of the lifestyles, beliefs and traditions of people from a variety of cultures, but particularly those represented in your local community

▶ organising and taking part in activities and events that celebrate the religious and cultural traditions of the local communities

▶ using non-discriminatory language

▶ promoting positive images of a diverse range of people and cultures

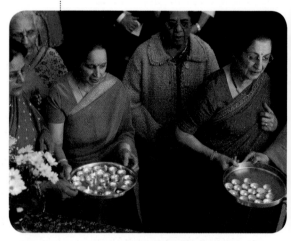

Awareness of religious and cultural traditions is a part of inclusive practice

▶ showing that you have high expectations of yourself and others

▶ adapting the physical environment of the setting so that people of all ages, abilities and disabilities can use the facilities easily

▶ asking questions, raising concerns and contributing to discussions about inclusion, discrimination and equality of opportunity

▶ becoming familiar with the inclusion and equal opportunities policies and procedures of the setting

▶ intervening if you witness people using discriminatory language, stereotypes, prejudices or discriminatory behaviour

▶ pointing out that such language or behaviour is not acceptable and can be hurtful to others, being clear that you object to the language or behaviour but are not rejecting the person who uses it

▶ providing an example of appropriate language to enable the person to avoid making the same mistake again

▶ providing appropriate support for people who have been subjected to discriminatory behaviour or hurtful language.

You may witness discriminatory behaviour or notice that the practices or procedures of colleagues in your workplace discriminate against some service

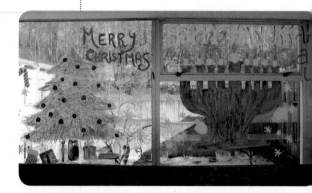

It is important to celebrate the religious festivals of all service users in a care setting

users or their relatives. It is always necessary to draw attention to discrimination – challenging it in a calm, constructive and clear way will help all those involved to learn from the situation and to promote changes in their thinking and behaviour so that it is less likely to occur again. Turning a blind eye to discriminatory practices allows it to continue and will compromise your own standards of practice. You should not let this happen.

Case study

Neil Sharma, aged 27, lives in a supported bungalow for people with learning disabilities. Neil is normally a very sociable, friendly and talkative person who enjoys the company of others and has good relationships with care staff. Janet, his main support worker for the last three years, recently left to begin a new job working in a day centre. Neil's dad, Jim, thought very highly of Janet and was quite upset about her leaving but seemed to gradually accept it. However, during recent visits to see Neil, Jim has been quite hostile to Josh, the new support worker who was appointed to replace Janet. Neil has established a good relationship with Josh and doesn't seem to share his dad's concerns. On a recent visit Jim shouted abuse at Josh for letting Neil hug him. Jim then told another care worker that he wanted to make a complaint because 'Josh is gay and keeps trying to touch Neil'. On his most recent visit to see Neil, Jim made an obscene gesture and directed homophobic comments towards Josh.

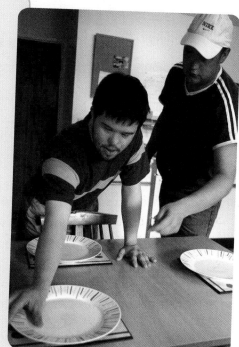

1. Identify the prejudice that is being expressed in this situation.

2. Suggest ways in which Josh's colleagues and his manager could provide support for him in this situation.

3. How could you respond in an anti-discriminatory way if you were present when Jim made homophobic comments towards Josh?

Practical Assessment Task   2.3

Discrimination can be deliberate and overt or inadvertent and covert. Practitioners in health and social care settings have a responsibility to challenge discrimination and to try and encourage people to adopt more positive, non-discriminatory ways of behaving and talking.

1. Describe how you have challenged, or would try to challenge, an instance of discrimination that occurred in your work setting.

2. Describe how your approach to challenging discrimination would encourage others to change their behaviour or way of talking so that they did not discriminate in future.

Your evidence for this task must be based on your practice in a real work environment and must be witnessed by, or be presented in a format that is acceptable to, your assessor.

Accessing information, advice and support about diversity, equality and inclusion

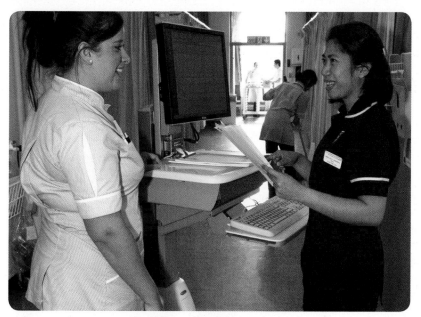

Senior colleagues and supervisors can be a useful source of advice, guidance and support on diversity issues

Where can you find information, advice and support?

You should now be aware of the need to take diversity, equality and inclusion issues seriously and will know that you should do your best to protect service users' rights, promoting equality for the individual. While you may be committed to inclusive practice, it can sometimes be challenging. You may be uncertain about the best way of dealing with some situations that arise. This is where accessing information, advice and support is necessary.

As you gain experience in health and social care practice, your ability to deal with the variety of situations and challenges that can occur will improve. However, even the most experienced care practitioners sometimes face unexpected situations and find themselves needing to seek information and advice about inclusion, diversity or equalities issues.

Health and social care practitioners can obtain information, advice and support about inclusion and equality issues from a variety of sources (see Figure 3.4).

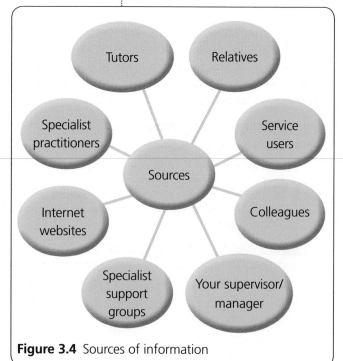

Figure 3.4 Sources of information

Relatives

Experienced health and social care practitioners recognise that a service user's husband, wife, partner or other close relatives are often the most accurate source of information or advice about an individual's needs, wishes and preferences. Wherever possible, and ensuring that you have the individual's consent, you should seek to include a service user's close relatives in discussions and decisions relating to diversity, equality and inclusion issues. As well as being good inclusive practice, this may also be the quickest and most effective way of finding out how you can best provide the kinds of support or assistance that a person needs.

Senior staff and colleagues

Your manager and other colleagues may be very good sources of information, advice and support when you are faced with difficult situations. They will almost certainly have greater experience and more training than you; it is a good idea to seek information, advice and support from more experienced people in your workplace whenever you can. You can do this by:

▶ asking questions during meetings or when chatting informally

▶ discussing issues you are unsure about with your supervisor or your manager

▶ identifying and discussing areas of practice that you find difficult with your supervisor, manager or a specialist practitioner or social worker, who spends time in your workplace.

Written resources

Information can also be obtained from a variety of resources that may be available in your health or social care setting, college resource centre or local library. These include:

▶ the policies and procedures written for your workplace

▶ codes of practice that provide guidance on professional standards and the implementation of laws

▶ books, magazines and journals that focus on health and social care practice and which regularly cover diversity, equality and inclusion issues

▶ the internet, particularly the websites of specialist care organisations, organisations focusing more generally on diversity, inclusion and equality issues, and reliable information providers such as the BBC.

Reflect

Can you think of an instance where you have needed additional information, advice or support in relation to a diversity, equality or inclusion issue? What did you do? Did you recognise you needed help and seek it? If you did not, think about whether getting assistance would have been more beneficial both to you and to the people involved.

When should you seek information, advice and support?

It is impossible to produce a definitive list of all of the situations in which you may need to obtain additional information, advice and support. To ensure you are well prepared for any challenges you might face, you could reflect on your knowledge and understanding of issues relating to:

▶ the cultural and religious needs of service users

▶ identity issues concerning ethnicity and race

▶ ways of including and supporting people with English as a second language

▶ gender differences

▶ forms of disability and how these impact on inclusion and equality

▶ the use of inclusive language

▶ ways of challenging incidents of unfair treatment or discrimination

▶ how to deal with bullying or other discriminatory behaviour by service users, relatives or visitors to the setting

▶ ways of helping people to learn from situations where discrimination or exclusion has occurred

▶ strategies for supporting people who have been subjected to discrimination or unfair treatment.

You may already have some experience of inclusion and equality issues in these types of areas. It is also possible that you can think of other inclusion and equality issues that are not mentioned here. In either case, once you are aware of an issue, the next step is to find ways of responding to it. It is at this point that you may need to access sources of additional information, advice and support.

Your assessment criteria:

3.1 Identify a range of sources of information, advice and support about diversity, equality and inclusion

3.2 Describe how and when to access information, advice and support about diversity, equality and inclusion

Key terms

Definitive: a final or complete list

Investigate

Review the resources available in your work setting to identify sources of advice, guidance and support on diversity issues. If none is available, ask your manager about the best way of accessing this type of support.

Knowledge Assessment Task   3.1   3.2

Imagine that you are about to take part in a performance and development review with the manager of your care setting. The review will focus on your learning and development needs in relation to your current role.

1. In preparation for the review, you have been asked to produce a short description of a diversity, equality or inclusion situation in which you needed additional information, advice or support. Ideally, your example should refer to a situation that you have already experienced or which you witnessed in your workplace. Alternatively, it could be a situation that you have thought about but which has not yet occurred.

2. How did you (or would you) demonstrate that you know how and when to access information, advice and guidance about this situation? Provide a brief explanation of what you did or would do.

Keep your written work as evidence towards your assessment.

Are you ready for assessment?

AC	What do you know now?	Assessment task	✓
1.1	The meaning of diversity, equality, inclusion and discrimination	Page 67	
1.2	The ways in which discrimination may deliberately or inadvertently occur in the work setting	Page 71	
1.3	How practices that support equality and inclusion reduce the likelihood of discrimination	Page 71	
3.1	A range of sources of information, advice and support about diversity, equality and inclusion	Page 84	
3.2	How and when to access information, advice and support about diversity, equality and inclusion	Page 84	

AC	What can you do now?	Assessment task	✓
2.1	Identify which legislation and codes of practice relating to equality, diversity and discrimination apply to your own work role	Page 77	
2.2	Show you can interact with individuals in ways that respect their beliefs, culture, values and preferences	Page 79	
2.3	Describe how to challenge discrimination in a way that encourages change	Page 81	

4 | Introduction to duty of care in health and social care (SHC 24)

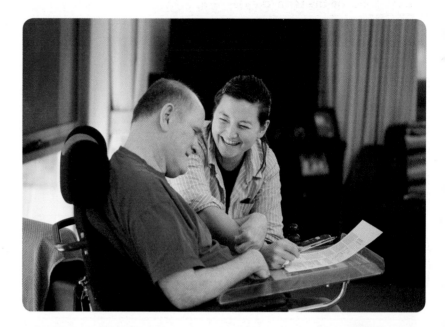

Assessment of this unit

This unit introduces the aspect of your work role and responsibilities referred to as a 'duty of care'. You will also need to be aware of the potential dilemmas or complaints that may arise as a result of having a duty of care for the people you support. You will need to:

- ▶ understand the meaning of duty of care
- ▶ be aware of dilemmas that may arise about duty of care and the support available for addressing them
- ▶ know how to respond to complaints.

The assessment of this unit is all knowledge based (things you need to know about), but it is also very important to be able to apply your knowledge practically in the real work environment.

In order to successfully complete this unit, you will need to produce evidence of your knowledge, as shown in the 'What you need to know' table opposite. Your tutor or assessor will help you to prepare for your assessment and the tasks suggested in the chapter will help you to create the evidence that you need.

CHAPTER 4

AC What you need to know

1.1	Define the term 'duty of care'
1.2	Describe how the duty of care affects your own work role
2.1	Describe dilemmas that may arise between the duty of care and an individual's rights
2.2	Explain where to get additional support and advice about how to resolve such dilemmas
3.1	Describe how to respond to complaints
3.2	Identify the main points of agreed procedures for handling complaints

There is no practical assessment for this unit but your tutor or assessor may question you about the points in the box below.

What you need to do

Apply your knowledge about duty of care to your practice in the real work environment.

Respond to dilemmas, difficulties and complaints relating to duty of care in the real work environment.

This unit also links to some other units:

SHC 22	Introduction to personal development in health and social care
HSC 025	The role of the health and social care worker
HSC 027	Contribute to health and safety in health and social care

Some of your learning will be repeated in these units and will give you the chance to review your knowledge and understanding.

Understanding what a duty of care means

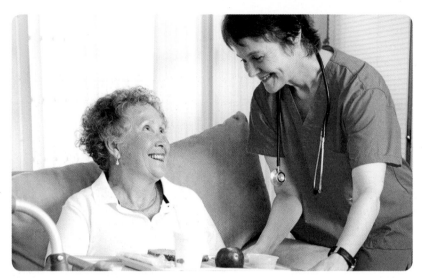

Care practitioners owe a duty of care towards each person they provide care for

Your assessment criteria:

1.1 Define the term 'duty of care'

1.2 Describe how the duty of care affects your own work role

What is a 'duty of care'?

The concept of duty of care is central to all roles within health and social care. Having a duty of care can be defined as doing all that you reasonably can, at all times, to ensure you act in the best interests of those you support. This means:

▶ putting the needs and interests of those you provide care for at the centre of your thoughts and actions

▶ always ensuring that what you do, or don't do, will not be harmful to the wellbeing of those you provide care for.

In practice, having a duty of care towards the people you provide care for means that you must:

▶ carry out care practice only within your own level of competence

▶ have the knowledge, understanding and skills needed to fulfil your work role and responsibilities at the standard expected in a health and social care setting.

The quality of care an individual would normally expect to receive is determined by:

▶ legislation

▶ standards of care

▶ professional standards

▶ codes of practice

▶ good practice guidance

▶ organisational policies and procedures.

Both you and your employer have a duty of care to meet those expectations.

Key terms

Competence: the knowledge, understanding, experience, personal attributes and training that give a person the ability to do something well, as measured against a standard

Legislation: written laws, such as Acts of Parliament

Code of practice: a set of rules or guidelines which describe how people in a particular profession are expected to behave

Grievance: a reason for complaint. It may be formal in cases where someone feels their rights have been breached

Your legal obligations

Health and social care practitioners must always work within the law. As part of your duty of care towards others (service users, colleagues and your employer) you must ensure that your actions do not break the law, even if that is what an individual or senior colleague asks you to do. For example, if an individual asks you to do something you are not appropriately trained or qualified to do, or which would be in breach of health and safety law, you must refuse. This might cause some difficulty or tension in your relationship with the person, but your duty of care towards others prevents you from acting in an unlawful way or in any way that puts others at risk of harm.

Your employer's responsibilities

The concept of duty of care extends beyond you putting service users' best interests first. Your employer, too, has a duty of care towards you as an employee. They must, for example, provide you with training and appropriate equipment to undertake your job safely and to the standard expected by service users. Your employer should also have a range of policies and procedures which explain how they will meet their duty of care towards you as an employee. These include, for example, policies and procedures relating to equality and diversity, harassment, grievances and confidentiality issues.

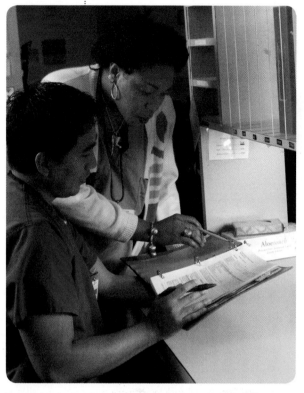

Employers have a duty of care towards all employees

Case study

One of your colleagues is off sick and your manager asks you to visit one of their service users. You read the care plan and discover that you will need to use a hoist to move the person. You have never used a hoist, only observed one being used, and only on one occasion. You tell your manager that you are not trained to use the hoist and don't feel you are able to visit the service user. They tell you that it's not a problem as the service user's partner is there and will explain how to use it. You tell them again that you are not happy to visit. The manager becomes angry and tells you that, if you don't visit, the service user will not receive a visit that day as there is no one else free to go.

1. What would you do in this situation?

2. Why would you take this action?

3. How does this relate to the duty of care?

Keep your notes as evidence towards your assessment.

Investigate

Do you know where the equality and diversity, harassment and grievance policies can be found in your work setting? Find out where they are and what they say, so that you understand the duty of care your employer has towards you as an employee.

Reporting on and recording care provision

Recording and reporting on the care that you provide for individuals is an essential part of providing health and social care services. Recording what, when, where and how care-related activities are carried out is a way of demonstrating that you have followed the policies and procedures of your work setting and that you have provided care to the expected standard. Ignorance of policies, procedures and expected standards of care is no defence in a situation in which a care practitioner is accused of failing in their duty of care. It is your responsibility to:

▶ ensure you are competent to do the tasks you carry out

▶ know and understand the policies, procedures and guidance that underpin your work activities

▶ speak out when you don't have the skills or are not competent to undertake particular tasks.

Similarly, you should let a senior colleague know when you:

▶ have concerns about the quality and standard of care being provided

▶ believe your duty of care towards others is threatened or compromised.

How does duty of care affect your work role?

Meeting your **obligations** in respect of a duty of care means that you need to keep your knowledge and skills up to date. You can do this by:

▶ attending training provided by your employer – for example, mandatory training for health and safety

▶ ensuring you understand changes in legislation, policies or procedures

▶ ensuring you can put changes in legislation, policies or procedures into practice.

Your assessment criteria:

1.2 Describe how the duty of care affects your own work role

Reflect

Have you ever felt that you should speak out about the quality or standard of care being offered in your work setting? Why did, or didn't, you decide to do this?

Key terms

Obligation: something that must be done; a duty which is either legally or morally correct

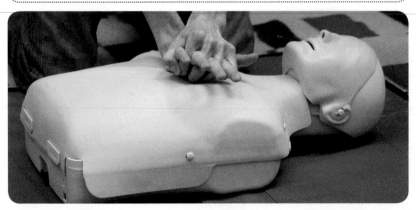

Attending training sessions will help you to meet your duty of care obligations

A duty of care applies to each and every aspect of your work. This includes, for example:

▶ making sure you keep accurate, complete and legible records within your workplace – these are legal documents and proof of the activities undertaken

▶ maintaining confidentiality of all information shared with you unless it conflicts with public interest or safety.

Health and social care practitioners have a duty of care to:

▶ the people they support

▶ themselves

▶ their employer.

Duty of care also means only doing those tasks that you have been properly trained to carry out safely. It also applies to the equipment you might use in the course of your work; for example, only using a fully functioning hoist that you have been trained to use by a competent person.

Reflect

Think about your understanding of the duty of care.

How was a duty of care explained to you during your induction to your current work role?

Are your clear about your responsibilities in relation to the duty of care?

What opportunities do you have to find out more about the duty of care and how it affects your daily work?

Knowledge Assessment Task

| 1.1 | 1.2 |

1. What does the term 'duty of care' mean for the following people:
   ▶ you as a health and social care practitioner?
   ▶ the people that you support in your service?
   ▶ your employer?

2. Copy and complete the table below, identifying four normal work activities and describing how your duty of care influences how you carry out the activity.

Work activity	How your duty of care influences this activity

Keep your notes as evidence towards your assessment.

Understanding support available for addressing dilemmas that may arise about duty of care

As British citizens many of our **rights** are described in legislation. For example, the Human Rights Act 1998 states that we have a right to:

▶ life

▶ a fair trial

▶ respect for private and family life, home and correspondence.

The rights of people receiving support from health and social services are outlined in legislation such as the Health and Social Care Act (2008). This Act includes the essential care standards, which specify the quality of support people can expect to receive. For example, Regulation 9, Outcome 4 relates to the care and welfare of people who use services, and demands that: 'People experience effective, safe and appropriate care, treatment and support that meets their needs and protects their rights'.

Although standards such as these provide clear guidance concerning both individuals' rights and the duty of care, there are times when the two conflict, and this often results in a **dilemma** for those providing support.

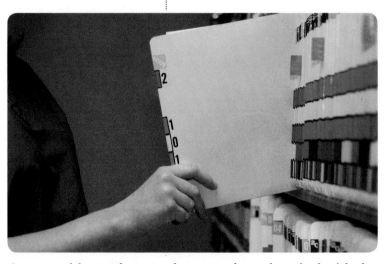

Care practitioners have to document how they deal with the dilemmas they face in practice

Individual rights

People receiving care and support have a right to:

▶ have their privacy, dignity and independence respected

▶ understand the options available so they can make an informed choice

▶ express their views

▶ be involved in decisions about their care, including how care is delivered

▶ protection from harm, danger and abuse.

Those providing health and social care services have a duty of care to:

▶ ensure individual rights are upheld, and

▶ always act in the best interests of the individual.

Conflicts and dilemmas can occur when a service user decides to do something that is considered by those providing support to be unsafe, dangerous, or not in their best interests.

Balancing rights and risks

Risk is a part in our everyday lives. Taking risks can help us to learn more about:

▶ ourselves – this builds confidence and self-esteem

▶ what we are capable of achieving

▶ our limitations

▶ the world around us.

For example, we take risks when we:

▶ form new friendships – risk of being hurt or disappointed

▶ take on a new challenge – risk of failure.

Taking a risk is something each individual has to consider carefully, weighing up what they could gain and what they could lose.

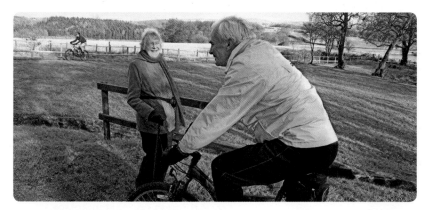

Individuals need to be able to weigh up the risks and benefits to themselves of the decisions they make

Some of the people you support will be able to think through the options and potential consequences of their actions. Others will, however, lack the **capacity** to do this. People may lack the ability to make informed decisions because of:

▶ failing health

▶ illness

▶ an inherited or acquired condition.

A lack of capacity may be:

▶ short-term and temporary; for example, due to confusion following an accident, infection or an anaesthetic

or

▶ long-term or permanent; for example, due to a condition such as a learning difficulty, a severe head injury or dementia.

Resolving dilemmas about the duty of care

Sources of advice and support

A dilemma arises when there are two or more alternative courses of action, none of which will provide a solution to suit everyone involved. Thinking through those alternatives and the potential consequences of each is often easier with the help of someone whose judgement we trust and respect. Another point of view will broaden your thinking and help you reach a decision about what action to take.

When dilemmas relate to work-related situations it is important to remember your duty of care in relation to maintaining confidentiality. Therefore, you must not discuss work-related information or dilemmas with anyone outside your work setting unless they are bound by confidentiality themselves; for example, a trade union or legal representative.

Gathering information to help you make decisions

You may need to identify and use sources of additional support and advice to deal with duty of care dilemmas that you face. Figure 4.1 identifies a number of different sources that may be helpful, depending on the dilemma.

Your assessment criteria:

2.1 Describe dilemmas that may arise between the duty of care and an individual's rights

2.3 Explain where to get additional support and advice about how to resolve dilemmas

Key terms

Confidentiality: keeping information private and only available to people who have a right and justifiable reason to have that information

Whistle-blowing: reporting concerns about bad or illegal practice to an external body, such as a regulatory organisation or the media. 'Whistle-blowers' often take this step when all attempts to resolve a situation through normal workplace procedures have failed

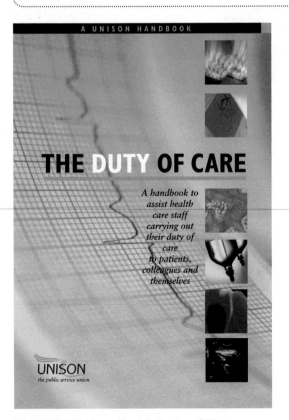

A UNISON HANDBOOK

THE DUTY OF CARE

A handbook to assist health care staff carrying out their duty of care to patients, colleagues and themselves

UNISON
the public service union

The UNISON handbook *Duty of Care*

To ensure we make sound or reliable decisions it is important to gather information related to the decision. You must then check that the information is:

- authentic – is it genuine?
- current – is it up-to-date?
- relevant – is it about the situation? Will it help you to reach a decision?
- reliable – does it come from a recognised and trusted source?
- complete – is there anything missing?

If your information meets all these criteria you will be more confident that you can use it to make decisions. Then take time to analyse the information to determine if it helps make the situation clearer. You may still find it difficult to reach a decision and would then need to seek support and advice.

There are a number of documents that could provide you with information and advice when you are faced with a dilemma regarding the duty of care. These might include:

- your job description
- your contract of employment
- a professional code of practice
- your employer's policies and procedures; for example, on **whistle-blowing** or on health and safety
- standards related to your area of work; for example, essential care standards
- legislation; for example, Health & Safety at Work Act (1974), Public Disclosure Act (1998)

There are also a number of people or organisations you could approach for advice and support (see Figure 4.1). These might include:

- your manager or supervisor
- a trusted colleague
- your employer
- a trade union representative
- the Care Quality Commission.

Reflect

Think about the people you work with.

- Who would you talk to if you were faced with a duty of care dilemma?
- Would you always choose the same person(s)? If not, why?
- How do you think talking to them could help you to resolve a dilemma?

Investigate

Do you know where to find the policies and procedures relating to raising concerns in your work setting? Find out which policies and procedures enable services users and carers to raise concerns. Find out how the procedure works in practice.

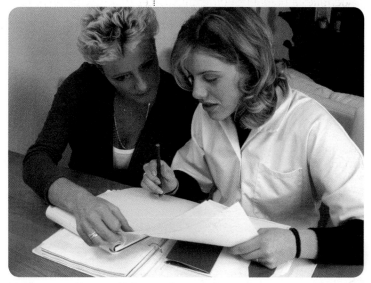

Understanding policies and procedures is part of your duty of care

Sometimes duty of care dilemmas result from being asked to do something which conflicts with good practice guidance. For example, your manager asks you to give a service user a bath using the hoist that you have reported as being faulty. You know that other staff members have been using the hoist even though you consider it to be unsafe. The dilemma is that if you refuse your manager's request this will reflect badly on you and you may be disciplined. However, if you use the hoist you potentially put yourself and the service user at risk of harm and the organisation at risk of litigation.

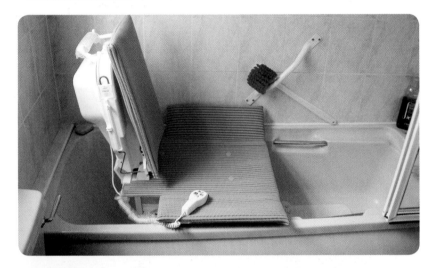

Case study

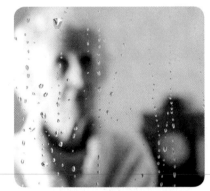

Harriet Palmer, 95, was admitted to a residential care home two days ago following a fall, and with evidence of self-neglect. It appears she has been struggling to care for herself at home following the death of her husband two months ago, and as a result has lost a considerable amount of weight and mobility. She is thin and frail and has a heart condition which is managed by medication. She has a left-sided weakness following several strokes and early signs of memory loss. She is grieving for her husband and is reluctant to be involved in any activities or interact with other residents. Since her admission Harriet has been refusing to eat and will only drink small amounts of liquid. Today she refused to take her medication and appears much weaker.

1. What dilemma does this situation present in relation to the duty of care?

2. What do you think you would do if you worked at the residential care home?

3. What are the potential consequences of the available options?

Keep your notes as evidence towards your assessment.

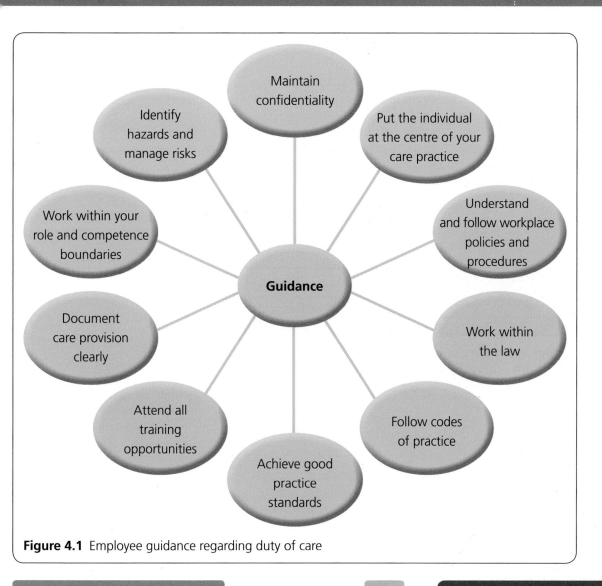

Figure 4.1 Employee guidance regarding duty of care

Knowledge Assessment Task   2.1

Describe how each of the following present a dilemma in relation to the duty of care:

1. You are asked to do a task you have not been trained to do.

2. You need to dispose of contaminated waste and there is no personal protective equipment available.

3. You have noticed that the cook never tests the temperature of the food before serving, even though the record has been completed to indicate it has been tested according to requirements.

4. You have heard the manager telling relatives a resident's diagnosis when you know that the resident specifically requested that no information be shared with their relatives.

Keep your notes as evidence towards your assessment.

Investigate

Do you know which policies and procedures relate to assessing and managing risk in your work setting? Find out which they are and what they say, so that you understand the duty of care your employer has towards you as an employee and towards service users.

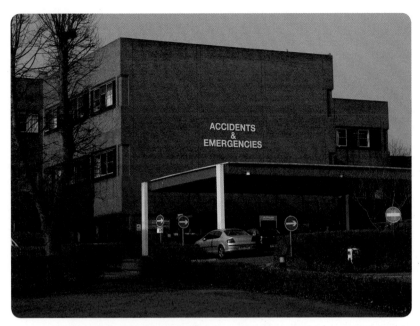

Your assessment criteria:

2.2 Explain where to get additional support and advice about how to resolve such dilemmas

Serious failures in the duty of care undermine public confidence and trust in health and social care institutions

Raising concerns

The consequences of not raising concerns about failures in the duty of care have resulted in situations of abuse and neglect going unnoticed and un-challenged.

For example, the independent inquiry into care provided by Mid Staffordshire NHS Foundation Trust January 2005 – March 2009 (chaired by Robert Francis QC, report published in February 2010) identified how concerns raised by patients, relatives and staff were ignored in a culture of intimidation. It is estimated that as many as 1,200 people died prematurely as a result of the 'appalling standards of care'. It is unknown how many patients experienced unnecessary pain and discomfort. Cases such as these represent not only a failure in the duty of care but a breach of trust between the public and those working in health and social care.

In cases where you have concerns about the duty of care, speaking out as a lone voice is difficult. Before raising concerns:

▶ be sure of the facts and/or evidence to support your concern

▶ seek advice, guidance and appropriate support

▶ maintain confidentiality

▶ ensure you know and understand how to use your organisation's whistle-blowing or confidential reporting policies and procedures.

Investigate

Find out how your organisation monitors to make sure that they are meeting their obligations in relation to the duty of care. How do they ensure all employees meet their obligations? Find out what action the organisation takes if they identify a failure in the duty of care. Find out how your organisation responds to recommendations that are made following failures in the duty of care.

Take the informal or formal route?

Most policies advise staff to first raise any concern informally; for example, by talking to a manager or supervisor. However, the seriousness and urgency of the situation may mean that it needs to be raised formally; for example, if there is a high risk of harm or death in the near or immediate future then this is clearly serious and urgent. Raising a concern formally requires that it is submitted in writing and subject to a clearly documented process. This provides evidence that a concern was raised so that it is harder to overlook or dismiss as unimportant.

Policies and procedures will provide information about what steps to take if the concern relates to your manager or employer, as this can present a difficult situation for an employee. The procedure should give guidance about whom to contact in these situations.

If you feel the response to the concern you have raised is inadequate then you need to know whom next to inform about your concern; for example, your employer or an inspection authority such as the Care Quality Commission. It is preferable when you raise a concern to put it in writing, as then you have proof that the concern was raised. You must also keep accurate records and copies of everything related to the concern as this provides evidence of your actions.

Case study

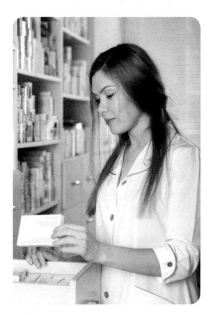

Your manager has asked you to check the medication delivery from the pharmacy. You tell the manager you are not sure about doing this because you have never done it before. The manager tells you it's easy, the pharmacy never makes mistakes, and so you should have no trouble with it. You are still not sure but do it as you are new to the job and want to create a good impression.

1. What is the dilemma in this situation?
2. Where could you get advice and support to resolve this dilemma?
3. Which policies and procedures could you use to deal with this situation?

Keep your notes as evidence towards your assessment.

Knowledge Assessment Task   2.2

1. List the people and organisational structures within your work setting who could provide support and advice to help you resolve a duty of care dilemma.
2. How would you access each of these?
3. What support and/or advice might you expect to receive from each of these?

Keep your notes as evidence towards your assessment.

Resolving complaints

How to respond to complaints

The right of individuals to make **complaints** is generally accepted in our society. People generally complain when:

- ▶ they are not satisfied
- ▶ something does not meet their expectations.

Making a complaint is one of the ways people tell us about the quality and consistency of a service, and how it is experienced by service users. To provide a good service and one which meets people's needs and expectations, it is important to know what they think. Knowing what works well and what doesn't work helps to identify potential changes and/or improvements. Without feedback things may continue to fall below expectations. This will only lead to further problems which are likely to worsen.

In the case of the duty of care, making a complaint is the formal process used to raise concerns. Making a complaint makes it harder to ignore concerns raised, as they become documented. Whether the complaint is made informally (verbally) or formally (written) any complaint must be recorded.

Responding to a complaint

Some people view any complaint as negative criticism, and as a consequence their response is defensive, making the complainant feel that they are wrong to complain. Many of us have experienced such a response when we have made a complaint, which may make us reluctant to do it again.

However, if our complaint has received a more positive response – the recipient has listened to our complaint, taken it seriously and taken action to resolve the problem – we feel justified and are more likely to feel able to complain on future occasions.

Your assessment criteria:

3.1 Describe how to respond to complaints

3.2 Identify the main points of agreed procedures for handling complaints

Key terms

Complaint: when we express dissatisfaction or unhappiness about a situation

Investigation: a procedure in which evidence is carefully and methodically examined to determine the facts about what has taken place

Intimidation: behaviour which creates a feeling of awe, inadequacy or fear (often through threats) to persuade or dissuade someone from doing something

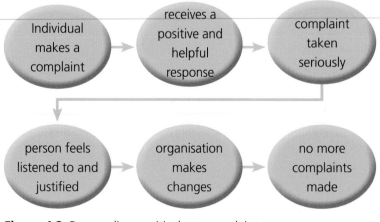

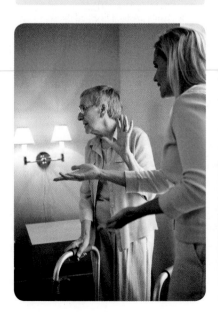

Figure 4.3 Responding positively to complaints

Complaints and failures in duty of care

Investigations into failures in the duty of care have found that significant factors include that:

▶ complaints have been often and routinely ignored

▶ **intimidation** was used to discourage, dismiss or hide complaints.

Investigations have concluded that had complaints been responded to appropriately – i.e. people treated with respect, their complaints taken seriously and procedures followed – those failures could have been addressed much quicker with fewer lives damaged or lost.

It is essential that you follow your organisation's complaints policy and procedure when someone makes a complaint. However, your initial response to a complaint also plays an important part in how well it will be resolved. When responding to a complaint it is what you do, how you do it, and what you say that makes the difference.

People will feel more able to complain and comment on what is happening if they are:

▶ responded to promptly

▶ listened to

▶ treated with respect

▶ taken seriously.

A more positive response to complaints is likely to mean that:

▶ complaints will be resolved quicker and more easily

▶ positive relationships will be maintained

▶ fewer complaints will be received

▶ people will feel able to complain

▶ the likelihood of people's rights being abused will be reduced

▶ people's vulnerability to abuse will be reduced.

Investigate

Think about two occasions when you have made a complaint: one when you received a positive response and one when you received a negative response – i.e. you were made to feel in the wrong for complaining.

▶ How were you made to feel in each situation?

▶ What did the person you complained to do differently to make it either a positive or negative experience?

▶ How can your experience help you in your work role when dealing with complaints?

▶ What would you do differently now if someone made a complaint to you?

Case study

Beth Perkins is a 45 year-old woman with advanced motor neurone disease. Her condition has deteriorated so much that she now needs help with all daily living activities. She is the youngest resident in a nursing home and her family visit daily. One day you go into Beth's room to find she is asleep and her husband is looking upset and angry. You ask him if there is anything you can do to help. He tells you that he is very unhappy because Beth hasn't been washed again and she is wearing someone else's clothes again. You start to apologise for this and ask if he has spoken to anyone about it. He then becomes more angry and upset and tells you it is pointless. He says he has lost count of the number of times he has complained and each time he does he is made to feel he is over-reacting and being ridiculous. He tells you he's had enough and this time he's going to make arrangements to move Beth to another home as he can't trust anyone here.

1. Why do you think Beth's husband is so upset?
2. What can you say to encourage him to raise his concerns and complain again before taking action?
3. What can you do to resolve the situation?

Keep your notes as evidence towards your assessment.

Ways of managing complaints

When someone makes a complaint we can feel that it's a personal criticism. People generally complain about:

▶ something they felt was incorrect or unfair

or

▶ something that was not done when it should have been.

The fact that someone feels able to complain to you shows that they believe you will listen to them and do something about their complaint.

Here are some suggestions to help you manage the situation and respond positively when someone makes a complaint:

1. Stay calm, respectful and polite.

2. If possible, take the person somewhere that is private and where you can sit down. This shows that you are taking their complaint seriously and are prepared to listen. It also helps to calm the situation.

3. Ask the person if they would prefer to speak to the person in charge:

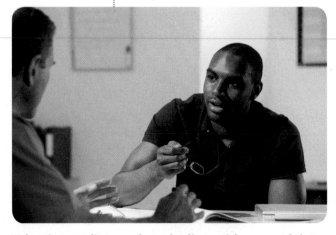

Take time to listen when dealing with a complaint

a. If yes, ask them to briefly explain their complaint so you can tell the person in charge when you go and get them. Don't get into the detail as they will only have to repeat this later.

b. If not, then you should be prepared to listen to the complaint yourself.

4. Ask the person to explain exactly what the problem is.

5. Listen without interrupting.

6. Ask questions to check you understand what they are saying.

7. Make notes to refer back to and to show that you are listening.

8. Apologise for the situation. Often people feel better when you say 'I'm sorry this has happened'. You are not admitting anything just acknowledging that they are upset.

9. Summarise how you think the person sees the situation. Again, you are not making any judgements or admitting anything.

10. Ask the person how they would like the situation to be resolved. Tell them what their options are. At this point you will need to refer to your manager or supervisor for advice and support.

11. You will need to give the person a copy of your organisation's complaints policy and procedure.

12. You should always record any complaints made according to your work place procedure and report it to your manager/ supervisor.

The complaints policy and procedure used in your work setting may indicate that all complaints should be immediately directed to the person in charge. If that is the case then you can still respond positively (points 1–3a, above, and point 8 if appropriate).

Reflect

Think of a situation when someone was making a complaint to you.

1. How did you feel when they first approached you?
2. How do you think your feelings affected your behaviour towards the person making the complaint?
3. How do you think your behaviour affected the person's actions/response?
4. What can you learn from this to improve how you deal with any future complaints?

Make accurate notes to ensure nothing is missed

Complaints procedures

All employers and organisations will have complaints policies and procedures in place. Leaflets explaining these policies and procedures should be given to everyone who accesses the services.

If an employee has a complaint about any aspect of their employment they will find details of the complaints procedure in their contract of employment.

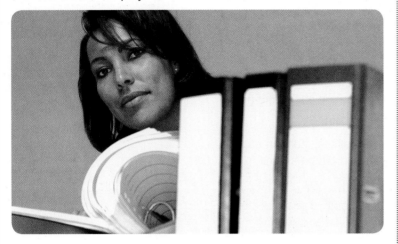

Generally, it is preferable to try and resolve complaints informally by following the actions described above.

Formal complaints

If the person making the complaint does not feel satisfied with the options being offered to resolve their complaint, or if the complaint is complex or there is serious risk of harm, the complaint needs to become a formal one.

When a complaint becomes formal it means that:

▶ it must be made in writing

▶ there are agreed timescales for actions; for example, the organisation must respond within five working days

▶ the complaint will be investigated by someone in authority and not directly connected to the complaint

▶ following investigation the person making the complaint is sent a formal letter with details of the outcome

▶ the person making the complaint has a right to appeal if unsatisfied with the outcome

▶ following appeal, if they remain unsatisfied, they can complain to the inspection and regulation authority; for example, the Care Quality Commission (CQC).

Your assessment criteria:

3.2 Identify the main points of agreed procedures for handling complaints

Investigate

Do you know where the complaints policies can be found in your work setting? Find out on what occasions these are given to service users. Find out how your organisation keeps a record of any complaints made and how they are resolved.

Knowledge Assessment Task — 3.1 3.2

You are visiting John, a tenant in the supported living accommodation where you provide support. As you are going in the front door you meet Mr Hedges, the father of one of the other tenants, Pam. You know both of them, as you occasionally provide Pam with support when her usual support practitioner is away. Mr Hedges appears upset and when you ask him why he tells you he has just seen Pam, who has told him she hasn't seen a support practitioner for a week. He tells you he wants to make a complaint as it is not the first time this has happened.

1. How would you respond to Mr Hedges's request to make a complaint?
2. What are the main points of your organisation's complaints policy and procedure?

Keep your notes as evidence towards your assessment.

Are you ready for assessment?

AC	What do you know now?	Assessment task	✓
1.1	Define the term 'duty of care'	Page 91	
1.2	Describe how the duty of care affects your work role	Page 91	
2.1	Describe dilemmas that may arise between the duty of care and an individual's rights	Page 97	
2.2	Explain where to get additional support and advice about how to resolve such dilemmas	Page 99	
3.1	Describe how to respond to complaints	Page 105	
3.2	Identify the main points of agreed procedures for handling complaints	Page 105	

5 | Principles of safeguarding and protection in health and social care (HSC 024)

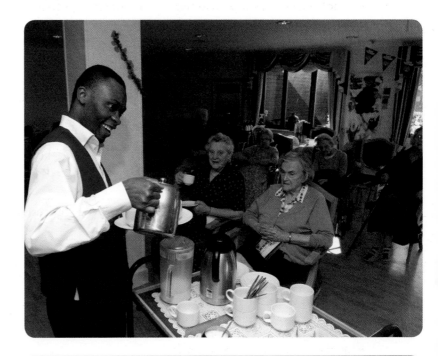

Assessment of this unit

This unit is relevant to people working in a wide range of health and social care settings. It introduces the importance of safeguarding individuals from abuse, identifies the different types of abuse that can occur as well as the signs and symptoms that might indicate a person is experiencing abuse. The unit also considers when individuals might be particularly vulnerable to abuse and what you can do if abuse is suspected or alleged. You will need to:

▶ know how to recognise signs of abuse

▶ know how to respond to suspected or alleged abuse

▶ understand the national and local context of safeguarding and protection from abuse

▶ understand ways to reduce the likelihood of abuse

▶ know how to recognise and report unsafe practices.

The assessment of this unit is entirely knowledge-based. To successfully complete this unit, you will need to produce evidence of your knowledge as shown in the table opposite. Your tutor or assessor will help you to prepare for your assessment, and the tasks suggested in this unit will help you to create the evidence that you need.

AC	What you need to know
1.1	Define the following types of abuse: • physical abuse • institutional abuse • sexual abuse • self-neglect • emotional/psychological abuse • neglect by others. • financial abuse
1.2	Identify the signs and/or symptoms associated with each type of abuse
1.3	Define factors that may contribute to an individual being more vulnerable to abuse
2.1	Explain the actions to take if there are suspicions that an individual is being abused
2.2	Explain the actions to take if an individual alleges that they are being abused
2.3	Identify ways to ensure that evidence of abuse is preserved
3.1	Identify national policies and local systems that relate to safeguarding and protection from abuse
3.2	Explain the roles of different agencies in safeguarding and protecting individuals from abuse
3.3	Identify reports into serious failures to protect individuals from abuse
3.4	Identify sources of information and advice about own role in safeguarding and protecting individuals from abuse
4.1	Explain how the likelihood of abuse may be reduced by: • working with person-centred values • encouraging active participation • promoting choice and rights.
4.2	Explain the importance of an accessible complaints procedure for reducing the likelihood of abuse
5.1	Describe unsafe practice that may affect the well being of individuals
5.2	Explain the actions to take if unsafe practices have been identified
5.3	Describe the action to take if suspected abuse or unsafe practices have been reported but nothing has been done in response

This unit also links to some of the other units:

SHC 24	Introduction to duty of care in health and social care
HSC 025	The role of the health and social care worker
CMH 02	Understand mental health problems

Some of your learning will be repeated in these units and will give you the chance to review your knowledge and understanding.

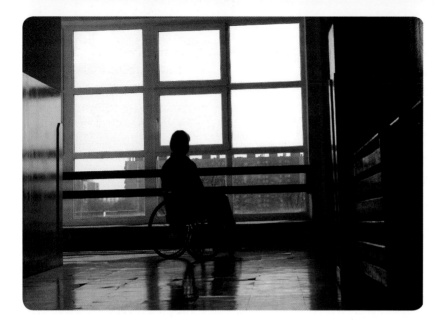

Your assessment criteria:

1.1 Define the following types of abuse:
- physical abuse
- sexual abuse
- emotional/ psychological abuse
- financial abuse
- institutional abuse
- self-neglect
- neglect by others

Key terms

Vulnerable: more prone to risk and harm

Adult at risk: any person aged 18 years and over who is or may be in need of community care services

Consent: giving informed permission for something to happen

Capacity: the mental or physical ability to cope with or to do something

Coerced: being forced to do something against your will

Omission: where something is either deliberately or accidently left out or not done

Commission: the deliberate act of doing something while knowing the implications and consequences

What is 'abuse'?

Abuse can occur when individuals are deprived of their rights to:

- privacy
- independence
- choose for themselves
- a decent quality of life
- protection and security.

Abuse is a significant and serious problem within society; anyone is potentially at risk of harm or abuse. However, most of us are able to take steps to protect ourselves. Most of us are not **vulnerable** to abuse. However, individuals accessing health and social care services have a greater level of vulnerability, and this places them at a greater risk of harm or abuse. This greater level of vulnerability is often associated with that individual's need for support. A key responsibility of every health and social care practitioner therefore is to safeguard and protect **adults at risk**.

In 2000 the Department of Health published *No secrets*, which provided guidance for organisations to enable them to develop and implement multi-agency procedures to protect adults at risk from abuse. In *No secrets* abuse is defined as: 'a violation of an individual's human and civil rights by any other person or persons'.

It goes on to add that abuse may:

- be a single act or repeated acts
- be physical, verbal or psychological

- ▶ be an act of neglect
- ▶ be a failure to act
- ▶ occur when a vulnerable person is persuaded to do something to which they cannot **consent** or have not consented
- ▶ occur in any relationship
- ▶ result in significant harm to or exploitation of the person subjected to abuse
- ▶ occur in situations in which the individual is unable to protect themselves or prevent abuse happening to them.

People can experience abuse in a number of different ways. It is more usual that a person will experience more than one type of abuse at the same time. For example, physical abuse or violence is generally accompanied by verbal threats and intimidation, so the person is both physically and emotionally abused.

Key terms

Norm: the standard pattern of behaviour accepted as normal

Investigate

What do you know about the different types of consent. Do you know what guidance there is regarding consent in your work setting? Find out how consent is established with the individuals you support in your work setting and what happens when an individual is unable to consent to care or treatment.

Figure 5.1 Types and examples of abuse

Type of abuse	Definition and examples of abuse
Physical	The deliberate use of physical force that results in bodily injury, pain or impairment. This includes the inappropriate application of techniques or treatments, involuntary isolation or confinement, misuse of medication.
Sexual	Direct or indirect involvement in sexual activity without valid **consent**. Consent to a particular activity may not be given because: the individual doesn't wish to consent; lacks **capacity** and is unable to consent; or feels **coerced** into an activity because the other person is in a position of trust, power or authority.
Emotional/ psychological	Any action by another that damages an individual's mental wellbeing. The use of threats, humiliation, bullying, swearing and other verbal conduct, or any other form of mental cruelty that results in mental or physical distress. It includes the denial of basic human and civil rights, such as choice, self-expression, privacy and dignity.
Financial	This is the theft or misuse of an individual's money or personal possessions to the advantage of another person.
Institutional	This is the mistreatment or abuse of an individual by a regime or people within an institution. It occurs when the routines, systems and **norms** of an institution override the needs of the people that they are there to support.
Self-neglect	This is where an individual fails to adequately care for themselves and meet their own basic needs for food, warmth, rest, medical care, personal care. This may be intentional or unintentional, due to physical or mental health issues.
Neglect by others	This is the deliberate or unintentional failure to meet an individual's basic needs for personal care, food, warmth, rest, medical care, social stimulation, cultural or religious needs. This can be either acts of **omission** (not doing something) or acts of **commission** (doing something on purpose).

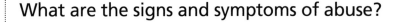

What are the signs and symptoms of abuse?

There are a number of ways you can recognise that an individual may have been abused, though the signs and symptoms are not always obvious. Knowing the individual and how they normally behave is an important part of being able to protect them, as changes in behaviour can be subtle and easily overlooked.

Physical abuse

Physical abuse is possibly the easiest to recognise as it is often more visible. However, it can also be missed, especially if explanations are accepted without questioning and careful monitoring. Some forms of physical abuse – such as denying an individual's needs or the misuse of medication – can be difficult to recognise. Any explanation that is inconsistent with an observed physical injury should raise concerns and prompt reporting and further investigation.

Signs and symptoms of **physical abuse**

- multiple or minor bruising of different areas with inconsistent explanations
- burns and scalds
- odd-shaped bruising/burns – such as the outline or shape of a weapon or cigarette end
- marks on the skin consistent with being slapped, scratched, bitten or pinched
- splits on the side of the lips consistent with the mouth being forced open
- broken bones
- evidence of old injuries, e.g. untreated broken bones
- black eyes and bruising around the mouth and ears
- smell of urine and faeces
- indicators of malnutrition or general signs of neglect
- misuse of medication, such as withholding pain relief or giving additional doses of sedatives
- bruising to wrists indicating forced restraint
- unexplained bruising to normally protected areas of the body – abdomen, fingertip marks on underarms or inside of the thigh
- unexplained falls
- guarding reactions by the individual when approached by anyone
- a reluctance to undress in front of others.

Sexual abuse

Sexual abuse can take many forms and can include contact or non-contact.

Sexual abuse through contact may be vaginal or anal rape; touching or forcing an individual to touch another in a sexual manner without consent.

Sexual abuse through non-contact can include: forcing an individual to watch pornographic or adult entertainment without fully understanding what this involves; subjecting an individual to indecent exposure, sexual innuendoes, harassment or inappropriate photography; and not giving choice regarding the gender of the carer giving personal care.

Sexual abuse is closely associated with power, and is generally accompanied by both physical and psychological abuse.

Signs and symptoms of **sexual abuse**

- anxiety and fear of physical contact
- injury, bleeding, irritation or infection of the genital area
- sexually transmitted disease
- bruising, bites, scratches on the breast or inner thigh
- inappropriate conversations of a sexual nature
- unexplained crying and distress
- withdrawal from social contact
- acute confusion
- depression
- nightmares
- torn clothes
- self-harm
- self-neglect.

Emotional/psychological abuse

Psychological abuse is often difficult to recognise as it is generally hidden, and happens over time. It may involve the removal or denial of the individual's right to make decisions and result in the restriction of their choices. The deliberate withholding of care, affection, companionship and love, as well as verbal threats, are often used by the abuser to intimidate and force the individual to do what the abuser wants.

Signs and symptoms of **emotional and psychological abuse**

- changes in appetite
- changes in sleep pattern, e.g. nightmares or insomnia
- attention-seeking behaviour
- self-isolation – especially when the individual was previously outgoing and sociable to others
- unusual weight gain or loss
- sadness or uncontrollable crying
- being passive, with no spontaneous smiles or laughter
- self-abuse or self-harm, e.g. misuse of alcohol, nicotine or illegal drugs; refusing food or medication
- withdrawal and disinterest
- depression
- avoidance of contact with others
- unexplained fearfulness or anxiety, especially about being alone or with particular people
- increased tension or irritability
- low self-esteem
- lack of self-confidence.

Financial abuse

Financial abuse can take many forms.

Signs and symptoms of **financial abuse**

- sudden, unexplained inability to pay bills
- unpaid bills resulting in utilities being discontinued
- a reluctance to spend any money (even when finances should not be a problem)
- no food in the house
- sudden, unexplained withdrawals of money from the individual's accounts
- missing money, chequebook, bank card, credit card or possessions
- being under pressure to make or change the terms of a will
- other people showing an unusual interest in the individual's assets.

Institutional abuse

In situations of institutional abuse, the policies and the way people work add to the risk of abuse rather than safeguard against it. For example, organisations that impose fixed care routines and which put pressure on practitioners and service users to just accept how things are done without question, are likely to be places where abusive practices occur.

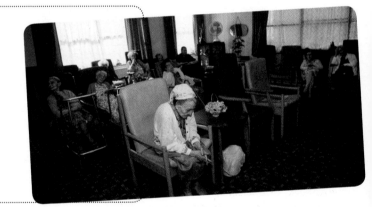

Signs and symptoms of **institutional abuse**

- rigid routines
- lack of choice offered
- activities arranged solely for the convenience of staff and the organisation
- cultural or religious needs not being met
- difficulty in relatives/friends accessing individuals – e.g. inflexible visiting times
- restriction of access to food and drink
- restriction of access to toilet, bathing facilities or a comfortable place to rest during the day
- inappropriate use of restraint
- misuse of medication, e.g. overuse of sedation to benefit staff not the individual
- lack of privacy, dignity or respect
- restriction of access to medical or social care
- inflexible mealtimes and bedtimes
- inadequate guidance, policies and procedures for staff
- inadequate access for individuals to complaints procedures
- inappropriate, inadequate and poor standards of care
- repeated examples of poor professional standards and behaviour.

Self-neglect

Self-neglect can be accidental as well as deliberate. An individual who is confused or has memory problems may neglect themselves unintentionally. Deliberate self-neglect can also be a way of expressing mental health problems or it may be a symptom of abuse, especially sexual abuse.

Reflect

How involved in making decisions about the support they receive are the people for whom you provide care? Do you think that the service you work in is flexible and responsive in meeting individuals' preferences about mealtimes, bedtimes and food choices, for example?

Signs and symptoms of **self-neglect**

- ▶ neglecting personal hygiene
- ▶ not seeking medical or social care
- ▶ not taking prescribed medication
- ▶ not eating
- ▶ overeating
- ▶ self-harm, e.g. misuse of alcohol, or illegal drugs, cutting themselves
- ▶ not taking exercise
- ▶ unsanitary living conditions that are a risk to health, e.g. presence of vermin.

Neglect by others

Neglect can be passive or active. An individual may experience neglect in a variety of ways: as a lack of attention; as abandonment; or as confinement by their family and by society. Whether neglect is intentional or unintentional, by acts of omission or commission, the result is the deterioration of the individual's wellbeing.

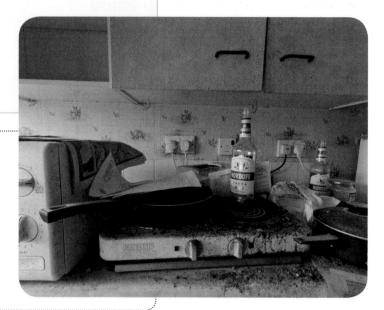

Signs and symptoms of **neglect by others**

- ▶ denial of access to health or social care
- ▶ denial of individual rights and choices
- ▶ the withholding of appropriate and adequate care to meet needs
- ▶ the withholding of medication
- ▶ isolation of the individual by denying others access
- ▶ failure to meet the individual's physical, emotional, social, cultural, intellectual and spiritual needs
- ▶ prevention of others from meeting the individual's needs
- ▶ failure to provide adequate and appropriate food, drink, warmth, shelter and safety
- ▶ failure in the 'duty of care'
- ▶ exposure of the individual to unacceptable risks and dangers.

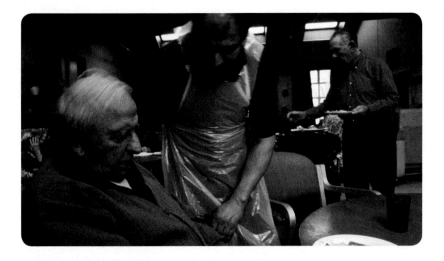

Your assessment criteria:

1.3 Define factors that may contribute to an individual being more vulnerable to abuse

Factors that contribute to abuse

There are a number of factors that contribute to an individual being more vulnerable to abuse. They may depend on physical, emotional, psychological or social support. If this support is either withdrawn or manipulated by an abuser, this will leave the individual more vulnerable to abuse as they become more isolated. Factors that may contribute to increased vulnerability to abuse include those related to the individual and those related to the situation or care-giver (see Figure 5.2).

Figure 5.2 Examples of factors contributing to abuse

Factors related to the individual	Factors related to the situation or care-giver
• Isolation	• Prejudice, resentment and hostility towards the individual
• Physical illness creating dependency	• High levels of care-giver stress
• Mental health issues, e.g. dementia	• Lack of support for care-giver
• Communication problems, e.g. speech or hearing impairments or a learning disability	• Care-giver is drug or alcohol dependent
	• Care-giver has physical or mental health issues
• Behavioural changes resulting from condition, e.g. following a stroke or head injury	• Care-giver has previously been abused themselves
	• Powerlessness and isolation of the care-giver
• Where violence is viewed as the norm within the environment or relationships	• Lack of understanding about the individual's medical condition
	• Lack of leadership and clear roles, responsibilities, policies and procedures
• Past history of accusations	• Lack of training and competence in giving care
	• Lack of or poor monitoring of care provision
	• Staff shortages
	• Lack of continuity of care, e.g. over-reliance on agency/ temporary staff

Environmental factors that contribute to abuse can lead to institutional abuse, especially those relating to inadequate management. These are likely to result in failures in the duty of care, as incompetence and poor practice becomes the norm within a given organisation. When this occurs, it constitutes an abuse of the fundamental rights of the individual. You have a **moral** and legal duty of care to raise your concerns using the appropriate mechanisms.

Key terms

Moral: moral issues are those concerned with deciding what is right and appropriate behaviour

Case study

Mrs Porter is a 73 year-old woman who lives alone in a large house. Her husband of 50 years died two years ago and since that time her health and memory have deteriorated. She has no other family. Mrs Porter receives two visits a day to provide personal care and support at mealtimes. You haven't visited Mrs Porter for two weeks and you are covering as the usual carer has had an accident. You are alarmed and shocked when you see Mrs Porter. She has lost a considerable amount of weight, her hair is matted, and her clothes are dirty. She is frail and appears very frightened. When you move towards her, she puts her arms up in front of her face as if to shield herself. You manage to reassure her and calm her. When you ask if she would prefer a wash or a shower, she tells you the usual carer doesn't normally bother. When you undress her in the bathroom, you are shocked to find her body is covered in bruises. You are particularly concerned about the bruising on the inside of her thighs. When you enquire about the bruising, Mrs Porter starts crying: 'I don't like him! I don't like him! He hurts me'. She then tells you that 'he' is the male carer who comes in at lunchtime visits. You also discover that there's no food in the fridge, and little in the cupboards. You know that shopping is part of Mrs Porter's care package.

1. What signs and symptoms lead you to suspect Mrs Porter is being abused?

2. What types of abuse may be taking place?

3. What factors have made Mrs Porter vulnerable to abuse?

Knowledge Assessment Task

1.1 **1.2** **1.3**

Part of your role and responsibility as a health or social care practitioner is to safeguard individuals from harm and abuse. To do this effectively you will need to be able to recognise the different signs and symptoms of abuse. You will also need to understand the factors that increase an individual's vulnerability to abuse. Complete the questions below to demonstrate your knowledge and understanding of this area of responsibility.

1. Define the different types of abuse.

2. Identify the signs and symptoms associated with each type of abuse.

3. Describe the different factors that may make individuals more vulnerable to abuse.

Keep the written work that you produce as evidence towards your assessment.

How to respond to suspected or alleged abuse

What to do if you suspect abuse

Your organisation will have an agreed policy and procedure for what to do in the event of suspected, actual or alleged abuse. You will need to follow the procedures as described by the organisation in charge of your workplace or placement.

If you suspect abuse YOU MUST:

▶ always raise an **alert** and report your suspicions

▶ follow the agreed procedures

▶ not be persuaded by others that it is 'unimportant' or 'minor', and not worth reporting

▶ seek advice and support from a trustworthy and more senior or experienced member of staff

▶ maintain confidentiality within your role and the procedures

▶ keep the individual safe

▶ remember that you have a duty of care and moral responsibility to act.

In cases where abuse occurs, it is often by linking together seemingly minor incidents that the pattern of abuse is uncovered. If these incidents go unreported, the pattern cannot be established, leading to systematic and repeated abuse becoming accepted practice.

So, if in doubt, always report. Reporting a manager, colleague, or someone who is a member of the individual's personal network, such as a family member or carer, is a highly sensitive and difficult task. It is important therefore to be sure of your facts, and to discuss these with either a more senior member of the team and/or Adult Social Care services before making a decision. However, you must raise the alert. Not doing so constitutes a form of abuse.

If you suspect abuse DO NOT:

▶ ignore it or hide it for fear of the consequences to you if you have unintentionally been involved in the abuse

▶ **collude** with colleagues or others and fail to report your suspicions

▶ make the situation worse by covering up for others

▶ confront the person you think is responsible for the abuse

▶ leave the individual in an unsafe situation or without appropriate support

▶ destroy anything that might be used as evidence.

Your assessment criteria:

1.1 Explain the actions to take if there are suspicions that an individual is being abused.

Key terms

Alert: make another person aware of a possible danger or difficulty

Collude: cooperate with somebody in order to do something illegal or undesirable, or to keep it secret

Adult at risk: the individual adult who may have been subject to, or at risk of, abuse

Investigate

Do you know where the safeguarding adults at risk policies and procedures can be found in your work setting? Find out where they are, and what they say, so that you understand what actions to take if you suspect an individual is being abused.

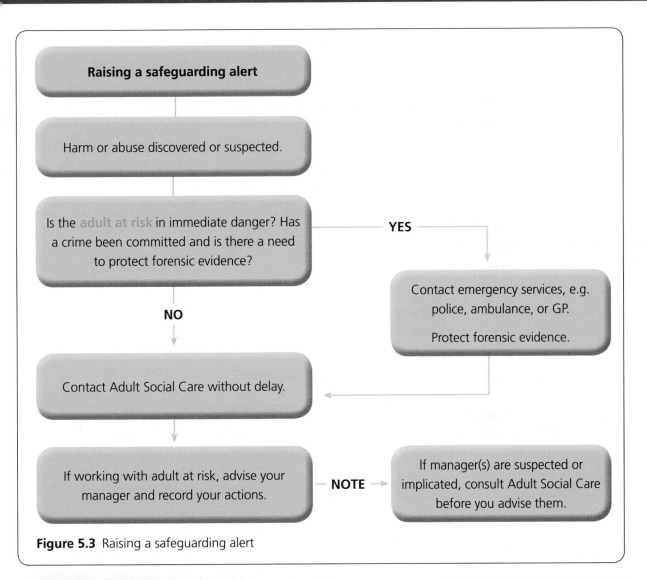

Figure 5.3 Raising a safeguarding alert

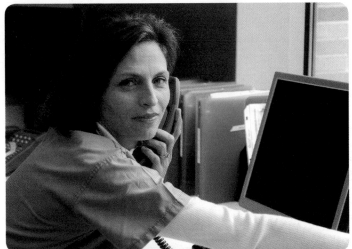

Incidents of suspected or actual abuse must always be documented and reported

Reflect

Think about the following in a situation where you witness an individual being abused by another worker and you fail to report it.

1. How do you think the individual might feel towards you, knowing you witnessed the incident and did nothing?
2. How do you think the abuser might feel towards you?
3. What is likely to happen to the individual being abused?
4. How you would feel about not reporting the incident?

What to do if an individual alleges abuse

If an individual makes an allegation of abuse remember what can and cannot be done. They are described in the previous section. In addition, ensure that you DO:

► follow agreed procedures

► take the individual's allegations seriously

► take them somewhere safe and private

► remain calm and try not to look shocked or angry

► listen without interrupting or prompting

► respect the individual's wishes

► offer reassurance and tell them they have done the right thing

► remember they are likely to feel shocked, frightened, distressed, blameworthy, ashamed or embarrassed

► be honest about your responsibility to act and the limits of this

► offer them the opportunity to talk to someone more senior (if appropriate)

► tell the individual what you are going to do to deal with the situation

► record what they tell you accurately and completely.

Ensure that you DO NOT:

► make assumptions or judge the individual

► put them in any further danger

► ask them any leading questions

► pressure them to talk or give you details they're not comfortable to give

► promise the individual a level of confidentiality beyond your role and responsibility

► discuss the information with anyone outside the individuals who need to be informed.

How to preserve evidence of abuse

In the event of an allegation of abuse, your first duty of care will be to the alleged victim. However, you must also take steps to preserve any evidence vital to a case where a criminal offence may have taken place.

Your assessment criteria:

2.2 Explain the actions to take if an individual alleges that they are being abused

2.3 Identify ways to ensure that evidence of abuse is preserved

Key terms

Leading question: a question which strongly suggests the answer the person asking the question wants to hear

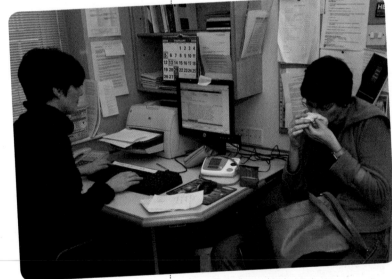

DO NOT:

▶ move or remove anything

▶ touch anything unless you have to make the area, thing or person safe

▶ clean or tidy up

▶ allow access to anyone not involved in investigating.

DO:

▶ record any visible signs of abuse, such as bruising, or physical injuries, torn clothing, signs of distress

▶ if you have to touch something, keep it to a minimum and try not to destroy fingerprints

▶ keep anything of interest dry and safe, especially anything that may have been used to injure the individual

▶ preserve clothing, footwear, bedding and other such items, and handle them as little as possible

▶ preserve anything used to keep the individual warm

▶ record in writing

▶ record any injuries

▶ preserve and record the state of the individual and the alleged abuser's clothing (if appropriate)

▶ record the condition and attitudes of the people involved.

If items need to be preserved, then this can be done by placing:

▶ most items in a clean brown paper bag or in a clean unsealed envelope

▶ liquids in clean glassware.

Reflect

An individual you support returns from a visit to the shops tearful and distressed. Their coat is torn and dirty. They are holding their arm as if it hurts and will not let you look at it. When you ask them what has happened they just mumble that they have 'lost' their bag and shopping. You suspect something more has happened. What would you do in this situation?

Who would you involve?

How would you preserve any evidence?

Knowledge Assessment Task | **2.1** | **2.2** | **2.3**

Having a good working knowledge and understanding of the reporting processes is part of a health and social care practitioner's responsibilities. Knowing what to do, what not to do and whom to report to are all important aspects of safeguarding individuals from abuse. Completing the following questions will help you to demonstrate your knowledge and understanding of this area of practice:

1. What would you do if you suspect abuse?

2. What would you do if someone tells you they have been abused?

3. How would you preserve any evidence of abuse to ensure it is not contaminated?

Keep the written work that you produce as evidence towards your assessment.

National and local policies and systems for safeguarding

Two key national policy documents that relate to safeguarding adults at risk are:

▶ *No secrets – guidance on developing and implementing multi-agency policies and procedures to protect vulnerable adults from abuse* (2000)

▶ *Safeguarding adults – a national framework of standards for good practice and outcomes in adult protection work* (2005)

Together, these two documents provide best practice guidance on establishing local multi-agency policies and procedures, and clearly outline multi-agency roles and responsibilities. They also reinforce the need for rigorous, transparent recruitment practices. As a result of the recommendations made, prior to being employed in health and social care all prospective employees and volunteers are required to undergo a Criminal Records Bureau (CRB) check. This check is repeated every three years. In addition, all health and social care employees and volunteers are required by law to be registered with the Independent Safeguarding Authority (ISA).

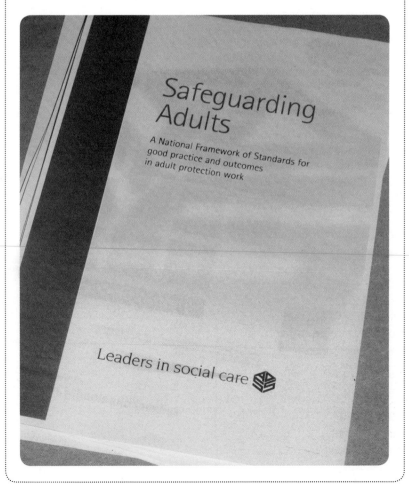

Your assessment criteria:

3.1 Identify national policies and local systems that relate to safeguarding and protection from abuse

Investigate

Do you know where the Safeguarding Adults at Risk policy and procedures can be found in your work setting? Does your workplace have a copy of *No secrets*? Find out if and when individuals using your service are given a leaflet/information about Safeguarding Adults at Risk procedures. If they are not given any information, find out why this is the case?

Figure 5.4 National legislation with regards to safeguarding

Legislation or national policy	Summary of key points
Legal powers to intervene	There are a range of laws that enable abusers to be prosecuted. These include: • Offences Against the Person Act 1861 – relates to physical abuse • Sexual Offences Act 2003 – relates to sexual abuse • Protection from Harassment Act 1997 – relates to psychological abuse • Section 47, National Assistance Act 1948 – relates to neglect.
Human Rights Act 1998	All individuals have the right to live their lives free from violence and abuse. Rights include: • Article 2: 'The right to life' • Article 3: 'Freedom from torture (including humiliating and degrading treatment)' • Article 8: 'Right to family life'.
Mental Capacity Act 2005	Provides the statutory framework to empower and protect adults at risk who are unable to make their own decisions. The five key principles are: • a presumption of capacity • the right for individuals to be supported to make their own decisions • individuals must retain the right to make what might be seen as eccentric or unwise decisions • anything done must be the in the individual's best interests • least restrictive intervention. The Act includes guidance regarding care and treatment and restraint and particularly relates to financial abuse.
Safeguarding Vulnerable Groups Act 2006	Resulted from the Bichard Inquiry in 2002 into the Soham murders. Recommendations led to creation of the Independent Safeguarding Authority (ISA) which is responsible for: • the Vetting and Barring Scheme (VBS) • maintaining children and adults barring lists.
Health & Social Care (HSC) Act 2008; HSC Act (Regulated Activities) Regulations 2010; CQC Regulations 2009	Established the Care Quality Commission (CQC) to regulate the quality and safety of health and adult social care services. Replaces National Minimum Standards. Introduced essential standards of quality and safety, which are 28 regulations and associated outcomes.

In February 2011 the UK government decided that the Criminal Records Bureau and the Independent Safeguarding Authority would merge to form a single streamlined authority to provide a barring and criminal recording checking service.

What roles do different agencies play in safeguarding?

Part of the duty of care remit requires a working knowledge of safeguarding procedures. Understanding how to use national and local safeguarding procedures is a crucial aspect of health and social care work. This responsibility includes volunteers as well as employees.

Your assessment criteria:

3.2 Explain the roles of different agencies in safeguarding and protecting individuals from abuse

3.3 Identify reports into serious failures to protect individuals from abuse

Figure 5.5 Agencies involved in safeguarding

Agency	Key responsibilities
Local authority adult social care services	These agencies: • receive safeguarding alerts • ensure action is taken to keep individual safe – may require immediate intervention/assessment/provision of additional care services • liaise with all individuals/agencies involved • provide information and advice • coordinate investigations • arrange, chair and record meetings and case conferences • remove the alleged abuser, if required • are represented at police interviews.
All agencies, including police, NHS, GPs, medical services, councils, emergency services, independent, voluntary, private providers, Trading Standards, CQC	These agencies: • implement and work to the agreed safeguarding adults policies and procedures • cooperate and collaborate with other agencies to ensure the safety of adults at risk • ensure all staff can recognise signs and symptoms of abuse • ensure all staff receive regular awareness training of safeguarding policies, reporting and recording procedures • provide information and advice to people who access services to ensure they understand how they can protect themselves and others • ensure all employees and others required by law are CRB checked and registered with the ISA prior to employment • inform the ISA of anyone who is unsuitable to work with adults at risk.

In addition to the above, the following have additional roles and responsibilities:

Police	The police: • investigate allegations of abuse if a crime is suspected • gather evidence • pursue criminal proceedings if appropriate • protect people in vulnerable situations.
Medical Services e.g. GP, NHS Acute Trusts	These agencies: • provide immediate treatment if required • undertake evidential investigations or medical examinations, if required and following consent.

What reports are available regarding serious failures in safeguarding adults at risk?

As a health and social care worker, it is important that you learn from the findings and recommendations of inquiries into failures in practice. You must also be able to relate these findings and recommendations to your organisation's policies and care practice.

In the past five years there have been a number of inquiries into failures in safeguarding. The following are just three of the resultant reports:

1. *Six lives – the provision of public services to people with learning disabilities* (2009): a report by Ann Abraham, Health Service Ombudsman, and Jerry White, Local Government Ombudsman. This inquiry was launched in response to complaints by Mencap on behalf of the families of six people with learning disabilities who died whilst in NHS or local authority care between 2003 and 2005. Details were initially highlighted in the Mencap report *Death by Indifference* (2007). As a result an urgent review of health and social care for people with learning disabilities was recommended.

2. *The Francis Inquiry Report* (2010): a report on the level of care provided by Mid Staffordshire NHS Foundation Trust (see page 98 in SHC 24 for more about this report).

3. *Care and Compassion?* (2011): a report by Ann Abraham, Health Service Ombudsman, on 10 investigations into NHS care of older people. The investigations highlighted the gaps between the actual experiences of older people and their families, and the principles and values of the NHS. The report identified that:

   ▶ fundamental needs were consistently neglected

   ▶ staff attitudes were dismissive

   ▶ staff had a total disregard for the older person's rights, dignity and privacy

   ▶ poor communication, planning, coordination and thoughtlessness left people in excessive pain and discomfort

   ▶ inflexible attitudes led to families being excluded at mealtimes, resulting in patients unable to feed themselves becoming malnourished and dehydrated.

Reflect

Read one of the inquiry reports mentioned in this last section. Think about the following:

1. How were the individuals involved in the failures abused?

2. What types of abuse did they experience?

3. Who else do you think was abused?

4. Could similar failures and abuses as those identified in the report happen in your work setting?

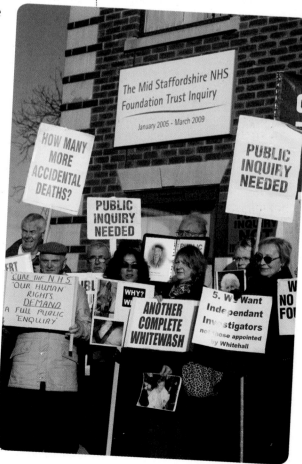

Your role in safeguarding and protecting against abuse

Where can you go to seek information and advice?

Advice and guidance on safeguarding procedures are available in your organisation's safeguarding policy and procedures document. Your employer will also provide training and updates on safeguarding and protecting adults at risk. Policies and procedures documents, training and updates will contain information about:

▶ types of abuse

▶ signs and symptoms

▶ how to respond to suspected, actual or alleged abuse

▶ what to do and who to go to if you suspect someone more senior than yourself

▶ how to report and record suspected, actual or alleged abuse

▶ a list of contact numbers and names.

Supervision meetings are a good opportunity for you to seek advice and guidance about your role. These should occur regularly. Your manager or a senior member of the team will provide you with advice and support at any time.

Your assessment criteria:

3.4 Identify sources of information and advice about own role in safeguarding and protecting individuals from abuse

4.1 Explain how the likelihood of abuse may be reduced by:
- working with person-centred values
- encouraging active participation
- promoting choice and rights

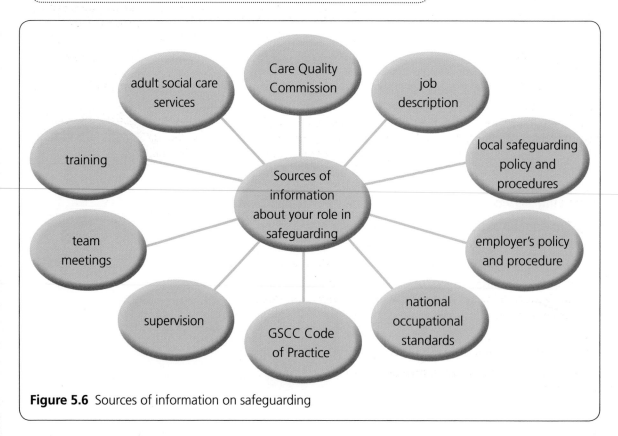

Figure 5.6 Sources of information on safeguarding

Person-centred approaches

Person-centred approaches have been successfully used in the support of adults with learning disabilities and individuals with dementia. Person-centred approaches place the individual at the centre of all activities. This kind of approach reduces the likelihood of abuse occurring by means of the following core values:

▶ **individuality** – planning support around the unique needs of the individual

▶ **rights** – never doing things that may ignore or go against the individual's rights

▶ **choice** – making sure choices are appropriate to the individual and in their best interests

▶ **privacy** – making sure the individual is free from unwanted intrusion by others

▶ **independence** – giving the individual time and opportunity to self-manage

▶ **dignity** – supporting the individual to maintain emotional control and sense of self-worth in difficult and sensitive situations

▶ **respect** – always treating the individual in a way that demonstrates their sense of self-worth and their importance to others

▶ **partnership** – working with others with a focus on achieving outcomes that are always in the best interests of the individual.

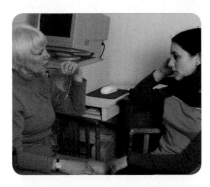

Investigate

Find out which policies and procedures underpin person-centred approaches in your work setting. Find out what advice and training is available to existing and new employees about person-centred approaches.

Reflect

Think about the individuals you support. Consider how you support them to ensure you work in a person-centred way.

1. How do you demonstrate that you see them as a unique individual?

2. What do you do to ensure you really understand their point of view, wishes and expectations?

3. How do you ensure they are involved in decisions about their support and care?

Knowledge Assessment Task   3.1 3.2 3.3 3.4

Safeguarding individuals from abuse is the responsibility of everyone involved in providing support. Understanding the roles and responsibilities of other agencies and how to clarify your role is an important way of learning from failures in practice that lead to abuse. Complete the following questions to demonstrate your knowledge and understanding about joint working, clarifying your role and what can be learnt from inquiry reports to improve safeguarding procedures:

1. What are the national policies and local procedures that relate to safeguarding and protecting adults at risk?

2. Outline the roles of different agencies in safeguarding and protecting adults at risk?

3. Identify at least two inquiry reports regarding serious failures in care practice that led to abuse taking place.

4. Where would you obtain information and advice about your role in safeguarding and protecting adults at risk?

Keep the written work that you produce as evidence towards your assessment.

How can working with active participation reduce the likelihood of abuse?

An impersonal support regime, which allows infringement of individual rights, generates the conditions in which abuse can occur. The individual is depersonalised, disempowered and ceases to be an active, social agent in their own right. Active participation is a way of working that recognises an individual's right to participate in the activities and relationships of everyday life. The individual is given as much independence as possible. Crucially, the individual is viewed as an *active* participant or partner, and not as the *passive* recipient of health and social support. The main result of an active participatory approach is the **empowerment** of the individual concerned. The individual is empowered to make choices about how their personal support is delivered. This way the individual's needs are met, and care regimes that are simply convenient to the provider are ended.

The increased access to, and use of, self-directed budgets, where individuals manage their own care package, is one example of how active participation has changed the way health and social care services are delivered. Being in control of how care and support is provided enables individuals to enter into more equal partnerships with providers. This further reduces the potential for an individual's rights to be disregarded.

In 2009 the government carried out a consultation process to review the effectiveness of *No secrets*. Of the 12,000 people involved, 3,000 were members of the public, and many were people to whom the guidance applied. The following recommendations with regards to procedure are a good example of active participation on a national scale. The process recommended that care organisations ensure:

▶ that the abused individual is empowered and listened to

▶ that the individual is fully involved in safeguarding decisions

▶ that the individual who lacks capacity to independently participate in the decision-making process is represented and able to participate as fully as possible.

Key terms

Empowerment: gaining more control over your life by being given greater self-confidence and self-esteem

Reflect

Think about the individuals you support.

1. How do the assessment and care planning processes used take account of the individual's life story?

2. How is understanding of their life experiences used to create a person-centred approach to supporting their needs?

3. How do you think taking a person-centred approach enables you to safeguard them from harm and/or abuse?

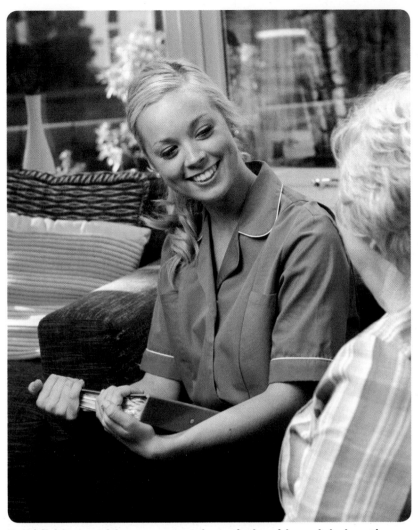

Investigate

Investigate all the different ways in which individuals being supported within your workplace are empowered. Find out how individuals are:

▶ supported to make their views and opinions known

▶ involved in the processes of assessment, care planning and reviewing care

▶ given easily understandable and accessible information about their rights and responsibilities.

Establishing positive, empowering relationships minimises the possibility of abuse happening in care settings

Case study

You work in a residential care home for individuals with dementia. The residents have moderate levels of dementia and many are still physically active. Most require frequent prompting when undertaking daily living activities. Most of the residents are in their 90s and very few have relatives who visit frequently.

1. What factors make the residents of the home vulnerable to abuse?

2. How can you apply person-centred values to working with the residents to reduce the likelihood of abuse?

3. How can you encourage the residents to actively participate in their support to reduce the likelihood of abuse?

How can promoting choice and rights reduce the likelihood of abuse?

In organisations where it is common practice to work in ways that actively promote individual choices and rights, the potential for abuse is reduced. This is because the way support is provided will be organised in such a way as to ensure the individual is actively involved in everything that happens. It encourages a culture of care based on listening to the individual, and making decisions based on the individual's expressed wants. Carers, family members and friends share the same beliefs and values; and understand the benefits of choice and the necessity of rights. Such a practice actively promotes the individual's rights, including the right to choose, on a daily basis. It is a transparent practice, and as such it is much more difficult to abuse. Finally, in the event that abuse does occur, the chances that it is discovered – and discovered early – are high.

How to actively promote individual choices and rights:

▸ Spend time getting to know the individual.

▸ Understand their needs and abilities.

▸ Understand how their situation/condition affects their day-to-day life and activities.

▸ Understand their likes and dislikes.

▸ Understand what is important to them and what their priorities are.

▸ Understand their values and beliefs.

▸ Understand how their past experiences impact on their view of life/their current situation.

▸ Respect their uniqueness.

▸ Understand the duty of care.

How can an accessible complaints procedure reduce the likelihood of abuse?

An organisation that is actively involved in reducing the likelihood of abuse occurring will be one that accepts complaints as a form of feedback. In this way, the organisation will be able to constantly review and improve its procedures for the detection of abuse. It is essential therefore that care organisations develop complaint procedures that are easily accessed – available, easy to understand and easy to use – and that remove the fear of retribution.

Your assessment criteria:

4.1 Explain how the likelihood of abuse may be reduced by:
- working with person-centred values
- encouraging active participation
- promoting choice and rights

4.2 Explain the importance of an accessible complaints procedure for reducing the likelihood of abuse

Key terms

Retribution: something done to injure a person in any way as punishment for something that person may have done

Making the complaints procedure accessible to all encourages openness. Providing individuals vulnerable to abuse with a user-friendly complaints procedure further diminishes the likelihood of abuse taking place. Accessible complaints procedures should:

- be written in plain English and made available in different formats – i.e. in pictures, other languages, on tape or in Braille

- be available as copies to anyone using the service

- include an explanation as to how to use the procedures

- include a way of checking that the user has understood the procedure

- be displayed in the public areas of the service

- be provided by staff trained to respond positively to a complaint

- encourage individuals to complain if they are dissatisfied with their support

- involve the use of a key worker system to ensure individuals are listened to and given the opportunity to complain informally

- confidentially inform individuals using the service when complaints have been dealt with

- confidentially inform individuals as to the outcome of individual complaints.

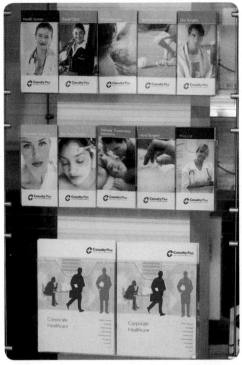

Information must be accessible, easy to understand and available in a variety of formats

Knowledge Assessment Task   4.1   4.2

As a health and social care practitioner the way that you support individuals will have a direct impact on how safe or vulnerable they are to abuse. Complete the questions below using examples to demonstrate how current approaches can improve safeguarding and reduce an individual's vulnerability.

1. Use examples to explain how the following reduce the likelihood of abuse:
   - working with person-centred values
   - encouraging active participation
   - promoting choice and rights

2. How is making sure the complaints procedure is accessible an important way to reduce the likelihood of abuse?

Keep the written work that you produce as evidence towards your assessment.

Recognising and reporting unsafe practices

What are unsafe practices?

Any practice that puts the service user or care worker at risk could be considered as unsafe. An **unsafe practice** can take place due to: poorly observed procedures; insufficient resources; operational difficulties.

Poor working practices include:

▶ not wearing personal protective equipment

▶ not following correct procedures

▶ not undertaking risk assessments

▶ ignoring strategies to manage risk

▶ lack of monitoring, supervision and guidance.

Insufficient resources may include:

▶ not having the appropriate equipment to undertake a task

▶ not having enough equipment or materials to undertake a task safely

▶ one person doing a task that should be done by two people

▶ not allocating enough time to safely carry out activities and tasks.

Operational difficulties may include:

▶ not having enough staff to adequately meet individuals needs

▶ lack of appropriate staff training

▶ lack of policies, procedures and guidance for staff

▶ lack of regular and appropriate staff supervision

▶ lack of leadership and management.

What action should you take if you identify unsafe practices?

When practices are unsafe it suggests that they are being carried out without due care and attention to the potential danger and harm that may result. You have a duty of care to make your employer aware of any unsafe practices, and to take action to protect yourself and others (see page 86).

An organisation's written procedures will outline the action to be taken in the event of unsafe practice. These procedures will differ from organisation to organisation, but all procedures concerning unsafe practice will share the same core elements:

Your assessment criteria:

5.1 Describe unsafe practices that may affect the wellbeing of individuals.

5.2 Explain the actions to take if unsafe practices have been identified.

Key terms

Unsafe practice: a level of care that puts individuals at risk

Reflect

Think about the individuals you support. Consider how you support them to ensure you work in a person-centred way.

1. How do you demonstrate that you see them as a unique individual?

2. What do you do to ensure you really understand their point of view, wishes and expectations?

3. How do you ensure they are involved in decisions about their support and care?

1. If possible and safe to do so, make the situation safe, e.g. identify an unsafe area with a hazard sign.

2. Report the situation without delay to the person in charge:

   ▶ verbally – to the senior person on duty

   ▶ in writing – in the daily record, and complete an incident form/maintenance form.

3. Ensure others are aware of the potential danger. If appropriate, remove and label broken equipment.

4. Follow up to check if the situation has been remedied. Keep your own records.

Safety is everyone's responsibility. In some situations unsafe working practices may have become normalised over time. In these situations, care workers who refuse to carry out a procedure they may deem unsafe can be made to feel incompetent or negligent. Should this occur, check the procedure against the organisation's written procedures. If you are correct, and it is unsafe, seek advice from a senior colleague, and if necessary register a complaint. Remember to act. Doing nothing supports the unsafe practice.

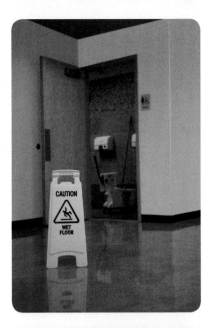

Investigate

Think about your work setting. Find out what the correct procedures are. How would you use the procedures to help report and record the following:

▶ unsafe working practices?

▶ unsafe equipment?

▶ suspected/actual abuse?

Find out the procedure for making a complaint, and what further steps to take if no action results from the initial complaint.

Case study

You have been working as a domiciliary care worker for nine months in a rural area. When you first started you had a two-week induction which included both the mandatory training and shadowing a more experienced worker for a week. You work in the evenings and one day at the weekend. During your five-hour shift you normally undertake eight 30-minute visits. However, for the past month your manager has allocated you ten visits in the same time. You have explained to your manager several times that this is not possible to do as your calls are all at least 10 minutes apart and each individual you visit has a 30-minute allocation to carry out the agreed care plan. Your manager has told you to ignore the care plan and just to do what you can. When you question your manager as to what should be recorded now that you don't have enough time to complete the care plan, your manager tells you to write that everything was done as stated on the care plan. You tell them you don't agree. You say that are unhappy about the situation. They indicate to you if you don't do as asked, your hours could be reduced.

1. What is unsafe about this situation?
2. What are the potential consequences of these unsafe practices for the individuals you visit?
3. What action can you take to resolve the situation?
4. Who is being abused in this situation?

What action should you take if there has been no response to reported suspected abuse or unsafe practices?

When you raise a concern and report either suspected abuse or unsafe practices always ensure you put this in writing, and that you keep a copy for your own records. This will protect you and the people you are trying to protect, and allow you to produce written detailed evidence when your alert or complaint is investigated.

Most procedures operate agreed timescales that stipulate when a complaint, concern or incident should be dealt with. These timescales will entail a number of time-related step-by-step procedures, one of which guarantees the time it will take to respond to an alert. However, depending on the severity of a case, or the danger posed by an incident, timescales may be overridden by senior care managers and other associated external services, such as the police. Make sure you know and understand which procedures apply.

In the event that you have been asked to carry out a task you deem unsafe, and have followed in-house procedures with regards to complaints and alerts, and the times within which the incident should have been responded to have passed, then you will need to follow your organisation's procedures for grievances. An employee or volunteer grievance procedure should provide details of persons and organisations to contact. These may include a more senior person within the organisation; an external body, such as the Adult Social Care Services; the Care Quality Commission (CQC). Depending on the nature of the grievance, you may also want to notify your trade union, which will provide information, advice and help (see also page 94).

Knowledge Assessment Task   5.1   5.2   5.3

As a health and social care practitioner you have a responsibility to recognise and take appropriate action when you become aware of unsafe practices that place you, individuals you support or other people at risk of harm or abuse. Complete the following questions to demonstrate your knowledge and understanding in relation to unsafe practices:

1. Use examples to describe unsafe practices that may affect the wellbeing of individuals.

2. Explain what you would do if you identified unsafe practices.

3. Describe what you would do if suspected abuse or unsafe practices had been reported but no action had been taken to respond to or resolve the situation.

Keep the written work that you produce as evidence towards your assessment.

Are you ready for assessment?

AC	What you know now	Assessment task	✓
1.1	Define different types of abuse	Page 115	
1.2	Identify the signs and/or symptoms associated with each type of abuse	Page 115	
1.3	Describe the factors that may contribute to an individual being more vulnerable to abuse	Page 115	
2.1	Explain the actions to take if there are suspicions that an individual is being abused	Page 119	
2.2	Explain the actions to take if an individual alleges that they are being abused	Page 119	
2.3	Identify ways to ensure that evidence of abuse is preserved	Page 119	
3.1	Identify national policies and local systems that relate to safeguarding and protection from abuse	Page 125	
3.2	Explain the roles of different agencies in safeguarding and protecting individuals from abuse	Page 125	
3.3	Identify reports into serious failures to protect individuals from abuse	Page 125	
3.4	Identify sources of information and advice about own role in safeguarding and protecting individuals from abuse	Page 125	
4.1	Explain how the likelihood of abuse can be reduced by working with person-centred values, encouraging active participation and promoting choice and rights	Page 129	
4.2	Explain the importance of an accessible complaints procedure for reducing the likelihood of abuse	Page 129	✓
5.1	Describe unsafe practice that may affect the wellbeing of individuals	Page 132	
5.2	Explain the actions to take if unsafe practices have been identified	Page 132	
5.3	Describe the actions to take if suspected abuse or unsafe practices have been reported but nothing has been done in response	Page 132	

6 | The role of the health and social care worker (HSC 025)

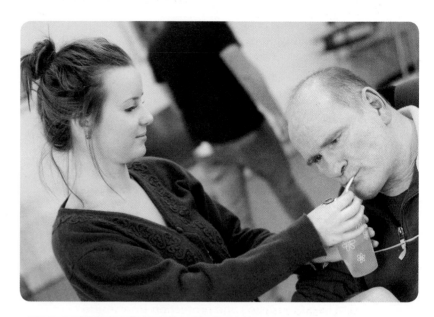

Assessment of this unit

This unit will introduce you to the knowledge and skills needed to understand working relationships in care settings, the importance of working in ways that are agreed with your employer, and the role that partnership working now plays in the health and social care sector. You will need to:

▶ understand working relationships in health and social care

▶ be able to work in ways that are agreed with the employer

▶ be able to work in partnership with others.

The assessment of this unit is partly knowledge-based (things you need to know about) and partly competence-based (things you need to do in the real work environment). To successfully complete this unit, you will need to produce evidence of both your knowledge and your competence. The tables on the page opposite outline what you need to know and do to meet each of the assessment criteria for the unit.

Your tutor or assessor will help you to prepare for your assessment and the tasks suggested in the unit will help you to create the evidence that you need.

CHAPTER 6

AC What you need to know

1.1 Explain how a working relationship is different from a personal relationship

1.2 Describe different working relationships in health and social care settings

AC What you need to do

2.1 Describe why it is important to adhere to the agreed scope of the job role

2.2 Access full and up-to-date details of agreed ways of working

2.3 Implement agreed ways of working

3.1 Explain why it is important to work in partnership with others

3.2 Demonstrate ways of working that can help improve partnership working

3.3 Identify skills and approaches needed for resolving conflicts

3.4 Demonstrate how and when to access support and advice about:
- partnership working
- resolving conflicts

Assessment criteria 2.1–2.3, and 3.1–3.4 must be assessed in a real work environment.

This unit also links to some of the other units:

SHC 22 Introduction to personal development in health and social care settings

SHC 24 Introduction to duty of care in health and social care

Some of your learning will be repeated in these units and will give you the chance to review your knowledge and understanding.

Understanding working relationships in health and social care

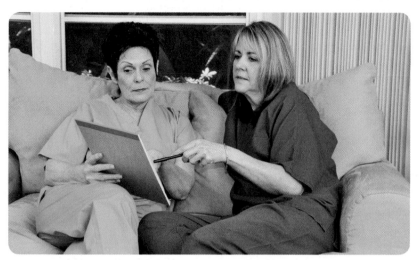

Relationships with service users and colleagues are a key part of care practice

Your assessment criteria:

1.1 Explain how a working relationship is different from a personal relationship

1.2 Describe different working relationships in health and social care settings

Reflect

Can you think of examples of different types of relationship in your own life? Which relationships are most important to you, and most influential in your life?

Different types of relationship

We all experience a number of different types of relationship throughout our lives. These include:

▶ family relationships (with partners, parents and siblings, for example)

▶ friendships

▶ intimate personal and sexual relationships

▶ working relationships.

These different relationships can have both a positive and a negative impact on our personal development and wellbeing. They each perform a different function and meet our needs in different ways. The nature and significance of the relationships we have depend on the life stage that we are in; the relationships change as we grow older.

Family relationships

Whatever type of family structure a person lives in (see Figure 6.1), their relationship with their parent(s) or main carers, and with their siblings, will play a big part in their personal

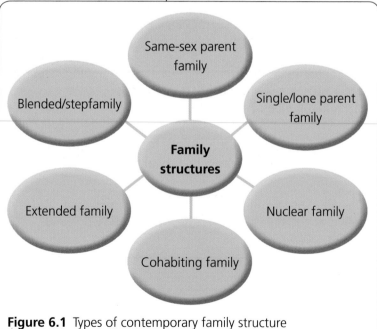

Figure 6.1 Types of contemporary family structure

development and wellbeing. An infant generally forms their first relationship with one or both of their parents. Close physical contact, the provision of food, and regular, reassuring care and communication between the child and their parents will create an **attachment relationship**. The child who feels loved, with complete trust in their parents' affection and support, develops a sense of emotional security and self-confidence.

A child's parents continue to play an important role in their development as they get older. Parents become role models, socialising the child, providing care and support, and helping them to learn how they should behave towards others. During this stage of life parents have a strong influence on their child's self-concept and self-esteem.

When a person moves into adolescence their relationship with their parents tends to change. In particular, there is less of a focus on **socialisation** and providing physical support, and more of a focus on emotional support. Despite the growing desire for independence, and the strains and tensions that this can bring to family relationships, adolescents need to feel that their parents love and support them. Adolescents who have a trusting, supportive and affectionate relationship with their parents will tend to have better self-esteem and be better equipped for the transition to adulthood than adolescents who lack this relationship.

A person's family relationships may change significantly during adulthood. The majority of people leave home and begin new relationships with people outside of their birth family, perhaps getting married or living with a partner and starting a family of their own. As a result, adults tend to alter the relationship they have with their parents. Whilst still being their parent's child, an adult is now independent, able to manage their own life and perhaps also committed to relationships in their new family. Despite this, parents can still play an important part in an adult's emotional life and may be consulted about important decisions or issues that the person faces.

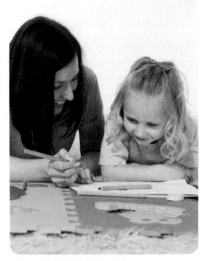

Parental relationships are based on attachment

Key terms

Attachment relationship: relationship based on strong emotional bonds

Socialisation: the process through which individuals learn the culture, norms and way of life of a group or society

Discuss

What impact do you think a person's early relationships have on them later in life? Share thoughts and ideas on this with a work colleague or a classmate. Do you think that a person's early, childhood relationships provide a 'blueprint' for the relationships they develop later in life?

Reflect

Have your family relationships changed over time? Think about how they have changed and the impact that this has had on you.

Intimate, personal and sexual relationships

People generally first start to become interested in more personal relationships in their early teens. Adolescents tend to fall in and out of love quite frequently as they experience 'crushes' (infatuations) during puberty. This can be emotionally painful but most teenagers use these experiences to learn more about the emotional aspects of relationships and to extend their understanding of their own needs and preferences. For many teenagers their first intimate relationship is an intense emotional experience rather than a sexual one. Intimate personal relationships tend to be short-lived during early adolescence but become longer and more emotionally and physically involved in later adolescence. Sexual relationships can be long- or short-term but tend to be seen as significant because of the level of physical intimacy and emotional closeness they involve. People usually establish longer-term intimate, personal and sexual relationships when they are emotionally mature and have a stronger sense of personal identity.

Friendships

Friends are people whom we generally see as likeable, dependable and with whom we can communicate easily. People form friendships for a variety of reasons, including: shared attitudes, values and interests; emotional support and companionship. Friendships tend to boost a person's self-esteem and self-confidence and help people to develop social skills. Friendships make an important contribution to an individual's emotional and social development and the formation of their self-concept.

Friendships play an important role in a person's social and emotional development. An individual will first learn how to behave and relate to others through family relationships during infancy. As they move into early childhood, the person will begin meeting other children and increase their range of friendships. Friendships can be especially important during adolescence, when young people are trying to forge an identity separate from their parents, and also in adulthood when friendships form the basis of our social lives outside of the family. Friendships in later adulthood can be a vital source of companionship and connection to a person's past. Throughout life, an individual's personality, social skills and emotional development are all shaped by their friendships. Friendships play a role in helping people to feel they belong, are wanted and liked by others, and that there are people to whom they can turn for support.

Investigate

What do the policies and procedures of your care organisation say about the intimate, personal and sexual relationships of service users? How are you advised to deal with issues relating to these types of relationships in your care setting?

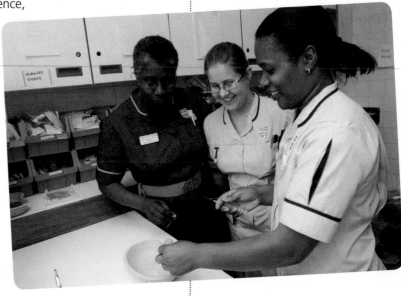

Working relationships

Working relationships are different to other forms of relationship because the relationship serves a particular, non-personal purpose to do with achieving tasks or coordinating roles in an organisation. Most working relationships are formed between individuals who are not of equal status, and have clear boundaries. A person's job description, and the line management arrangements that exist in the work setting, often define these boundaries. As a result, one person usually has more power or authority in the relationship than the other. Relationships between students and teachers, between employers and employees, and between colleagues, are examples of working relationships. Effective working relationships tend to be based on good communication, trust and respect between the people involved. Figure 6.3 identifies some other qualities of good working relationships.

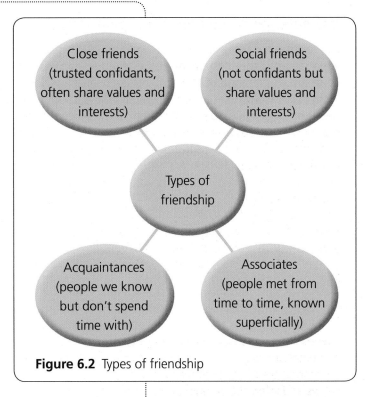

Figure 6.2 Types of friendship

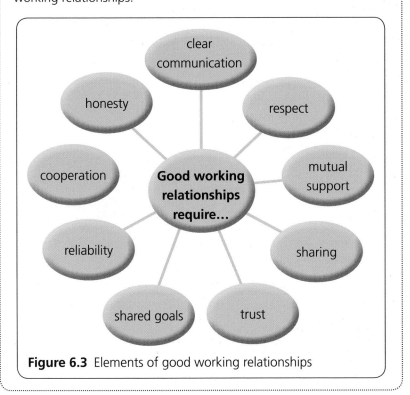

Figure 6.3 Elements of good working relationships

Reflect

What qualities or skills do you have, and what strategies do you use, which contribute to the effectiveness of your working relationships?

Employer/employee relationships

The relationship that you have with your employer has a very important influence on your role as a health or social care worker. There are a vast range of different roles in health and social care. Many, such as adult social worker, paramedic and occupational therapist, involve giving care directly to service users. Some other roles, such as care manager or residential home manager, have a significant but usually indirect impact on the care that people receive.

The employer-employee relationship is an example of a **formal relationship**. That is, it is based on a set of rules and expectations about how people should relate to each other because of their employment relationship. The employer has the most power and authority to direct the activities of the employee in these situations. Employment relationships can affect an individual's self-image, their social skills and their intellectual development, depending on the type of work they do and the development opportunities they are given. A person's relationship with their employer may also influence their attitudes, values and behaviour as well as their self-concept.

Relationships with colleagues

Care practitioners need to form effective working relationships with colleagues as they tend to work in teams or in collaborative partnerships, such as multi-agency arrangements, when providing care and support. Trust, mutual support and cooperation are important features of team working. However, each health and social care team is different and relationships within a team often change or need to be adapted each time someone joins or leaves the team. Within your work setting, some of your colleagues will also be your peers. That is, they will be people of equal status and similar background to you. Being supported, liked and valued by your work colleagues will have a positive effect on your self-confidence and self-esteem as well as your effectiveness as a team member. Key points for effective team work include:

▶ understanding communication processes within your workplace (and in your team in particular) and knowing how you can contribute to effective communication

▶ recognising and valuing the contributions of others

▶ valuing and accommodating individual differences

▶ carrying out your own role effectively so that you make an appropriate and expected contribution to the team.

Key terms

Formal relationship: relationship based on agreed, formal terms, such as that between colleagues in a workplace

Reflect

Think about the different people you work with. Why are some of your relationships stronger and more supportive than others? Are there any colleagues with whom you would like to have a better or more effective working relationship? What could you do to improve this?

There will be numerous occasions when you have to communicate effectively in order to provide high quality care to service users or information to others regarding an individual's care. In addition, you and your colleagues are likely to meet and communicate as a team in:

▶ planning and review meetings

▶ staff support meetings

▶ staff development meetings

▶ training and education sessions

▶ handover or report meetings.

You can use these occasions to develop your knowledge and understanding of care and team working issues, share best practice or discuss different approaches, and resolve any disputes or concerns about practice in your care setting.

Reflect

Which of these meetings take place in your work setting? Do you attend and make a contribution to team discussions? Think about how you might be able to improve or increase your involvement in the different kinds of team meetings that take place in your work setting.

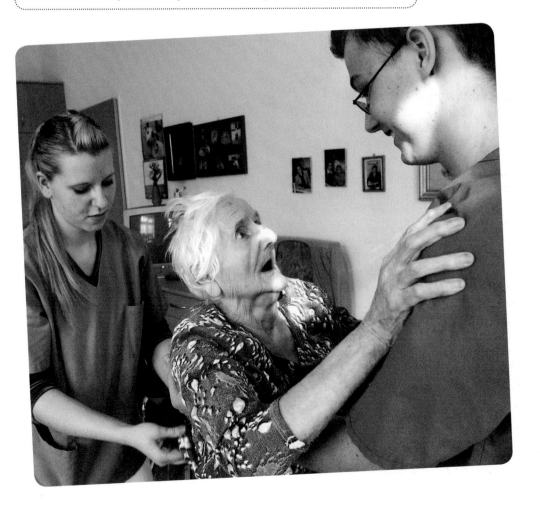

Supportive relationships

It is important that relationships between colleagues are supportive. You can promote this by recognising when individuals are:

- ▶ feeling stressed by personal or professional matters

- ▶ performing their work effectively

- ▶ over-stretched, struggling to cope with their workload and needing help.

Effective health and social care teams tend to involve colleagues who are supportive of each other. Sharing information, showing new or less experienced colleagues how to do things, and being available when a colleague needs practical or emotional support, all contribute to this supportive environment. Supportive relationships tend to be mutual so the support that you provide for others should be reciprocated (returned) to help make your work life a little easier and less stressful.

Relationships with service users

The relationship that a health or social care practitioner has with the individuals for whom they provide care or support plays a crucial part in their professional work. Care relationships are different to the other types of relationship that the care practitioner may have. One of the unusual and defining features of a care relationship is that it can involve a higher level of non-sexual physical contact and an emotional closeness with the person than is present in other relationships. As a result, care relationships depend heavily on the development and maintenance of trust and mutual respect between care practitioners and service users.

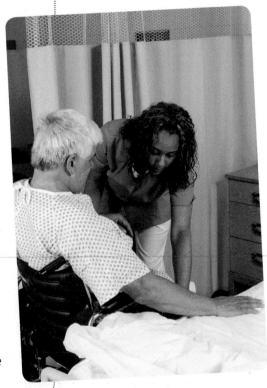

Providing personal and physical care, and listening and responding to the often very personal problems and difficulties that a service user has, puts the care practitioner in a powerful and privileged position in the care relationship. It is vital that care practitioners do not abuse or misuse the power or privileged position that the care relationship gives them. Because the relationship with the service user is the cornerstone of all the work that they do as a care provider, it must be based on trust. Good care relationships must also promote and support service users' rights to make their own decisions and to have their safety and security protected during care interventions and when they are most vulnerable and unable to care for themselves.

Reflect

Who are the supportive people in your work setting? Why do you find these people more supportive than others? Think about what it is that makes these people more supportive than others.

Case study

Geraldine is 32 years old and a single parent. Since the age of 25 she has suffered from multiple sclerosis. Her condition has left her without the ability to walk, has impaired her eyesight and has reduced her energy to care for herself and her two children, Eddie (10) and Sara (13).

Geraldine's children provide all the home care their mother needs when she has an episode of illness and is unable to care for them or herself. These periods of ill health are becoming longer as Geraldine's condition progresses. During the week Eddie and Sara take it in turns to cook, wash the dishes, clean the house, wash and dress their mum, make her comfortable and make sure that she has her medication. They also go to school most days. At weekends Eddie and Sara take their mum out to see friends of the family, push her around the local park so that she gets fresh air, wash their clothes at the launderette and do the shopping at the supermarket.

Claudette Gidens, the district nurse who comes to see Geraldine, has got to know Eddie and Sara very well. They try to do the things she says and ring her when they feel worried about their mum. Geraldine wants to stay at home with her children as long as she can. She feels loved and cared for by her children but now feels they are under too much pressure to keep meeting her needs. Eddie and Sara say it's tiring but they don't want their mum to go away to hospital or a home.

1. How might Eddie and Sara's relatiosnhip with their mum be changed by her periods of illness?
2. List some of the positive and negative feelings and responses that carer like Eddie and Sara may experience when caring for a close relative at home.
3. How might Claudette's relationship with Geraldine be different to the relationship that Eddie and Sara have with their mum?

Knowledge Assessment Task   1.1   1.2

Imagine that you are applying for a new job in your health or social care organisation. Your employer has asked all applicants to complete an application form detailing their qualifications, skills and experience. As a final way of selecting the most suitable candidates for interview, your employer has included a written task. You are required to:

▶ describe examples of different working relationships in health and social care settings
▶ explain how a working relationship is different from a personal relationship.

Write an account of 300–500 words that demonstrates your understanding of working relationships in health and social care. You should also be prepared to answer any questions that your assessor may ask you about the work you produce. Keep a copy of your work as evidence towards your assessment.

Working in ways agreed with your employer

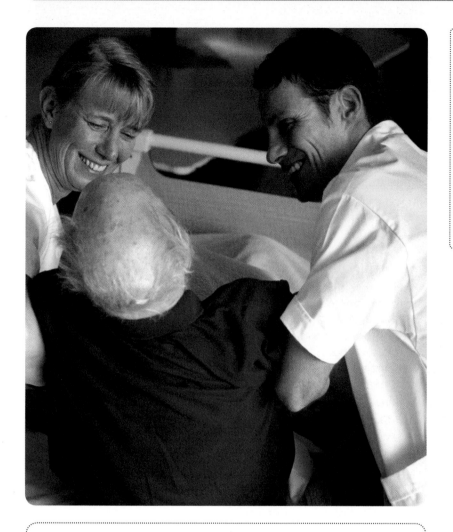

Adhering to the scope of the job role

Everybody who works in your work setting has been employed to work within a particular role. If you are a student on placement in a care setting you should also have a clear role, even if you are **supernumerary**. Service users and your colleagues will expect you to work within the boundaries of your particular role, and these boundaries should be clear from your job description. The job description should refer to the:

▶ responsibilities of your job

▶ supervision and line management arrangements for your job

▶ setting where you will work

▶ management or supervisory responsibilities attached to your work role, if appropriate.

Health and social care organisations usually produce a job

Key terms

Supernumerary: a member of staff, usually a student or trainee, who is not counted in the number of people required to staff a care setting

description outlining the expectations and tasks associated with each job. This is typically produced when a job vacancy occurs and is given to all applicants for the post, so that people are very clear about what is expected of them from the beginning of their employment. A job description may include a clear, detailed and structured set of duties and responsibilities associated with a work role. Alternatively, it may consist of a much looser set of tasks and responsibilities that are described in a general way. If this is the case, it is important to clarify with your employer any aspects of the job description that seem vague, confusing or unclear.

Your employer will expect you to fulfil all aspects of your work role because they have identified a need for somebody to carry out the range of tasks or activities associated with it. That is, your job has been designed and created as part of a broader **workforce planning** process within your care organisation. Your role covers work tasks and duties that need doing. Each of your colleagues will also have a job description associated with their work role, and will also be expected to complete particular work tasks and duties. You therefore need to do your job at the prescribed level and in the expected way to fit in with others. If you ensure that you always meet your own responsibilities and your colleagues do the same, service users should receive appropriate care and support. Taking over other people's responsibilities or doing random tasks not expected of you can disrupt workload management and the daily allocation of tasks. However, your manager or supervisor may occasionally request that you undertake work not normally associated with your work role. Where you agree to do this you should always ensure that you work within the boundaries of your own level of competence, qualifications and experience.

Reflect

Can you remember what your job description says? When was the last time that you looked at this document? Think about whether your job description actually describes the role and responsibilities that you undertake in the work setting.

Key terms

Workforce planning: the planning carried out by employers to determine the size of their workforce, the different work roles, and the management structure

Case study

Alice Bell is 79 years old and lives alone. She has some memory impairment and forgets what time of day it is, whether she has eaten, and the names of all but her closest relatives and Betty Edwards, her community nurse. Betty visits Alice every other day. She knows that this is a little bit too often but she says that Alice likes (and needs) to see a friendly face. Betty is supposed to monitor Alice's physical and mental health and change the dressing on a leg ulcer that Alice has recently developed. Betty says that she is doing these things but she has also started to take shopping for Alice and washes and styles her hair once a week. Alice doesn't complain about this but has now become very dependent on Betty's help.

1. Do you think that Betty is adhering to the scope of her job role?

2. Which activities described in the case study are likely to be outside of her job description?

3. Explain why Betty's approach to providing care for Alice may be seen as problematic and inappropriate.

Agreed ways of working

The policies and procedures designed and written by your employer set out how you should provide care and support for others and how you should deal with specific issues in your work setting. These should include policies and procedures relating to:

▶ health and safety

▶ equal opportunities

▶ confidentiality

▶ data protection

▶ supervision

▶ waste management

▶ moving and handling

▶ managing medication

▶ security and safeguarding.

The workplace policies produced by your employer identify the general approach that the organisation takes towards an issue. For example, the moving and handling policy may outline a 'no manual lifting' approach to moving and supporting service users. The procedures that accompany the policy would then outline the detailed way of putting the 'no manual lifting' approach into practice, such as through the use of lifting aids and equipment. You should know about and understand all of the procedures that affect your work role. For example, there should be detailed procedures explaining how to:

▶ respond to a fire incident

▶ deal with the receipt of medication

▶ deal with an accident or a death in the work setting

▶ assess and manage risks.

The policies and procedures written by your employer should incorporate all of the legal requirements affecting care work and should reflect the safest and most effective ways of carrying out particular tasks. It is essential that you understand and follow these policies and procedures to ensure that you are working in ways agreed by your employer.

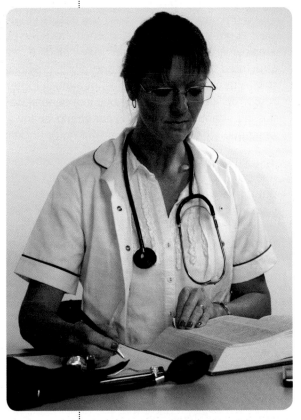

It is important, and your responsibility, to make sure that you know about agreed ways of working in your work setting

Reflect

Do you know where to find copies of these policies and procedures in your work setting? When was the last time that you consulted or read through one of these documents? Could you explain how the different policies and procedures used in your work setting impact on your particular work role?

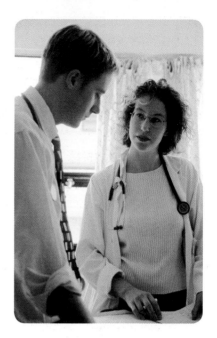

Case study

Daniel McClaren is a residential support worker in a care home for older people. he works shifts on a rota system which means that he works two weekends per month, three months of nights and day shifts in between. Daniel is very keen to progress in his career and hopes to become a residential home manager one day. However, at his recent appraisal, Daniel's line manager drew attention to reports that she had received about Daniel's work practices. Despite having residents' best interests at heart, Daniel has a habit of taking short cuts 'to get the job done' as he explained to his line manager. This has recently involved lifting an individual into the bath on his own and not checking the water temperature before doing so. Daniel has also been reminded on several occasions that he should not take residents out for walks on his own.

1. In what ways is Daniel failing to follow the agreed ways of working in his care setting?

2. How could Daniel clarify what the agreed ways of working are?

3. Explain why it is important that Daniel does know about and actually follows the agreed ways of working for his care setting.

Practical Assessment Task   2.1   2.2   2.3

The duties and responsibilities of your health or social care work role should be set out in your job description. In signing a contract of employment you have stated that you will work in ways agreed with your employer, which are described in the policies and procedures that apply in your work setting.

For this assessment task you need to:

▶ describe why it is important to adhere to the agreed scope of your job role

▶ show that you can access full and up-to-date details of agreed ways of working

▶ implement agreed ways of working in your care setting.

You may want to make notes to help you to prepare for your assessment. The evidence that you produce for this assessment task must be based on your practice in a real work environment.

Working in partnership with others

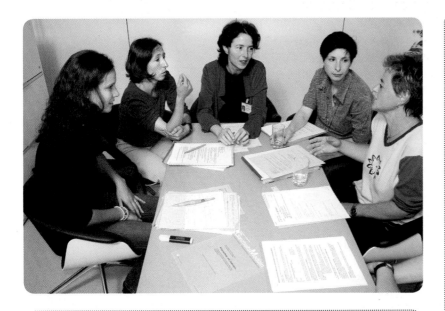

Your assessment criteria:

3.1 Explain why it is important to work in partnership with others

3.2 Demonstrate ways of working that can help improve partnership working

3.3 Identify skills and approaches needed for resolving conflicts

3.4 Demonstrate how and when to access support and advice about:
- partnership working
- resolving conflicts

How would you describe your role as a care practitioner to someone you have just met? What would you say? Would you describe your role as *working with* people or *doing things for* people? In the past, there was a general expectation that care practitioners would do things *for* people. Now the emphasis has changed and you are expected to work in partnership with the people you care for or support. There are, in fact, many different types of partnership in the health and social care field. These include partnerships with:

▶ colleagues

▶ practitioners from other agencies

▶ people receiving care or support

▶ the partners and families of the people you are caring for.

Partnerships with individuals

Part of your role as a care practitioner involves providing people with enough care and support to enable them to get on with their daily life. The relationship that you develop with an individual, and the approach that you take to providing support for them, should be based on the idea of partnership. Partnership is all about working together in a relatively equal and collaborative way. Within the care partnerships that you develop you should enable and support individuals to make as many decisions as possible and to do as much as they can for themselves. An individual's problems may well be made worse by a care practitioner who provides too much care and support even though this may be given with the best of intentions.

Reflect

What different kinds of partnerships are you involved in within your work role? Think about the range of other people with whom you work.

Discuss

In a small group, discuss examples of how you work in partnership with the individuals for whom you provide care or support. Does this actually happen in your care setting or does pressure to 'get the work done' lead to a lack of collaboration and partnership working with service users?

Care practitioners are sometimes tempted to do too much for individuals because they are trying to compensate for skills and abilities that people have lost or because they do not like to see people struggle, take risks and sometimes fail in their efforts to be self-caring. However, encouraging and supporting individuals to be involved in their own care and to take as much control as possible is a crucial way of helping them to maintain their skills and their self-esteem.

Team work and partnerships

Effective partnerships are based on teamwork. Health and social care practitioners increasingly work in integrated multi-agency and multi-disciplinary teams, bringing different skills and specialisms together to provide the range of services and high quality care that service users often require. They provide a way of pooling resources and expertise and are an efficient means of reducing duplication or overlap of service provision.

Multi-agency teams working in partnership with each other and with the individual need to have a clear understanding of and approach towards issues such as:

- ▶ communication
- ▶ information sharing and confidentiality
- ▶ decision-making procedures
- ▶ each practitioner's role and responsibilities
- ▶ ways of resolving conflicts
- ▶ agreeing objectives.

It is important that people working in partnership situations all have a clear, common understanding of the problems or needs of the individual and of the shared goal they are all seeking to achieve.

Key terms

Multi-agency: collaboration between practitioners employed by different agencies or organisations

Multi-disciplinary: arrangements that involve practitioners from different care professions working together in the same team

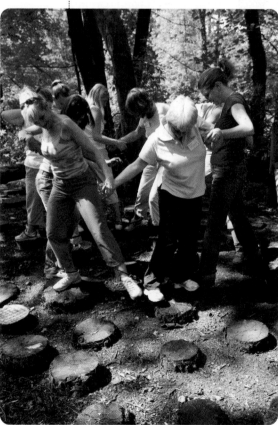

Partnership working requires cooperation, collaboration and a willingness to compromise

Investigate

Is your care setting a multi-disciplinary or multi-agency environment? Find out about the roles and specialist skills or responsibilities of other people who practise within your work environment.

Investigate

What role do the care or support plans written for individuals in your work setting play in coordinating the work of different care practitioners?

149

Improving partnership working

Good communication is essential for building trust and establishing efficient working arrangements. Trust and goodwill are needed to make partnerships work, as are respect and appreciation of others' involvement. As a care practitioner you should:

▶ value equally the different skills, contributions and approaches of others

▶ acknowledge the efforts and contributions of other people.

Clear decision-making that follows agreed processes and procedures enables practitioners working in partnership teams to feel more confident about the process of working together. It is important to ensure that you do not exclude any practitioners or team members from taking part in the decision-making process, as they may well then feel rejected, demotivated and less committed to a shared, team-based approach to providing care.

Resolving issues and difficulties

Partnership and team-based working can produce conflicts between individual practitioners or between practitioners from different agencies. This can result from the fact that practitioners with different professional training and backgrounds may approach situations differently or have different priorities. A community-based health care support worker may, for example, want to focus on completing particular tasks each day. A community nurse or social worker may have a longer-term view and may wish to work in a way that promotes active participation and independence.

To avoid potential problems, there need to be ways of resolving problematic relationships and conflict within teams and partnerships. Cordial, professional working relationships must be established even if people are not as cooperative or compatible on a personal level. Professional, not personal, standards apply to these situations. It is essential that you communicate and relate to others effectively and courteously, even when you have a different perspective on what ought to happen or on how a procedure should be carried out.

Accessing support and advice

You may need advice and support about partnership working in relation to:

▶ sharing information

▶ issues of confidentiality

▶ clarification of roles and responsibilities, including professional boundaries

▶ understanding agreed ways of working.

Reflect

Have you ever become involved in a conflict or disagreement over a practice-related issue in your work setting? How did you resolve this? Did you seek out or make use of any support or advice services?

Reflect

How do people resolve sensitive issues or personal difficulties in your work setting? What would you do if you became involved in a dispute or had cause to complain about a colleague or a practitioner from another agency?

Advice and support on issues such as these can be obtained from several different sources – firstly, from your manager or supervisor. You also need to know about and understand your organisation's policies and procedures relating to partnership working. These should provide detailed information and guidance on a range of issues. Seeking advice from senior colleagues and your manager will also be helpful.

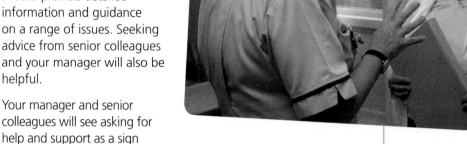

Your manager and senior colleagues will see asking for help and support as a sign that you have a conscientious, professional approach, not as a sign of weakness or incompetence. Other sources of advice and support include mentoring organisations, independent advisory organisations, trade unions and the occupational health service provided by your employer. Whenever you are considering whether you need to seek support or advice, you should always prioritise the needs of people for whom you provide care and support. Asking for help when you need it is usually in everyone's best interests.

Practical Assessment Task   3.1   3.2   3.3   3.4

Health and social care practitioners are increasingly likely to be working in partnership with others. This assessment task requires you to engage in some form of partnership working activity and to:

▶ explain why it is important to work in partnership with others

▶ demonstrate ways of working that can improve partnership working

▶ identify skills and approaches needed for resolving conflicts

▶ demonstrate how and when to access support and advice about:
  ▶ partnership working
  ▶ resolving conflict.

The evidence that you produce for this assessment task must be based on your practice in a real work environment. Your assessor may wish to observe you in practice and may ask you questions relating to the way you work in partnership with others.

Are you ready for assessment?

AC	What do you know now?	Assessment task	✓
1.1	How a working relationship is different from a personal relationship	Page 143	
1.2	How to describe different working relationships in health and social care settings	Page 143	

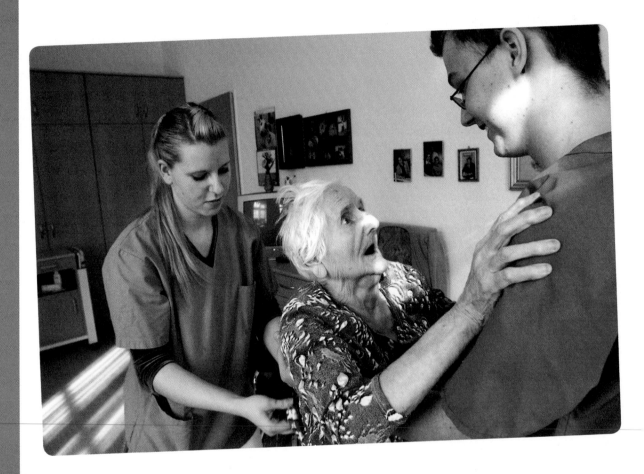

AC	What can you do now?	Assessment task	✓
2.1	Describe why it is important to adhere to the agreed scope of the job role	Page 147	
2.2	Access full and up-to-date details of agreed ways of working	Page 147	
2.3	Implement agreed ways of working	Page 147	
3.1	Explain why it is important to work in partnership with others	Page 151	
3.2	Demonstrate ways of working that can help improve partnership working	Page 151	
3.3	Identify skills and approaches needed for resolving conflicts	Page 151	
3.4	Demonstrate how and when to access support and advice about: • partnership working • resolving conflicts	Page 151	

7 | Implement person-centred approaches in health and social care (HSC 026)

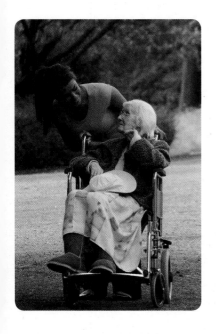

Assessment of this unit

This unit introduces you to the person-centred approach to care practice. The unit is relevant to people working in a wide range of health and social care settings; it will provide you with the knowledge and skills you will need to apply person-centred approaches in your work setting. You will need to:

▶ understand person-centred approaches to care and support

▶ be able to work in a person-centred way

▶ be able to establish consent when providing care or support

▶ be able to encourage active participation

▶ be able to support the individual's right to make choices

▶ be able to promote the individual's wellbeing.

The assessment of this unit is partly knowledge-based (things you need to know about) and partly competence-based (things you need to do in the real work environment). To successfully complete this unit, you will need to produce evidence of both your knowledge and your competence. The tables below and opposite outline what you need to know and do to meet each of the assessment criteria for the unit.

Your tutor or assessor will help you to prepare for your assessment, and the tasks suggested in the unit will help you to create the evidence that you need.

AC	What you need to know
1.1	Define person-centred values
1.2	Explain why it is important to work in a way that embeds person-centred values
1.3	Explain why risk taking can be part of a person-centred approach
1.4	Explain how using an individual's care plan contributes to working in a person-centred way

AC	What you need to do
2.1	Find out the history, preferences, wishes and needs of the individual
2.2	Apply person-centred values in day-to-day work, taking into account the history, preferences, wishes and needs of the individual
3.1	Explain the importance of establishing consent when providing care or support
3.2	Establish consent for an activity or action
3.3	Explain what steps to take if consent cannot readily be established
4.1	Describe how active participation benefits an individual
4.2	Identify possible barriers to active participation
4.3	Demonstrate ways to reduce the barriers and encourage active participation
5.1	Support an individual to make informed choices
5.2	Use agreed risk assessment processes to support the right to make choices
5.3	Explain why a worker's personal views should not influence an individual's choices
5.4	Describe how to support an individual to question or challenge decisions concerning them that are made by others
6.1	Explain how individual identity and self-esteem are linked with wellbeing
6.2	Describe attitudes and approaches that are likely to promote an individual's wellbeing
6.3	Support an individual in a way that promotes a sense of identity and self-esteem
6.4	Demonstrate ways to contribute to an environment that promotes wellbeing

Assessment criteria 2.1–6.4 must be assessed in a real work environment.

This unit also links to some of the other units:

DEM 204	Understand and implement a person-centred approach to the care and support of individuals with dementia
HSC 2013	Support care plan activities

Some of your learning will be repeated in these units and will give you the chance to review your knowledge and understanding.

What are person-centred values?

The principle underlying any person-centred approach to care or support is that the individual plays a central role. This means they are involved in every aspect of their care or support, including needs assessment, care delivery or support planning. If an organisation's activities are based on a person-centred approach, all policies, procedures and care practices should put the people receiving care or support at the centre of day-to-day activity. Person-centred approaches are underpinned by **values** that guide how individuals are treated.

The person-centred approach is based on the values of:

▶ individuality – recognising the uniqueness of the individual

▶ rights – ensuring individual rights are maintained

▶ choice – ensuring care or support is led by the individual's choices

▶ privacy – ensuring the individual's life is free from unwanted intrusion by others

▶ independence – enabling the individual to achieve maximum independence

▶ dignity – supporting the individual to maintain emotional control and their sense of worth in difficult and sensitive situations

▶ respect – recognising and valuing the individual's sense of worth and importance to others

▶ partnership – working with others to achieving the best outcomes possible.

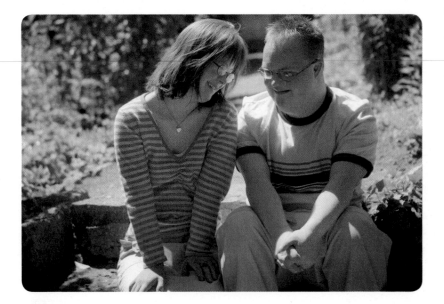

Your assessment criteria:

1.1 Define person-centred values

1.2 Explain why it is important to work in a way that embeds person-centred values

Key terms

Values: the beliefs, principles or standards of a person or a group

Social model of disability: the approach that explains disability as being the result of wider factors within society (for example, systems or negative attitudes) that directly or indirectly disable some people

Inclusion: being a part of something; in this case, it means the individual being involved in their own care

Social inclusion: means ensuring that marginalised groups and those in poverty have opportunities to participate in society and improve their wellbeing

Working to embed person-centred-values

Person-centred approaches build on a social model of disability and inclusion. Traditional models view people with disabilities as being helpless and therefore needing to have things 'done for them'. A social model of disability sees the way that society is organised as having a 'disabling' effect on some people. This creates helplessness. Helplessness is *not* an inevitable consequence of disability.

The social model of disability has had a significant influence on attitudes to disability. For example, people with disabilities are no longer hidden away and separated from society. Equal rights have led to improved access to education, employment and all aspects of life for disabled people. Changes in attitude have also challenged health and social care practitioners to provide care and support in ways that put the individual more in control of their life.

Person-centred approaches are about sharing power, so the emphasis is on 'doing things with' the individual: this means including the individual in decision-making. Person-centred approaches focus on:

▶ who the person is

▶ who the important people are in their lives

▶ what all members of the care team – including the individual concerned – can do together to achieve a better life for that person, in the present and in the future.

If people with disabilities are to be empowered and seen as equal partners, then person-centred values have to be embedded in every aspect of care provision. In reality, this means all organisational policies and procedures and ways of working need to reflect person-centred values.

Key terms

Power: the ability, strength or capacity to do something or to control or influence others

Empowered: means that a person has gained more control over their life by gaining greater self-confidence, self-esteem or access to resources

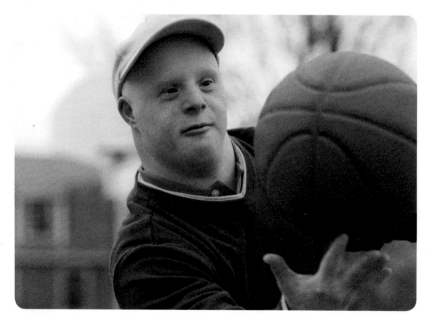

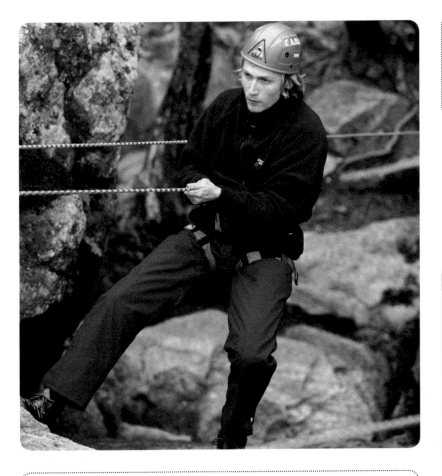

Key terms

Risk: the possibility or likelihood of something negative happening

Investigate

Find out how person-centred values are embedded in your workplace practices, policies and procedures. Do any policies or procedures specifically refer to person-centred values? You could also find out whether any individuals who use your service have been involved in developing the policies and procedures for recruiting new employees.

Risk taking in a person-centred approach

Risks in practice

Person-centred approaches are about enabling the individual to achieve their potential through exercising choices and developing independence. If this is to be achieved then **risk** must be included as a factor in decisions over care or support. Care practitioners should recognise that each person for whom they provide care or support has their own:

► views and opinions

► attitude to risk

► likes, dislikes and choices

► wishes and aspirations.

People who want to be fully involved in decision-making regarding their care or support are likely to want to try new things, to realise their potential and achieve their wishes and aspirations. They must be supported to do this, even if it involves an element of risk. Part of any planning process will involve risk assessment. This helps to keep risk in perspective, whilst at the same time maintaining the safety of the individual (see pages 174–177).

Reflect

How are service users currently involved in decision-making in your workplace? For example, how are service users involved in:

► designing their living environment (e.g. their own room as well as shared spaces)

► planning meals

► planning activities

► providing comments and feedback on what is provided?

Case study

Bethan has learning disabilities and has lived in a residential care home for four years. She has been working with her key worker, Jane, to develop a person-centred plan. Over the past three years Bethan has had four different key workers and so information about her past, her likes and dislikes is incomplete. Jane has developed a good relationship with Bethan, and has been working with her to put together Bethan's personal profile. During this process, Bethan said that she wanted to try some new activities and to meet two people, Philip and Karen, with whom she had lost touch. Bethan used to meet Philip and Karen at a weekly friendship club, but stopped going about a year ago. This was because there had been no one to accompany her, and since then it had been forgotten. Bethan loves to sing and dance and she really missed being able to do this. Bethan also wanted to get a job working with people as she is very sociable. She likes things to be neat and tidy, so she and Jane looked at jobs that would suit Bethan's character and likes. They found a volunteer job in a local charity shop two afternoons a week, which Bethan has said she would like to try.

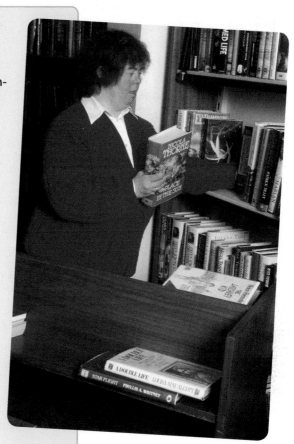

1. Which person-centred values are being demonstrated by Jane?
2. What are the potential risks in Bethan's choices?
3. What do you think Bethan could gain by taking these risks?

Reflect

Think about the last time you were involved in undertaking a risk assessment with an individual you support.

1. How did you establish the individual's understanding of potential and actual risks involved?
2. How did you involve the individual in assessing the risks?
3. How did you involve the individual in making the decision regarding the activity being risk-assessed?
4. How can the process be more person-centred?

The person-centred approach to care planning

Care plans often reflect a service approach to the provision of care or support with 'needs' identified in terms of what can be provided rather than what the individual really requires. The care plan should, however, present a key opportunity for using a person-centred approach. This can be achieved by involving the individual at every step of the care planning process to ensure that the care plan reflects their individuality and responds to their particular needs. A care plan should always contain information on:

▶ an individual's assessed care needs

▶ the person's circumstances and current level of support

▶ required outcomes (what they need to keep them safe and healthy)

▶ the individual's views about desired outcomes (what they want)

▶ planned forms of support or interventions

▶ timescales for implementing and reviewing the care plan.

A person-centred care plan will also contain information about the:

▶ individual's views regarding their needs and circumstances

▶ priorities and needs the person considers to be most important

▶ individual's strengths, interests, likes and dislikes

▶ way the individual want to live their life

▶ ways the individual prefers to have their needs met

▶ people who are important to and contribute to the person's life and provide their support network.

Your assessment criteria:

1.4 Explain how using an individual's care plan contributes to working in a person-centred way.

Key terms

Care plan: a document that details an individual's care needs and wishes, how these will be met, and who is involved in meeting those needs

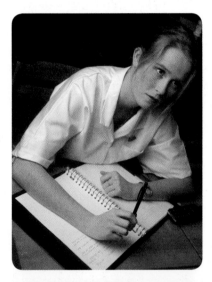

Knowledge Assessment Task | 1.1 | 1.2 | 1.3 | 1.4

Person-centred approaches to care practice are seen as progressive and positive because of the way they focus on and involve service users in care planning and delivery processes. In this activity you are required to produce some information that introduces and explains the person-centred approach to a group of care practitioners who do not currently use this way of providing care. The information that you produce should:

▶ define what is meant by the term 'person-centred values'

▶ explain why is it important to work in a way that embeds person-centred values in care practice

▶ explain why risk taking can be a part of a person-centred approach

▶ explain how using an individual's care plan contributes to working in a person-centred way.

Keep your written work as evidence towards your assessment.

Reflect

Are people who receive care or support services involved in care planning processes in your workplace? How person-centred do you think the current care planning process used in your workplace is?

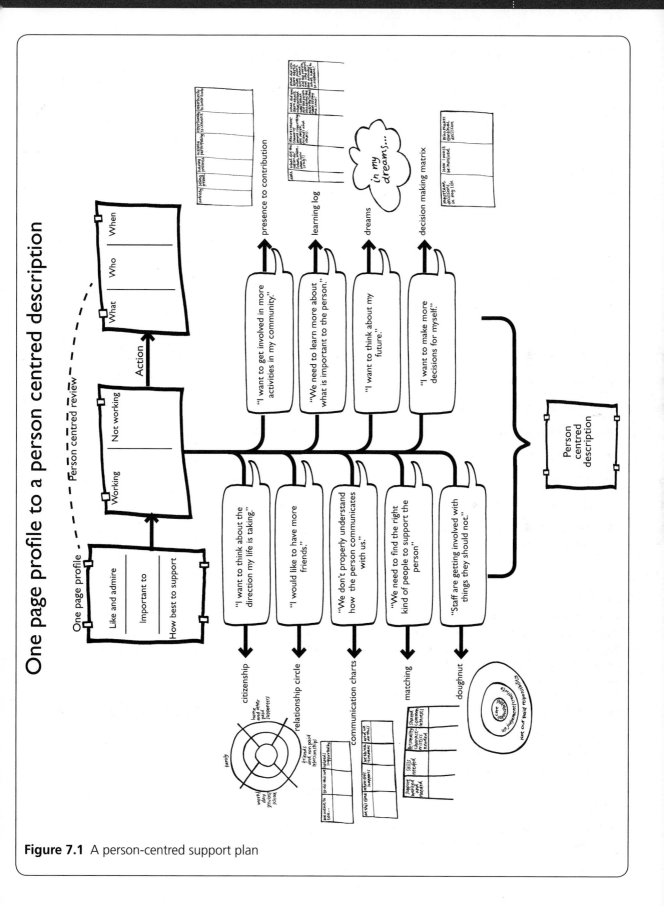

Figure 7.1 A person-centred support plan

Working in a person-centred way

In deciding to work a person-centred way, you place the individual at the centre of all your thinking and activities. To do this effectively you need to really understand the individual. And to do that, you need to know something about their personal history (life story).

Personal history

When a person is admitted to an inpatient or residential setting, or becomes part of a care practitioner's caseload, care workers tend to focus on the person's current situation. However, past experiences are a strong influence on a person's behaviour and functioning, and it is important to understand these too if care or support is to be appropriate and beneficial.

It is easy to lose sight of the individuality of the person in care. A medical diagnosis may create a label behind which the individual person 'disappears'. The list of needs can override the individual's wishes and aspirations. It is important to remember that the person's present circumstances are only a part of the person they are, and not the whole picture. Finding out about an individual's life – their experiences, culture and values – will help you to understand what is important to them, and what their likes and dislikes are. It may also provide important information to help you understand how past experiences have influenced their current behaviour or situation.

Preferences, wishes and needs

Finding out about an individual's preferences, wishes and needs is key to working in a person-centred way. This can be done by:

▶ talking and listening to the individual

▶ asking the people who are significant to them (their family and friends) about the person

▶ observing behaviour – especially if the individual has limited verbal communication

▶ monitoring how the person responds to you – especially if they have communication difficulties

▶ offering choices and observing responses

▶ reading the case notes and information provided by other practitioners or services.

It is useful to remember that an individual's preferences, wishes and needs may change. You should never assume that because an individual liked something a month ago, they still do. So, if in doubt ask, watch and listen.

Your assessment criteria:

2.1 Find out the history, preferences, needs and wishes of the individual

Investigate

Find out what processes are in place in your workplace to understand an individual's life history. Who is responsible for gathering this information? How and where is this information recorded? How is this information shared with other members of the team? How is it used to inform and enhance the support provided?

Reflect

Think about yourself: your life story to date; the past experiences that have influenced who you are today; your likes and dislikes; your preferences and expectations about how you would like your life to be.

Now imagine that you are in a situation where you need to be supported by others.

How do you think it would feel if the people supporting you only knew about your support needs and not these personal things about you?

How do you think this would affect the way they supported you?

How do you think this would affect how you felt about them and being in the position of needing support from others?

How would you like the people supporting you to get to know you and to understand who you really are as a person?

Think about how you can use what you have learnt from this reflection in your practice.

Case study

George is an 84 year-old man with dementia. He is physically fit, but finds communication difficult. George appears happiest when moving about, and is constantly walking the corridors of the home where he lives. Other residents find this disturbing and shout at him to sit down. George can become quite distressed by this, and if anyone tries to get him to sit down he can get very agitated. On occasions, he has been quite aggressive. George regularly goes missing, as he waits by the front door of the home and slips out when someone opens the door. He is always found walking in the nearby park.

The new manager has asked Paul to become George's key worker. George's previous key worker recently moved jobs and left little information about George's personal history. Paul arranged a meeting with George, his wife and his son, to find out more about him. Paul found out that prior to his retirement, George had been a postman for twenty years. He was also a keen cyclist and a prize-winning gardener, with roses as his special interest. George's son told Paul that he was researching their family tree. Paul talked to him about putting together a life story book that could be used to help George remember and to encourage him to communicate. George's family are keen to help with this.

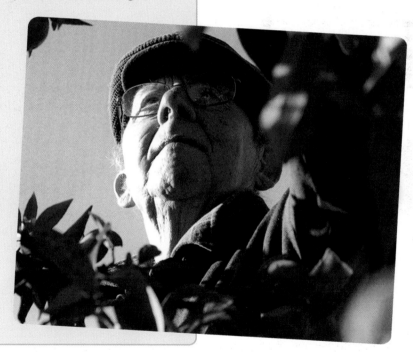

1. How do you think George's personal history may be influencing his current behaviour?

2. How could you use George's interests and likes to plan his day-to-day activities?

3. How do you think a better understanding of George's life history could enable care practitioners to improve the quality of his life?

Reflect

Is care practice in your workplace based on these values? How do you put these values into practice yourself?

Applying person-centred values in day-to-day work

To apply person-centred values you have to embrace person-centred thinking. You need to:

▶ think about your role in the individual's life

▶ think about how you can bring about change for that individual

▶ think about and analyse what life is like for the person now, including what is and is not working for the person, and what needs to change so that it does work.

This process will help you to learn what is important *to* and *for* an individual, and what needs to happen to balance these two priorities. To ensure that the people you support are treated as individuals whose rights, choices, preferences, wishes and dignity are respected, you need to actively participate in a continuous process of listening, learning and acting upon what you learn. This may require you to make some changes in your practice.

Applying person-centred values

In the example below, a care worker has made notes, using person-centred values (see page 156), on the wishes, needs and preferences of Helen, a service user:

▶ individuality – *Helen likes to wear clothes that are red or blue.*

▶ rights – *She only wants information about her care to be shared with her close family.*

▶ choice – *She is a vegetarian.*

▶ privacy – *She listens to Classic FM Radio alone in her room each day between 2 and 4pm.*

▶ independence – *Helen asks for help when she needs it; she doesn't like being 'taken over'.*

▶ dignity – *She likes people to ask her how she would like to be addressed.*

▶ respect – *She likes to talk about her life as a teacher and enjoys telling stories about working abroad.*

▶ partnership – *She is involved in every decision affecting her daily life.*

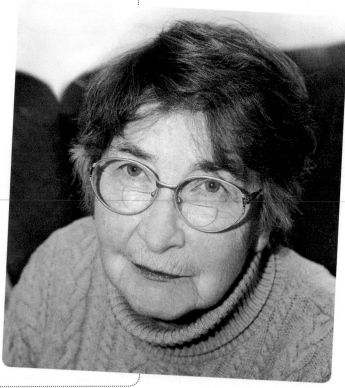

Your assessment criteria:

2.2 Apply person-centred values in day-to-day work, taking into account the history, wishes and needs of the individual.

Reflect

How could you change your care practice to be more person-centred?

Case study

Hamish is a 45 year-old retired solider. He is visually impaired and a bilateral amputee as a result of serious injuries sustained while on active service in Afghanistan. He spent a year in rehabilitation and has been back home with his wife, Ellen, and two children, Sam (14) and Lilia (10) for the past three months. Hamish is keen to return to full-time working and to build up his involvement in playing sports as he was very physically active prior to his injuries. His home has been adapted to meet his needs. He works at the local military base 10 miles away where he is also involved in various sports. He continues to have physiotherapy twice a week at the local hospital. He manages his own Self Direct Support personal budget which funds his care and support needs. His wife Ellen works full time at the local school as a teacher. Hamish is independent and is determined to continue supporting his family. He also wants to use his experiences of overcoming adversity to encourage others, and is involved in a charity which works with disadvantaged young people promoting sport as a way to build confidence and self-esteem.

You have been working as Hamish's personal assistant now for the past two months.

Using what you know about Hamish, think about how you can apply person-centred values when supporting him. Consider:

▶ individuality
▶ rights
▶ choice
▶ privacy
▶ independence
▶ dignity
▶ respect
▶ partnership.

Practical Assessment Task 2.1 2.2

Working in a person-centred way involves putting the individual at the centre of the care or support you provide, and ensuring that you work in ways that best meet their wishes, needs and preferences. Using an appropriate format, such as a care study that describes your practice with an individual, describe how you were able to:

▶ find out the personal history, preferences, wishes and needs of the individual
▶ apply person-centred values in your day-to-day work with the person, taking into account the history, preferences, wishes and needs of the individual.

Your evidence for this assessment activity must be based on your practice in a real work environment. Keep the work that you produce as evidence towards your assessment.

Establishing consent when providing care or support

What is capacity and consent?

A person who consents agrees to something taking place or to a decision being made. A person needs **capacity** to give consent. This means they are able to:

▶ understand the information they are being given that is relevant to the decision

▶ retain that information long enough to make a decision

▶ analyse (use and weigh up) the information

▶ communicate their decision to others (verbally or using sign language or pictures, for example).

Different types of **consent** apply within health and social care work. These are:

1. *Informed consent:* the individual has capacity, has access to all relevant information, and is fully aware of the implications of the decision. There is a formal agreement, usually in writing.

2. *Implied consent:* The actions of the individual give the impression that they are consenting. There is no formal agreement. An example is an individual attending their GP. The implication is they are consenting to the GP making a diagnosis and offering treatment.

3. *Continued consent:* Informed consent continues during a period of treatment, care or support.

4. *Consent by proxy:* If the individual is unable to provide informed consent there may be times when decisions are made in their best interests by an appropriate person (such as a relative, next of kin).

Legally, practitioners have to establish consent before any intervention or care-giving takes place. For example, consent is frequently sought verbally by asking an individual if they are ready to be moved. Obtaining consent demonstrates respect for the individual's dignity, and is likely to establish their trust and co-operation. The person is then more likely to work with you to achieve the intended action. Doing something to an individual without their consent is an infringement of their rights and, if it involves physical contact, may be viewed as assault.

Key terms

Capacity: the mental or physical ability of a person to do something

Consent: means giving informed permission for something to happen

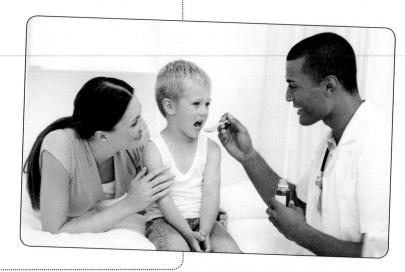

How to establish consent

Part of your role and responsibility is to make sure that you support individuals to make informed decisions. To establish consent to undertake an action or activity with an individual you must ensure that you:

▶ understand the person's needs and circumstances in relation to capacity and decision-making

▶ have all the relevant information available relating to the decision, including the options available to the person

▶ understand and can clearly explain the options and any potential or actual risks.

If the person lacks the capacity to make informed decisions alone then you will need to establish who else needs to be involved. This information is usually found in the person's care plan or in a communication chart established to cover a range of circumstances.

To establish consent to an action or activity:

▶ explain what it is, using language familiar to the individual

▶ describe what the action or activity involves

▶ explain the benefits to the individual

▶ explain any potential or actual risks involved in doing it

▶ explain any potential or actual risks involved in not doing it

▶ listen to and observe the individual's response

▶ encourage the individual to ask questions

▶ give the individual time to process the information

▶ confirm consent again immediately prior to any action or activity.

In day-to-day activities, consent is very often verbal and informal. If the action or activity involves serious consequences, such as a treatment, medical procedure or legal process, then consent is generally formal, and needs to be recorded in writing on a consent form.

Your assessment criteria:

3.2 Establish consent for an activity or action

Reflect

Reflect on the type of consent that may be required in the following situations:

1. Emergency treatment in the Accident and Emergency department
2. Participating in research by completing a questionnaire
3. Receiving medical treatment following a consultation with a specialist
4. A child of 6 years having their tonsils removed

Reflect

How do you find out about the capacity to consent of the people for whom you provide care or support? What do you do to establish their consent to actions and activities that you undertake with them?

Case study

When Debbie arrives at Mr Klein's house for her usual morning visit, she finds that Mr Klein (72 years old) is feeling unwell and lethargic. Debbie suspects that Mr Klein could have a chest infection as his breathing is poor and he has a raised temperature. Debbie thinks that she should call his GP straight away and request a visit.

1. What kind of consent is needed in this kind of situation?
2. Explain why it is important to establish consent when providing care or support.
3. What might be the consequences of acting without gaining Mr Klein's consent in this situation?

What to do if consent cannot be readily established

Your assessment criteria:

3.3 Explain what steps to take if consent cannot readily be established

Before deciding on whether or not to seek consent on behalf of an individual, it is important to remember that when a person is tired, in pain or discomfort, hungry, thirsty or anxious, they may not be able to concentrate sufficiently, or may find the information overwhelming. In these situations they may *appear* unable to give consent to your requests to provide care. In non-emergency situations, it is worth addressing these issues before making a decision to obtain consent on the individual's behalf.

However, there are some circumstances where individuals are unable to give consent. This can be as a result of congenital or childhood problems, such as a learning disability, a head injury, illness or disease (such as dementia). An individual may temporarily or permanently lack capacity as a result of this. The Mental Capacity Act (MCA) 2005 outlines the circumstances in which another person can make a decision or take action on behalf of an individual who lacks capacity. The action or decision taken must relate to care or treatment. The person making the decision must apply the principles of the MCA, and:

▶ reasonably believe the individual lacks the capacity to make a decision in the circumstances and at that time

▶ act in the individual's best interests

▶ make sure the action is the least restrictive alternative available in the circumstances.

In these circumstances, consent details will be formally recorded in the individual's care plan, or in another document within their records. Even in circumstances where the individual is incapable of giving consent, it is important to continue to attempt to communicate directly with the individual. Talking the individual through the process dignifies the action of having to make a decision on that person's behalf. Use other forms of communication, such as pictures or signs, with individuals used to communicating non-verbally. In many circumstances, where consent (especially informal) cannot readily be established, it is useful to ask the next of kin or family about the individual's preferences and wishes.

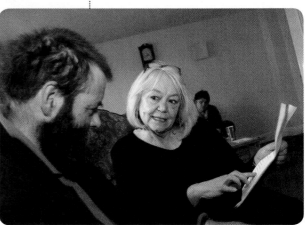

An independent advocate can be used to make an informed decision

A person's ability to give consent may change from time to time. If a person has dementia, for example, their ability to make decisions may fluctuate due to their disease. In this case, care plan strategies should have been previously negotiated and set down in writing, enabling you to take steps to establish consent. This may include repeating requests, moving the individual or choosing the best time to make a request.

Case study

Phillipa 'Pip' Norris is a 54 year-old woman with learning disabilities and early signs of dementia. She lives with her younger sister who is her main carer. Pip's disability means that her capacity to make decisions fluctuates during the day. She becomes particularly anxious when she is given too much verbal information at once. Pip finds it difficult to concentrate unless the person talking to her is facing her, and likes to be spoken to using a soft tone of voice. She likes to be called 'Pip' not Phillipa, as she associates the name Phillipa with her grandmother, who brought her up very strictly. Pip is a morning person and this is the best time to plan her day with her. She has a pin board in her room, and her sister uses pictures to remind Pip of the things she is doing that day. Pip has a support worker visiting three times a week to give her sister a break.

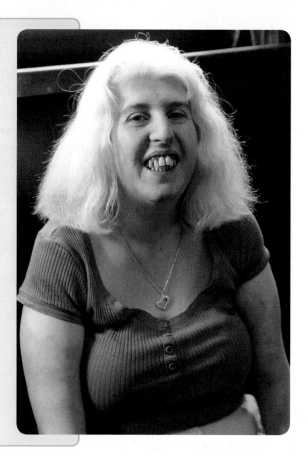

1. What strategies could you use to establish Pip's consent to actions or activities?

2. What would you do if it was difficult to establish Pip's consent?

3. How can a person-centred approach help when supporting Pip?

Practical Assessment Task   3.1   3.2   3.3

Health and social care practitioners should always establish consent before undertaking care or providing forms of support. Produce evidence to show that you are able to:

▶ explain the importance of establishing consent when providing care or support

▶ establish consent for an activity or action that you undertake in your work setting

▶ explain what steps to take if consent cannot readily be established.

The work that you produce should be based on your practice in a real work environment. Your assessor may wish to observe you establishing consent for care delivery with an individual who uses your care setting, and may also ask you questions about establishing consent. You should retain any notes, witness statements or other written work you produce for this activity as evidence towards your assessment.

How does active participation benefit an individual?

Active participation is a way of working that treats people in need of care or support as active participants or partners, rather than as passive recipients of care or support services. A person-centred approach is one of the most effective ways to encourage active participation, as the focus is on the individual, their wishes and abilities and on using these to maximise their independence. Finding out about an individual's personal history, likes, dislikes, abilities and wishes is an important starting point for encouraging active participation. Taking a person-centred approach to care or support means looking for ways to meet the individual's needs and wishes. This is quite different from trying to make the person fit in to available services, whether they are right for them or not.

Being made to 'fit' into something that isn't shaped for your particular needs and wishes means you are unlikely to enjoy it or want to make it work. You are likely to fight against it, and may be unhappy and uncooperative. You may feel unimportant, or a burden. Adapting services to the person to create a 'best fit' – tailoring services to meet an individual's specific needs – is more likely to result in a positive outcome for all involved.

Your assessment criteria:

4.1 Describe how active participation benefits an individual

4.2 Identify possible barriers to active participation

Key terms

Active participation: this means being directly involved in activities and decision-making relating to your own life

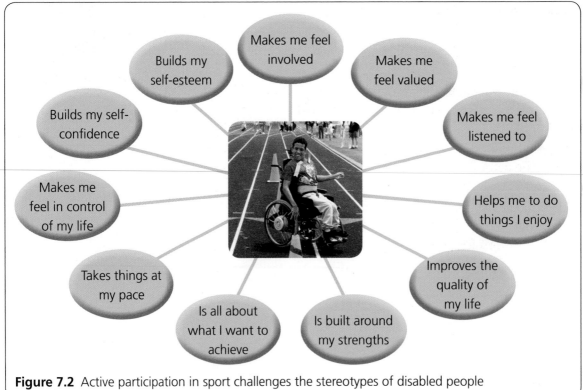

Figure 7.2 Active participation in sport challenges the stereotypes of disabled people

Potential barriers to active participation

Putting active participation into practice means being able to recognise and reduce the potential barriers to its implementation. Active participation benefits the individual as it enables them to achieve their potential and improve their life experience, rather than being a passive recipient of care or support. Encouraging active participation challenges:

▶ the individual to believe they can be active rather than passive

▶ family/friends to view the individual as an equal with the same capacity for wishing and aspiring

▶ health and social care workers to work with the individual as an equal partner in care or support

▶ health and social care organisations to provide flexible, personalised care or support

▶ society to view people with disabilities as 'givers', as individuals able to contribute, and not as 'takers' or dependents.

Barriers to implementing an active participation approach can occur where the health or social care practitioner:

▶ lacks understanding of the individual's personality, history, health and cognitive status and social abilities

▶ views the person as a passive recipient of care who is always dependent on others

▶ has low expectations of the person's ability to develop, change and achieve

▶ is not committed to making an active participation approach work

▶ lacks creativity and flexibility in thinking about ways of providing care or support – they are 'stuck' in old ways and old solutions

▶ lacks patience and tenacity when pursuing active participation goals

▶ has an inconsistent approach, and doesn't integrate active participation into their care practice to the extent that it becomes part and parcel of their daily care practice.

Reflect

Is active participation encouraged in your work setting? Can you think of some examples of active participation or of ways you could encourage all individuals to actively participate?

Investigate

With permission, investigate how active participation has benefied at least two individuals in your workplace.

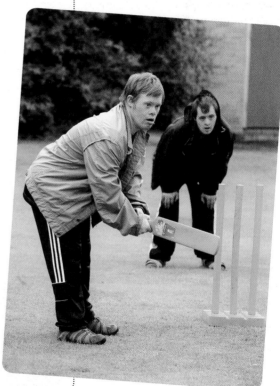

Reducing barriers to active participation

Changing attitudes is key to reducing barriers to active participation. Improving society's attitudes to, and expectations of, people with disabilities is an important part of this. The social model of disability has already created a shift in thinking. Information, education and training will help to move that further. Involving the individual and all those people who are significant to them is also crucial to success. To encourage active participation you will need to:

▶ keep the individual's goals central to planning using a person-centred approach

▶ focus on what the individual *can do*

▶ work in partnership with the individual and the other important people in their life

▶ maintain a positive approach

▶ break goals down into smaller, more achievable steps

▶ celebrate every small achievement as being significant to the individual

▶ set longer timescales for reaching goals

▶ monitor and review more frequently

▶ get into the habit of a 'review, adjust, review, adjust' approach

▶ not be afraid to make changes and move in a different direction if something does not work

▶ find out what is available to support the individual's goals

▶ be creative and flexible in your thinking

▶ think of risk assessment as a means of making an activity possible.

Your assessment criteria:

4.3 Demonstrate how to encourage active participation and reduce any potential barriers

Reflect

How are choices presented to the people you support or care for? What kinds of choices are service users offered in your work setting each day? How are people helped to make informed choices?

Active participation means doing, not just watching

Case study

Carla is 34 years old, has physical and learning disabilities, and lives at home with her parents. She attends a day centre each day. One weekend a month, and for one week every two months, she stays at a local residential care home to give her parents a break. Carla's mobility is limited and she tires quickly, so she uses a wheelchair when she is outside. Carla uses signing to communicate and has some verbal skills. The people who know her say that she has a good sense of humour, is great fun to spend time with, becomes cranky when she is tired, is determined and patient, has a meticulous approach to detail, and is creative. Her key worker has been working with Carla and her parents on her person-centred support plan.

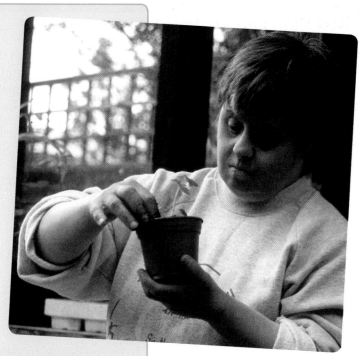

Carla has expressed a wish to get a job working with plants as she loves growing things. She knows that to do this she will need to get a qualification. Carla's key worker and her parents have helped her to research this and they have found a course at a local college.

1. What strengths, skills or interests does Carla have that her key worker could focus on as part of an active participation approach to working with her?

2. What barriers do you think there may be to Carla actively participating? How could Carla's care worker help reduce the chances of Carla being subjected to social exclusion?

3. How could you overcome those barriers?

Key terms

Social exclusion: the process of pushing some people or groups to the margins of society – normally for reasons of their poverty, lack of education, minority status or inadequate life skills

Practical Assessment Task 4.1 4.2 4.3

In your work setting, do you promote and encourage active participation in the planning and provision of care and support? Produce evidence to show that you:

▶ are able to describe how active participation benefits an individual with whom you work

▶ can identify possible barriers to active participation in your work with the individual

▶ are able to demonstrate ways to reduce the barriers and encourage active participation.

The evidence that you produce should relate to your practice in a real work setting. Keep any written work as evidence towards your assessment. You may be observed by your assessor and questioned about your practice.

Supporting the individual's right to make choices

Having the opportunity to make choices is something most of us take for granted. However, for many of the people you support, being presented with choices may be confusing or a new experience for them. Part of your role is to provide and promote choice for the people you provide care or support for.

Making informed choices

In order to support an individual to make a choice you need to:

► understand the individual's needs and abilities

► provide the person with relevant information

► explain how each choice may benefit or suit the individual

► explain what the person may lose by making each choice

► ensure that you are objective in the way you present each choice

► give the individual time to consider their options

► check the person understands each choice available to them.

How can risk assessments support the right to make choices?

Risk assessments are often viewed in a negative way, as a means to justify stopping an individual from doing something. Viewed in a positive way, however, risk assessment can support choices and enable an individual to do something. Person-centred risk assessments:

► explore the hazards and risks to an individual in an area of their life

► enable individuals to carry out tasks and activities more independently and safely.

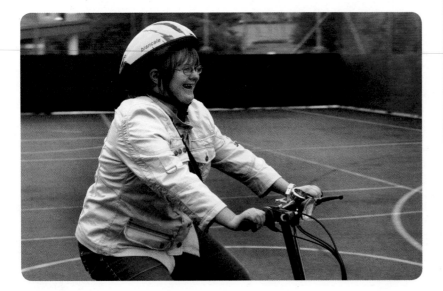

Your assessment criteria:

5.1 Support an individual to make informed choices

5.2 Use agreed risk assessment processes to support the right to make choices

Reflect

Read the list of ways to reduce barriers to active participation on page 171. Reflecting on your own experience, can you think of any other barriers to active participation?

Think of examples that would illustrate how you have worked with individuals to overcome barriers to active participation.

Investigate

Find out what the risk assessment policies and procedures of your workplace are. Look at a selection of completed risk assessments and evaluate them using the following criteria:

1. How person-centred are they?

2. Who was involved in the risk assessment?

3. Was risk assessment carried out to enable the individual to do something or to justify them not doing something?

4. How often are risk assessments monitored and reviewed?

Case study

Kathy is 61 years old and lives in a small group home with three other people. The group home is part of a community complex with workshops, a cafe and a horticulture centre. The adults who live and work there all have learning difficulties. Kathy works in the cafe during the week. She is finding the work more tiring these days. Kathy is quite independent and manages her daily activities, including her finances, with minimal support from her key worker, Tina.

After watching a report about retirement ages on television, Kathy told Tina that she thinks it's unfair that she has to continue working now she is over 60 years old. Tina said that she would speak to the manager about this. When Tina raised this, however, the manager told her that they didn't have the funding to support Kathy during the day and so they didn't have any option but for her to continue working in the cafe where she could be supervised. They were also concerned that she would get lonely in the house on her own when everyone was at work. Kathy was not happy with this decision. She has asked Tina what she can do as she feels the decision is unfair.

1. How are Kathy's rights and choices being overridden in this situation?

2. How can Tina support Kathy in this situation?

3. Who else could Kathy and Tina involve?

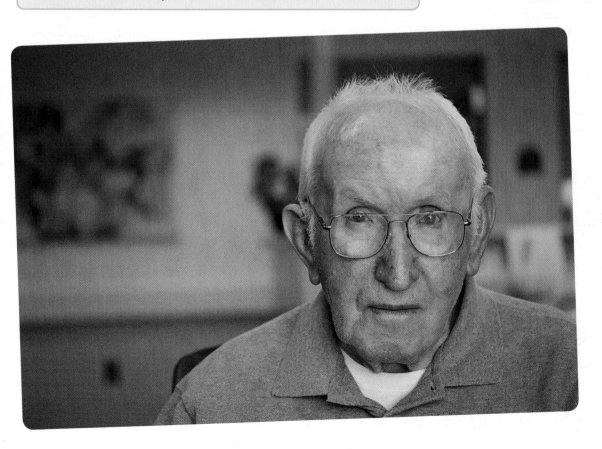

How can you ensure risk assessments are objective?

Everyone has had past experiences of risk, and this tends to influence our attitude towards it. If past experience has taught you that there is a great deal to be gained by taking a risk, then you are more likely to view risk as something to welcome. If, however, taking a risk has resulted in negative experiences and memories, then it is likely that you will view risk as something to be wary of and avoided if at all possible.

Supporting an individual to challenge decisions made about them by others

There may be times when an individual is unhappy about decisions that have been made about them or for them. This may occur because:

▶ others believe the individual is not capable of making complex decisions

▶ others do not agree with the individual's decision

▶ others use 'duty of care' and risk assessment to override the individual's choices

▶ others believe it is their right to make the decision on the individual's behalf (for example, as parents, carers or next of kin)

▶ others believe their decision is in the individual's best interests

▶ the individual's decision does not suit other people because, for example, they feel it creates more work for them

▶ it has become normal for others to make decisions without really involving the individual

▶ others have coerced the individual into making a decision that suits them and not the individual.

Your assessment criteria:

5.3 Explain why a worker's personal views should not influence an individual's choices

5.4 Explain how to support an individual to question or challenge decisions concerning them that are made by others

Reflect

What has influenced your attitude towards risk? How does that affect the way you assess risk in relation to care practice and the active participation of service users?

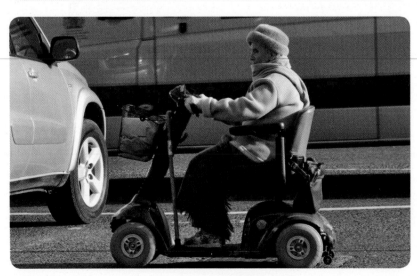

Age shouldn't be a barrier to independence

In situations where an individual's right to make their own choices and decisions has been infringed, the person also has a right to question or challenge the decisions made by others concerning them.

An individual who wishes to question or challenge decisions concerning them can be supported in a number of ways. For example, a health or social care practitioner could:

▶ work with the individual to help them decide what they want to do, how they want to raise their concern and who they wish to involve

▶ identify how the individual's views were not considered or listened to

▶ identify others who can support the individual's view

▶ arrange an informal meeting to raise the individual's concerns

▶ use the complaints procedure if informal processes don't work

▶ involve an independent advocate if this is the best option for the individual.

Investigate

Find out how your workplace policies and procedures enable people to question or challenge decisions concerning them that have been made by others.

Key terms

Advocate: a person responsible for communicating the views, wishes and feelings of an individual on their behalf

Practical Assessment Task   5.1   5.2   5.3   5.4

Health and social care practitioners have an important role to play in supporting the right of individuals to make choices in relation to their care and lifestyle. Produce evidence to show that you are able to:

▶ support an individual to make informed choices

▶ use agreed risk assessment processes to support the right to make choices

▶ explain why a worker's personal views should not influence an individual's choices

▶ describe how you would support an individual to question or challenge decisions concerning them that are made by others.

Your work for this assessment activity should be based on your practice in a real work setting. Your assessor may want to ask you questions about this or to observe you in practice. Keep any written work that you produce for this activity (such as a case study of a person with whom you work) as evidence towards your assessment.

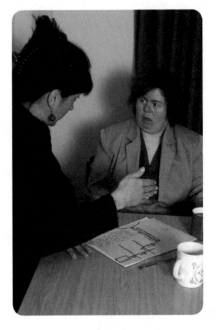

Promoting individual wellbeing

What are identity and wellbeing?

A person's **identity** is something that develops throughout their life and is closely linked to their emotional and social development. It expresses what we think and feel about ourselves as individuals and also takes into account how others see us.

An individual's identity is a combination of their **self-image** and their **self-esteem**. Self-image is a kind of mental picture a person has of themselves. It gradually develops as the person becomes aware of their own physical, intellectual, emotional and social abilities, qualities and attributes. This awareness is developed through interacting with others. When a person talks about their self-image, they will often compare themselves to others.

Self-esteem also results from the way we compare ourselves to other people. People who compare themselves negatively to others, thinking they are not as good, not as attractive or not as capable as others, for example, are more likely to have low self-esteem. People who are confident but not arrogant, who accept that they have both strengths and weaknesses, and who feel encouraged, loved and wanted, tend not to undervalue themselves so much and usually have higher self-esteem as a result.

Your assessment criteria:

6.1 Explain how individual identity and self-esteem are linked with well-being

Key terms

Identity: how a person sees, feels about and defines themselves

Self-image: the way a person views themselves

Self-esteem: the way a person values themselves

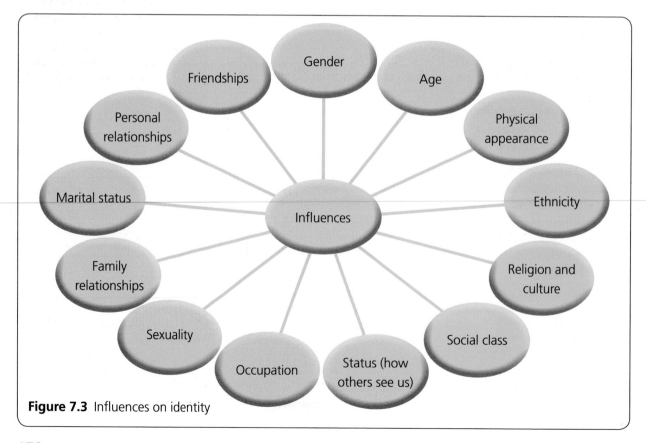

Figure 7.3 Influences on identity

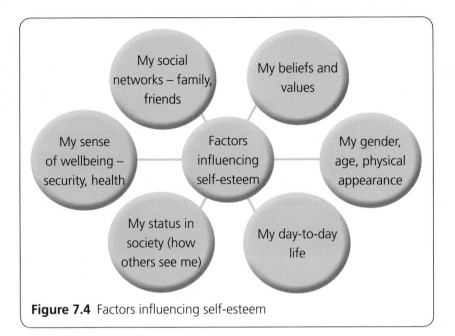

Figure 7.4 Factors influencing self-esteem

Linking identity and wellbeing

'Wellbeing' is a concept or idea that is very closely related to health. In fact, health and social care practitioners tend to think of wellbeing as combining an individual's health, their quality of life, and their satisfaction. In short, wellbeing is often considered as being a state in which the individual feels good and believes they are doing well. The term 'quality of life' is sometimes also used to assess an individual's wellbeing. An individual who has a clear self-image, robust identity and positive self-esteem, and who believes they are valued and respected by others, is likely to enjoy a positive sense of wellbeing. An individual whose sense of identity is threatened by illness, bereavement or other forms of 'loss', and who has negative self-esteem and perhaps even feels rejected by or worthless to others, is likely to have a poor sense of wellbeing.

Health and social care practitioners need to be able to recognise and support the identity and wellbeing needs of each individual they work with. An individual's values, beliefs, preferences and personal history all contribute to their sense of identity and define 'who' they are. People can feel disrespected, devalued and as though they, as an individual, don't matter anymore if their identity and wellbeing needs are not recognised, respected and nurtured.

Reflect

How would you sum up your view of the 'essential you' at this point in your life? Using both words and pictures, describe your identity. Think about your main features and characteristics. Consider your appearance, your gender, where you live, your personality and what you think others think about you as a person, for example.

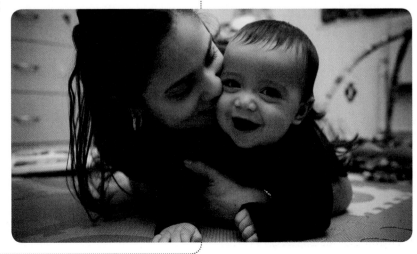

Attitudes that promote identity and wellbeing

If an individual feels worthless and has low self-esteem this will impact on how they view themselves. This negativity may also affect how they interact with others. A lack of self-worth and self-esteem may serve to demotivate an individual, and so reduce their chances of achieving their potential or of improving their sense of self and wellbeing: it is a vicious cycle. However, a vicious cycle can become a virtuous cycle if the attitudes and behaviour of the people around the individual are positive and nurturing.

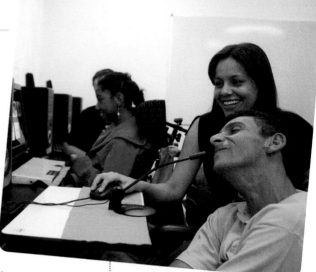

Promoting wellbeing

Wellbeing is an important part of being healthy. It is about being in a positive physical, social and mental state. Wellbeing is not just about having no pain, discomfort or incapacity. An individual with a positive sense of wellbeing will:

▶ have their basic needs met

▶ have a sense of purpose in their life

▶ feel able to achieve important personal goals

▶ feel able to participate in society, e.g. through work and by undertaking leisure activities

▶ have supportive personal relationships, e.g. with family, friends

▶ feel included in their community, e.g. able to access and participate in local activities

▶ experience good health

▶ have financial and personal security, e.g. provided with a secure income and a safe place to live, and having the ability to plan for the future

▶ have rewarding employment or meaningful daily activity

▶ live in a healthy and attractive environment.

One important way of promoting wellbeing is through supporting the individual to undertake meaningful daily activities. This is anything that involves a purposeful and valued outcome for the individual, including paid or unpaid employment, helping with domestic tasks, gardening or art and crafts activities. Promoting and supporting an individual's participation in purposeful activity will:

▶ encourage the use and development of their knowledge and skills

▶ maintain the individual's interest and give them a sense of purpose

---

Your assessment criteria:

6.2 Describe attitudes and approaches that are likely to promote an individual's wellbeing

6.3 Support an individual in a way that promotes a sense of identity and self-esteem

---

▶ create a sense of achievement which will build self-worth

▶ enable the individual to use and develop their creativity

▶ enable the individual to develop their resilience

▶ enable the individual to interact with others which will build their self-esteem.

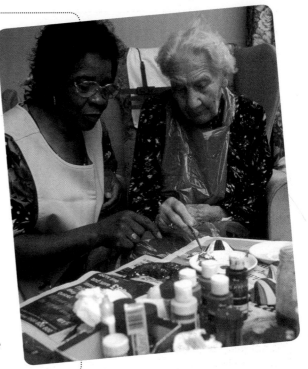

Finding out about individuals' interests and past history will help you to understand those activities which gave a sense of purpose to their lives prior to their need for care or support. Wellbeing can be improved by involving the individual in these activities. You may need to modify them or provide additional support for the individual to participate in certain activities again. For example, an individual who has always been a keen gardener, and who now uses a wheelchair to move around, will find it easier to continue growing plants if they are at a more accessible height or are grown in pots

Case study

Rachel is 25 years old and has a background of poverty, abuse and domestic violence. She spent her early life in and out of children's homes and has a long history of drug and alcohol misuse. As a result of a particularly violent assault and her drug use, Rachel has some cognitive impairment and needs support managing her money and planning daily activities. Since leaving rehabilitation Rachel has made good progress and is now beginning to feel more positive about her future. Rachel's key worker, Caro, has been working to build Rachel's self-esteem, confidence and resilience. Rachel has expressed a wish to use her experiences in a positive way to help others. Caro has been encouraging Rachel to look at youth work and has been supporting her to volunteer at a local youth centre. As a result of her progress, the youth centre has contacted a charitable foundation, which has agreed to support Rachel to gain experience and qualifications in youth work.

1. How do you think Rachel's background might have affected her sense of identity and wellbeing?

2. What factors have influenced a change in Rachel's self-esteem?

3. How have the attitudes and behaviour of other people in Rachel's life had:

   ▶ a negative impact?

   ▶ a positive impact?

Creating an environment that promotes wellbeing

An individual's wellbeing can be improved by those around them demonstrating nurturing, respectful and positive 'can do' attitudes. However, the physical environment in which the person lives, and the systems that operate within it, also play a part in promoting wellbeing. The physical environment can contribute to wellbeing by being:

▶ accessible

▶ welcoming

▶ well maintained

▶ comfortable

▶ light and airy

▶ appealing to the senses – colourful, pleasant to look at; tactile surfaces; noise controlled; well ventilated with fresh air

▶ designed to accommodate the individuality of service users

▶ temperature controlled

▶ safe and secure

▶ well equipped to meet individual needs

▶ designed with areas that provide privacy and quiet as well as space for large groups.

Your assessment criteria:

6.4 Demonstrate how to contribute to an environment that promotes wellbeing

Investigate

Look around your workplace. How does the environment promote individuals' wellbeing? What else do you think could be done to improve the environment and promote wellbeing?

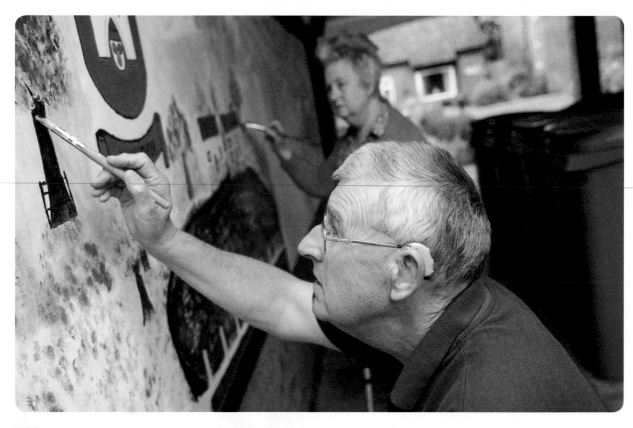

The systems and structures within an environmental can contribute to wellbeing by using:

▶ person-centred approaches to care or support

▶ risk assessments which focus on enabling activities

▶ creative and flexible approaches to meeting needs and enabling individuals

▶ user feedback and involvement to make decisions about how and what services are provided

▶ good evidence-based practice to develop services

▶ staff supervision and training to develop positive attitudes to care or support

▶ monitoring and review processes to make changes and improvements.

Investigate

Find out how individuals make suggestions to your employers about the service being provided. Find out what happens to their suggestions. Is this process informal (i.e. they make a verbal comment which is not recorded) or formal (i.e. they submit suggestions in writing or present them at a meeting)? Identify changes that have been made as a direct result of service user suggestions. How have changes improved individuals' wellbeing?

Practical Assessment Task   6.1 6.2 6.3 6.4

The care and support provided by health and social care practitioners should promote and support the health and wellbeing of the people they work with. Produce evidence that shows you are able to:

▶ explain how individual identity and self-esteem are linked with wellbeing

▶ describe attitudes and approaches that are likely to promote an individual's wellbeing

▶ support an individual in a way that promotes a sense of identity and self-esteem

▶ demonstrate ways to contribute to an environment that promotes wellbeing.

Your work for this assessment activity should be based on your practice in a real work setting. Your assessor may want to ask you questions about this or to observe you in practice. Keep any written work that you produce for this activity (such as a case study of a person with whom you work) as evidence towards your assessment.

Are you ready for assessment?

AC	What do you know now?	Assessment task	✓
1.1	How to define person-centred values	Page 160	
1.2	Why it is important to work in a way that embeds person-centred values	Page 160	
1.3	Why risk taking can be part of a person-centred approach	Page 160	
1.4	How using an individual's care plan contributes to working in a person-centred way	Page 160	

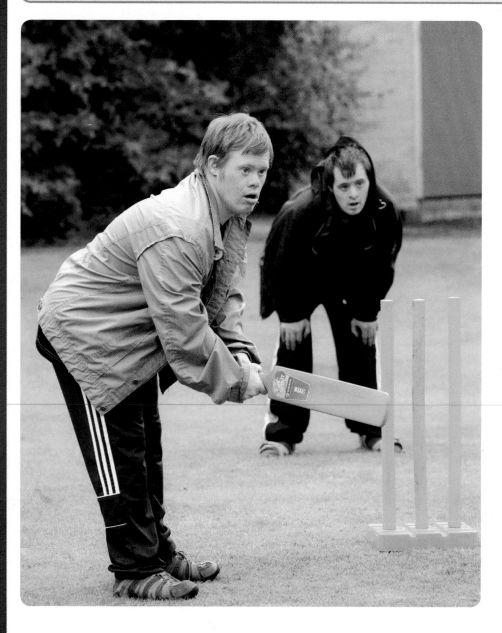

AC	What can you do now?	Assessment task	✓
2.1	Find out the history, preferences, wishes and needs of the individual	Page 165	
2.2	Apply person-centred values in day-to-day work, taking into account the history, preferences, wishes and needs of the individual	Page 165	
3.1	Explain the importance of establishing consent when providing care or support	Page 169	
3.2	Establish consent for an activity or action	Page 169	
3.3	Explain what steps to take if consent cannot readily be established	Page 169	
4.1	Describe how active participation benefits an individual	Page 173	
4.2	Identify possible barriers to active participation	Page 173	
4.3	Demonstrate ways to reduce the barriers and encourage active participation	Page 173	
5.1	Support an individual to make informed choices	Page 177	
5.2	Use agreed risk assessment processes to support the right to make choices	Page 177	
5.3	Explain why a worker's personal views should not influence an individual's choices	Page 177	
5.4	Describe how to support an individual to question or challenge decisions concerning them that are made by others	Page 177	
6.1	Explain how individual identity and self-esteem are linked with wellbeing	Page 183	
6.2	Describe attitudes and approaches that are likely to promote an individual's wellbeing	Page 183	
6.3	Support an individual in a way that promotes a sense of identity and self-esteem	Page 183	
6.4	Demonstrate ways to contribute to an environment that promotes wellbeing	Page 183	

3 | Contribute to health and safety in health and social care (HSC 027)

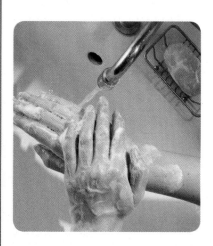

Assessment of this unit

This unit will introduce you to the knowledge and skills health and social care practitioners need to work safely and to manage the security of themselves and others in care settings.

The tables below outline what you need to know and do to meet each of the assessment criteria for the unit.

Your tutor or assessor will help you to prepare for your assessment and the tasks suggested in the unit will help you to create the evidence that you need.

AC	What you need to know
1.1	Identify legislation relating to general health and safety in a health or social care work setting
1.2	Describe the main points of the health and safety policies and procedures agreed with the employer
1.3	Outline the main health and safety responsibilities of: • self • the employer or manager • others in the work setting
1.4	Identify tasks relating to health and safety that should not be carried out without special training
1.5	Explain how to access additional support and information relating to health and safety
2.1	Explain why it is important to assess health and safety hazards posed by the work setting or by particular activities
2.2	Explain how and when to report potential health and safety risks that have been identified
2.3	Explain how risk assessment can help address dilemmas between rights and health and safety concerns
3.1	Describe different types of accidents and sudden illness that may occur in own work setting
3.2	Outline the procedures to be followed if an accident or sudden illness should occur
6.1	Identify hazardous substances and materials that may be found in the work setting

6.2	Describe safe practices for:
	• storing hazardous substances
	• using hazardous substances
	• disposing of hazardous substances and materials
7.1	Describe practices that prevent fires from:
	• starting
	• spreading
7.2	Outline emergency procedures to be followed in the event of a fire in the work setting
7.3	Explain the importance of maintaining clear evacuation routes at all times
9.1	Identify common signs and indicators of stress
9.2	Identify circumstances that tend to trigger own stress
9.3	Describe ways to manage own stress

AC   What you need to do

4.1	Demonstrate the recommended method for hand washing
4.2	Demonstrate ways to ensure that own health and hygiene do not pose a risk to others at work
5.1	Identify legislation that relates to moving and handling
5.2	Explain principles for moving and handling equipment and other objects safely
5.3	Move and handle equipment or other objects safely
8.1	Use agreed ways of working for checking the identity of anyone requesting access to:
	• premises
	• information
8.2	Implement measures to protect own security and the security of others in the work setting
8.3	Explain the importance of ensuring that others are aware of own whereabouts

Assessment criteria 4.1, 4.2; 5.1, 5.2, 5.3; 8.1, 8.2, 8.3 must be assessed in a real work environment.

This unit also links to some of the other units:

HSC 024	Principles of safeguarding and protection in health and social care
IC 01	Principles of infection prevention and control
HSC 2028	Move and position individuals

Some of your learning will be repeated in these units and will give you the chance to review your knowledge and understanding.

Health and safety responsibilities in care settings

The health and safety responsibilities of employers and employees in health and social care settings result from the wide range of legislation that governs health and safety in all workplaces, and other laws which are specific to care settings. Legislation is necessary to ensure that safe working practices are followed when caring for people, and to protect the health and safety of both service users and care workers.

The Health and Safety Commission and Executive

The Health and Safety Executive is the body that monitors standards and enforces health and safety law in the workplace in England, Wales and Scotland. The Health and Safety Executive Northern Ireland has this responsibility in Northern Ireland. The Health and Safety Executive was created by the Health and Safety at Work Act 1974. One of its key tasks is to investigate all accidents in the workplace. The website of the Health and Safety Executive (**www.hse.gov.uk**) states that: 'Our mission is to prevent death, injury and ill-health in Great Britain's workplaces'. The Health and Safety Executive can:

- enter premises to conduct investigations or carry out spot checks on health and safety
- conduct investigations into accidents and safety compliance
- take samples and photographs to assess health and safety risks
- ask questions about health and safety procedures and risk control
- give advice on how to minimise risk
- issue instructions that must, by law, be carried out
- issue improvement and prohibition notices.

The Health and Safety Executive is most likely to visit care settings where:

- there is evidence that health and safety is poor
- there are hazardous substances that should be properly stored and controlled
- a specific incident (accident, death or illness, for example) has occurred.

The purpose of Health and Safety Executive visits and investigations is to check that standards of workplace health, safety and welfare are satisfactory and to give advice on how risks to people being injured or becoming ill in the workplace can be minimised.

Your assessment criteria:

1.1 Identify legislation relating to general health and safety in a health or social care work setting

1.2 Describe the main points of the health and safety policies and procedures agreed with the employer

1.3 Outline the main health and safety responsibilities of: self; the employer or manager; others in the work setting

Key terms

Legislation: written laws, usually Acts of Parliament

Health and Safety Executive: the government agency responsible for monitoring and enforcing health and safety laws in the workplace

Compliance: doing what others want

Prohibition: prevention; stopping something from happening

The Health and Safety at Work Act 1974

The Health and Safety at Work Act 1974 is the main piece of health and safety law in the UK. It affects both employers and employees. Under this **statute**, care practitioners share responsibility for health and safety in care settings with the care organisation that employs them. The care organisation is responsible for providing:

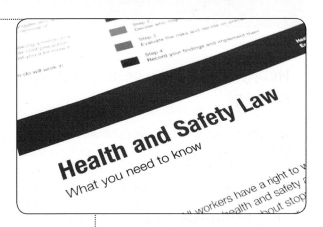

▶ a safe and secure work environment

▶ safe equipment

▶ information and training about health, safety and security.

In short, care organisations must provide a work environment that meets expected health and safety standards. They must make it possible for health and social care practitioners to work safely. Health and social care practitioners in turn have a responsibility to:

▶ work safely within the care setting

▶ monitor their work environment for health and safety problems that may develop

▶ report and respond appropriately to any health and safety risks.

To meet their legal responsibilities, health and or social care organisations must:

▶ carry out health and safety risk assessments

▶ develop health and safety **procedures**, such as fire evacuation procedures

▶ provide health and safety equipment, such as fire extinguishers, fire blankets and first aid boxes

▶ ensure that health and social care settings have appropriate safety systems, such as smoke alarms, fire exits and security fixtures (electronic pads on doors and window guards, for example)

▶ train their employees to follow health and safety **policies** and procedures, and to use health and safety equipment and safety features appropriately

▶ provide a range of health and safety information and warning signs to alert people to safety features such as fire exits and first aid equipment, and to warn them about prohibited areas and activities (no smoking, for example).

Key terms

Statute: a form of written law, also known as an Act of Parliament

Procedure: a document that sets out in detail how a particular issue should be dealt with or how particular tasks should be carried out

Policy: a written document that sets out an organisation's approach towards a particular issue

Reflect

Have you received any health and safety training relating to your work role? How did you find out about the health and safety procedures of your work or placement setting?

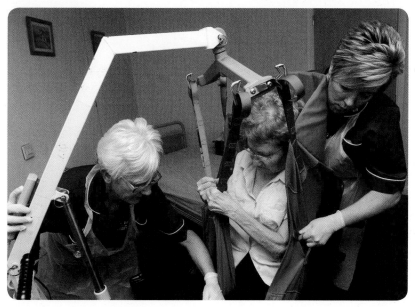

Health and safety training is vital for everyone who uses specialist care equipment

Your assessment criteria:

1.1 Identify legislation relating to general health and safety in a health or social care work setting

1.2 Describe the main points of the health and safety policies and procedures agreed with the employer

1.3 Outline the main health and safety responsibilities of: self; the employer or manager; others in the work setting

Health and safety regulations

The Health and Safety at Work Act 1974 enforces minimum standards of workplace health and safety and establishes a framework for safe working. In practice, a range of regulations that apply to care settings also extend and supplement this Act (see Figure 8.1).

Key terms

Regulations: legal rules that are created using the authority of a statute

Figure 8.1 Health and safety regulations

Regulations	Effects on practice
Management of Health and Safety at Work Regulations 1999	This places a responsibility on employers to train staff in relation to health and safety legislation, fire prevention, and moving and handling issues. Employers must also carry out risk assessments, remove or reduce any health and safety hazards that are identified, and write safe working procedures based on their risk assessments.
The Manual Handling Operations Regulations 1992 (amended 2002)	These regulations cover all manual handling activities, such as lifting, lowering, pushing, pulling or carrying objects or people. A large proportion of workplace injuries are due to poor manual handling skills. Employers have a duty to assess the risks surrounding any activity that involves manual handling. They must put in place measures to reduce or avoid the risk. Employees must follow manual handling procedures and cooperate on all manual handling issues.

continued...

Regulations	Effects on practice
Health and Safety (First Aid) Regulations 1981	These cover requirements for the provision of first aid in the workplace.
Reporting of Injuries, Diseases and Dangerous Occurrences Regulations (RIDDOR) 1995	These regulations require employers to notify the Health and Safety Executive, or other relevant authorities, of a range of occupational injuries, diseases and dangerous events.
Control of Substances Hazardous to Health Regulations (COSHH) 2002	These regulations require employers to assess the risks from hazardous substances and take appropriate precautions to ensure that hazardous substances are correctly stored and used.

Health and safety policies and procedures

A health or social care organisation's policies and procedures should always incorporate the key points of health and safety law. This means that a care practitioner will be able to put health and safety laws into practice simply by following their employer's policies and procedures. Health and social care organisations need to develop a range of policies to ensure all aspects of the legal framework of care are covered. These will include policies on:

▶ health and safety

▶ safeguarding

▶ reporting of accidents

▶ waste disposal

▶ fire prevention and evacuation procedures

▶ security

▶ cleaning

▶ food safety

▶ dispensing and storing medicines

▶ lone working.

The way health and safety-related policies and procedures are used should be monitored to check that employees are actually using them appropriately in practice. Employees are under a contractual obligation to implement their employers' policies and procedures and may face disciplinary action and possible dismissal for not doing so. You should know what the health and safety-related policies and procedures used in your work setting say and how they affect your work role.

Key terms

Safeguarding: the protection of vulnerable people

Care Quality Commission: the independent organisation that inspects and regulates all health and social care services in England

Discuss

How do these health and safety laws affect the way people practice in your work or placement setting? With a couple of colleagues, discuss the different ways in which legislation impacts on the way care is provided where you work.

Investigate

Go to the website of the Care Quality Commission (**www.cqc. org.uk**) and find a report on a health or social care organisation near to where you live or a report on the organisation you work for. What does the report say about standards of health and safety in the organisation?

Working within own limits

Health and safety law makes every health and social care practitioner responsible for working in ways that protect their own and other people's health, safety and security. A key part of this is recognising the limits to your own competence and ensuring that you always work within these limits. You must undertake all of the health and safety training relevant to your work role and cooperate fully with others on health and safety issues. Where personal protective clothing or specialist equipment is provided to carry out care-related tasks, you should ensure that you know how to use this properly. You must always let a senior member of staff know when you do not have the knowledge, skills or experience to carry out particular tasks or use particular items of equipment. Acknowledging and working within your own limits protects the health and safety of the people you provide care for, your colleagues and yourself. You should ensure that you receive specific training and health and safety guidance if your work role involves any of the following:

▶ using specialist equipment

▶ providing first aid

▶ administering medication

▶ carrying out health care procedures (bandaging, changing catheters)

▶ preparing or handling food.

Reflect

Have you ever been in a position where you were asked to carry out work beyond your capabilities or competence? How did you deal with this?

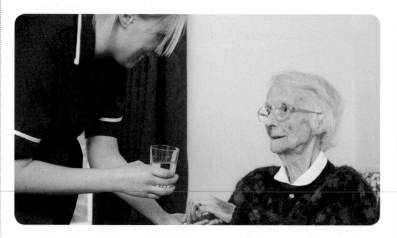

Accessing additional health and safety support and information

Information about health and safety should be provided in the health and safety policies and procedures relating to your workplace. You should be able to obtain additional information relating to specific health and safety issues from:

▶ the manager of your workplace

▶ your supervisor or mentor

- ▶ the health and safety representative for your workplace
- ▶ your tutor or assessor
- ▶ specialist websites such as the Health and Safety Executive (**www.hse.gov.uk**).

Health and safety issues are a priority in all health and social care settings. You should receive basic health and safety training when you first begin your work role. You should also have opportunities to learn more and to update your knowledge and skills on a regular basis through workplace or external training opportunities.

Investigate

Go to the Health and Safety Executive website and search through the different forms of advice and guidance that are relevant to your job role and your care setting. Print off and summarise any information that is particularly relevant to your setting.

Case study

Natasha has recently started a job as a support worker at Edward Watson House day centre. On her first day, Natasha was given the health and safety file to read. This was full of leaflets and complicated explanations of health and safety laws that apply to care settings like Edward Watson House. Natasha feels a bit overwhelmed. Sharon, the day centre manager, says she will ask Natasha to explain:

1. what her health and safety responsibilities (as an employee) are
2. what health and safety responsibilities she thinks Edward Watson House has (as her employer)
3. how RIDDOR and COSHH might apply to the care setting.

What would you say in response to each of these points if you were in Natasha's position?

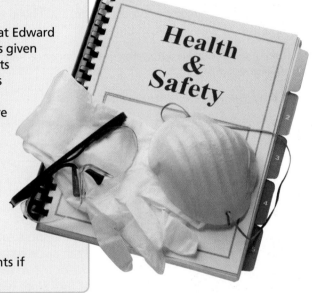

Knowledge Assessment Task | 1.1 | 1.2 | 1.3 | 1.4 | 1.5

Health and social care practitioners need to understand their own responsibilities, and the responsibilities of others, relating to health and safety in their work setting. Summarise your understanding of health and safety by carrying out the following tasks:

1. Identify examples of legislation relating to general health and safety in your work setting.
2. Describe the main points of the health and safety policies and procedures that are used in your work setting.
3. Outline the health and safety responsibilities that apply to yourself, your employer and others in the work setting.
4. Identify tasks relating to health and safety that should not be carried out without special training.
5. Explain how to access additional support and information relating to health and safety in your work setting.

Keep the work you produce for this activity as evidence towards your assessment.

What is risk assessment?

By law, health and social care organisations are required to carry out formal risk assessments of their workplaces and outside areas that employees or service users may use. **Risk assessment** aims to identify potential **risks** to the health, safety and security of service users, health and social care practitioners and anybody else who uses the care setting. The aim is to minimise risk by identifying **hazards** and putting measures in place to protect people from harm. You have an important role to play in contributing to and using risk assessments appropriately. You will need to understand and use risk assessments in order to:

▶ protect yourself and others from danger or harm in the work setting

▶ ensure you are working within the law

▶ reduce the risk of injuring yourself or others through your care practice

▶ reduce the liability and costs your employer may face if they are sued as a result of your reckless or unsafe actions.

The risk assessment process

Risk assessment recognises that health and social care provision, equipment and the care setting itself can all be hazardous. However, steps can be taken to remove or minimise the level of risk to people. All of the activities that take place within your workplace must be risk-assessed. Similarly, all of the equipment and facilities have to be checked for hazards. The ultimate aim of a risk assessment is to ensure that people can use care settings without coming to any harm. The Health and Safety Executive has identified five stages of a risk assessment process. These stages and their purpose are identified in Figure 8.2.

Key terms

Risk assessment: the process of evaluating the likelihood of a hazard actually causing harm

Risk: the chance of harm being done by a hazard

Hazard: anything that can cause harm

Figure 8.2 The five stages of risk assessment

Stage	Key questions	Purpose
1. Identify the hazards	What are the hazards?	• to identify all hazards that could cause a risk
2. Estimate the risk	Who is at risk?	• to evaluate the risk of hazards causing harm
3. Control the risk	What needs to be done? Who needs to do what?	• to identify risk control measures and responsibilities for reducing or removing the risk

continued...

Stage	Key questions	Purpose
4. Monitor risk control measures	Are the risk control measures being implemented?	• to monitor the implementation and effectiveness of risk control measures
5. Reassess the risk	Is the risk controlled? Can the risk be reduced still further?	• to evaluate the effectiveness of current risk control strategies • to identify new risks or changes to risk levels • to consider new strategies for controlling risk

The risk assessment process is a continuous one. Hazard identification and risk reduction are an ongoing process because circumstances, people's behaviour and care practices change on a regular basis in health and social care settings.

The Management of Health and Safety at Work Regulations 1999

These regulations place a legal duty on employers to carry out risk assessments in order to ensure a safe and healthy workplace. The risk assessments that are produced should clearly identify:

▶ the potential hazards and risks to the health and safety of employees and others in the workplace

▶ any preventive and protective measures that are needed to minimise risk and improve health and safety.

Many larger organisations employ people as health and safety officers to carry out their risk assessments and manage health and safety issues generally. In smaller organisations this might be the responsibility of one or more of the managers, or of a senior practitioner. Risk assessments must be:

▶ communicated to all health or social care practitioners and users of the setting

▶ implemented through the way practitioners work

▶ monitored and reviewed on a regular basis

▶ linked to health and safety policies and to staff training.

Reflect

Have you seen any of the written risk assessments that are used in your work setting? Who carried out or produced these risk assessments? How might you contribute to the risk assessment process in your work setting?

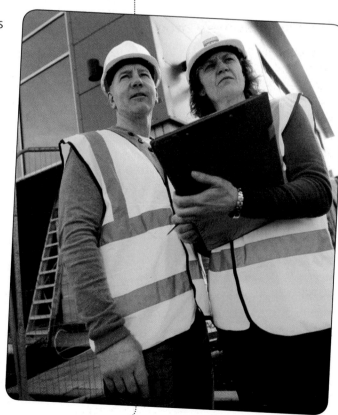

195

Reporting health and safety hazards and risks

You have an important role to play in contributing to health and safety risk assessment, in using the risk assessments that are produced for your workplace, and in ensuring that you minimise risk to yourself and others in the way that you work. You should be alert to all potential hazards to yourself and others and the need to report these, and any changes in risk, to your supervisor, manager or employer. Reporting hazards and risks ensures that the organisation you work for is aware of them and also places the responsibility for dealing with them onto the organisation.

Health and social care organisations generally have accident and incident books or forms that must be completed as part of the reporting procedure. You should know where these can be found and what kinds of information they require you to provide. Your employer has a legal obligation to report certain types of accident or incident to the Health and Safety Executive or the local authority environmental health department.

Reporting of Injuries, Diseases and Dangerous Occurrences Regulations (RIDDOR) 1995, (amended 2008)

These regulations require your employer to report all deaths, accidents, dangerous incidents or outbreaks of infectious diseases to the Health and Safety Executive's Incident Contact Centre. The Centre will then pass this information to the local authority or the Health and Safety Executive for an investigation to be carried out. This may result in further risk assessments being carried out or the existing risk assessments and procedures being modified.

Addressing dilemmas between rights and health and safety concerns

Risk assessment needs to be a part of every health or social care practitioner's approach to their work with service users. One of the challenges faced by care practitioners is to achieve a balance between providing a safe, stimulating environment for service users and minimising health and safety hazards and risks within it.

People who are unwell, infirm, disabled or who require assistance with everyday living activities may be less capable of identifying potential hazards than adults who are in good physical and mental health. An individual in receipt of care may not realise that an activity may be too challenging for them or may not understand why an area of the care environment is risky for them. In these circumstances, care practitioners need to find ways of promoting health, safety and security whilst also encouraging people to make choices and take appropriate risks in their life. Planning and organising care provision, creative activities or leisure situations carefully will enable you to identify potential hazards and work out

Your assessment criteria:

2.2 Explain how and when to report potential health and safety risks that have been identified

2.3 Explain how risk assessment can help address dilemmas between rights and health and safety concerns

Investigate

Do you know what the reporting procedure is for health and safety issues or incidents in your work setting? Obtain a copy of the policies and procedures relating to this and also find out which forms have to be completed to make a report.

ways of minimising risks to each individual you work with. Good planning should take into account the:

▶ developmental abilities and understanding of the individual

▶ physical and intellectual demands of an activity or task

▶ potential hazards involved in an activity or task

▶ level of risk an activity or task poses for a particular individual.

It is important to recognise that there are often no simple or easy solutions to the dilemmas that care practitioners face between promoting an individual's rights and ensuring health and safety concerns are addressed. People who receive care and support must be allowed to take some risks in life but everything should be done to minimise the likelihood of them experiencing harm or damaging their health by doing so.

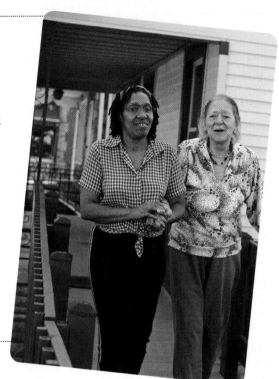

Knowledge Assessment Task   2.1   2.2   2.3

There are lots of myths and stories about health and safety and the way this affects practice in health and social care settings. Often the myths and stories present health and safety concerns as a barrier or hurdle that care practitioners have to overcome to provide people with the care or support they need. By contrast, professional care practitioners tend to prioritise health and safety issues and risk assessment processes in order to safeguard themselves and service users whilst providing effective care. In this knowledge assessment task you are required to produce a short report that explains:

▶ why it is important to assess health and safety hazards posed by the work setting or by particular activities

▶ how and when to report potential health and safety risks that have been identified

▶ how risk assessment can help address dilemmas between rights and health and safety concerns.

You should keep a copy of the report that you produce for this task as evidence for your assessment.

Understanding procedures for responding to accidents and sudden illness

Would you know what to do in an emergency?

Health and social care practitioners need to know how to react when an accident or sudden illness occurs in the care setting. Accidents can happen unexpectedly in all health and social care settings and adults can suddenly become unwell for a variety of reasons. In either of these situations, a person may need medical help. Part of your work role is to monitor individuals in the setting for signs of illness or injury, and to respond appropriately by getting help when necessary. The types of accidents and illnesses that you need to be prepared for are described in Figure 8.3.

Your assessment criteria:

3.1 Describe different types of accidents and sudden illness that may occur in own work setting

3.2 Outline the procedures to be followed if an accident or sudden illness should occur

Figure 8.3 Causes and possible effects of different types of accident

Type of accident	Causes and possible effects
Slips and trips	Wet floors, loose carpets or rugs, ill-fitting shoes or slippers. The effects can include fractures (hips, collar bones, arms, ankles) sprains and bruising.
Falls	Tripping over objects, standing suddenly and experiencing a drop in blood pressure, loss of strength or stamina. The effects can include fractures, sprains and head injuries.
Needle stick injuries	Failing to dispose of a used needle safely – don't try to re-sheath it! This can lead to the transfer of infection from one person to another.
Burns and scalds	Excessively hot baths, hot water bottles or wash basins of water, spilled hot drinks, pans that fall or are pulled from a stove, sitting too close to a heat source (e.g. open fire or very hot radiator). Severe skin damage can result.
Injuries from operating machinery or equipment	Lack of guards on equipment, poorly maintained or malfunctioning equipment or incorrect use/technique may result in injury. The nature of the injury will depend on the type of equipment but could include electrocution, fracture or lacerations.
Electrocution	Poorly wired electrical equipment, contact between electrical equipment and water, and overloaded sockets, can lead to electrocution. The effects include burns, altered heart rate/heart attack and death.
Accidental poisoning	This can result from ingestion of chemicals or other toxic fluids or overdose of medication, for example. Retching and vomiting, loss of consciousness and organ failure leading to death can result.

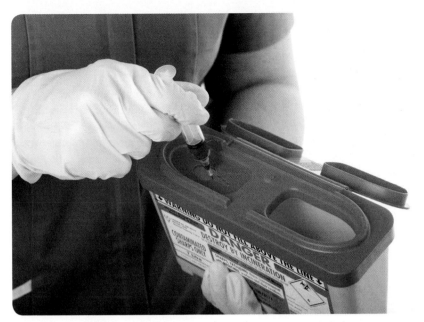

Correct disposal of sharps is an important health and safety procedure

Reflect

Can you think of any recent situations in which you noticed a person exhibiting the signs or symptoms of illness or injury? What was it you noticed and what were the causes of these signs or symptoms?

Identifying signs and symptoms of sudden illness

The **signs** of sudden illness are those things that you can *see*, such as a visible change in a person's normal appearance and behaviour – becoming pale in colour or not having the energy to respond in their usual way. People often know when they are unwell and will tell you about **symptoms** that they feel, such as feeling sick or having a headache. Observing and talking to people in the care setting should enable you to identify when they are unwell or have an injury.

Figure 8.4 Signs and symptoms of sudden illness

Type of sudden illness	Signs and symptoms
Heart attack	Chest pain: the chest can feel like it is being pressed or squeezed by a heavy object, and the pain can radiate from the chest to the jaw, neck, arms and back; shortness of breath; overwhelming feeling of anxiety
Diabetic coma	Increased thirst, the need to urinate frequently and tiredness; can be followed by a sleep-like state in which the person slips into a coma. They will be unresponsive and must be treated in hospital quickly.
Epileptic convulsion (seizure)	A tonic-clonic seizure has two stages: • stiffness in the person's body • twitching of the person's arms and legs The person loses consciousness and some people will wet themselves. The seizure normally lasts between one and three minutes but they can last longer.

Procedures to be followed

All health and social care settings have to be prepared for emergency situations and must have appropriate procedures in place so that staff can respond and people can be kept safe. You should know about and understand these and should take part in any accident or emergency response training that is provided by your employer. It is important to follow the correct procedure as soon as you realise that an accident or incident has occurred or that a person has suddenly become unwell. In general this will require you to:

▶ remain calm

▶ raise the alarm or call for help

▶ assess the situation and prioritise the safety of yourself and others

▶ clear the area of people, furniture and, wherever possible, equipment

▶ assess the individuals affected by the accident, incident or by sudden illness, for injuries and other symptoms of ill health

▶ administer first aid but only if you are trained to do so

▶ stay with the person until help arrives

▶ reassure and observe the person or people involved, noting any changes in their condition

▶ provide a clear verbal report of what happened and the state of any casualties to medical staff or others who arrive to provide assistance.

Recording accidents and incidents

You should know where the accident and incident forms are kept in your work setting. You will need to complete one of these if you are involved in or witness any kind of accident or incident. This must happen even if there are no injuries to the people involved.

Your assessment criteria:

3.2 Outline the procedures to be followed if an accident or sudden illness should occur

Discuss

Discuss with a work colleague or your supervisor what you think your role would be if an emergency, such as a fire or flood, occurred in your work setting. You may also want to consult the health and safety policies to find out what it says about care practitioners' roles in emergency situations.

Remaining calm and giving details concisely and clearly will ensure that appropriate help is sent in emergency situations

Sending for help

All members of staff in a health and social care setting should know whom to call for help and how to contact the emergency services when assistance is required. The names and telephone numbers of first aiders should be displayed on posters or on notice boards in public areas of the workplace. If a situation is serious, a 999 call should be made. The emergency operator will ask for the following information:

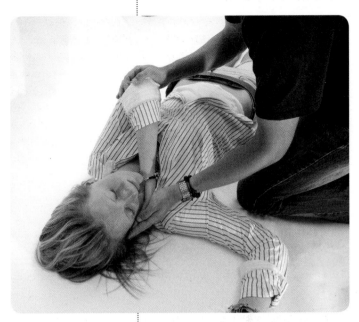

► which services are required (police, ambulance and/or fire service)

► the caller's name and the number of the phone they are calling from

► the location of the accident or incident

► if relevant, the number of casualties involved

► what has happened (including signs, symptoms and state of any casualties)

► whether any of the casualties are unconscious.

You should only administer first aid to accident casualties if you are trained to do so

It is important for the caller to listen carefully to the emergency operator, to provide the information they ask for and to remain as calm as possible, even though this may be difficult in the circumstances.

Knowledge Assessment Task   3.1   3.2

Accidents and sudden illness are, by definition, unexpected occurrences in a care setting. Despite this, care organisations and the practitioners they employ must be prepared for the unexpected. In this task you are required to prepare some teaching notes and a handout for students who are about to begin a placement in the care setting where you work or are on placement. These notes and the handout should:

► describe different types of accidents and sudden illness that may occur in your own work setting

► outline the procedures that people working in the setting (as employees or students on placement) need to follow if an accident or sudden illness should occur.

Keep a copy of the work you produce for this task as evidence for your assessment.

Investigate

What do the emergency procedures in your work setting say about the following:

► raising the alarm

► getting help and assistance from the emergency services

► evacuating the building

► the assembly point outside of the building

► protecting and reassuring people during emergency incidents?

Reducing the spread of infection

Infection control procedures aim to prevent bacteria and viruses from being passed from one person to another, causing illness. The **bacteria** and **viruses** that cause infections are present in everyday life. In most cases people gradually build up **immunity** to common infections and only suffer minor illnesses in the process. However, the weaker, sometimes impaired immune systems of people who are sick, frail or disabled can make them more vulnerable to both new and existing strains of infection that lead to significant health problems.

Infection control procedures

Health and social care practitioners should always follow basic infection control procedures. These include:

- ▶ maintaining good standards of personal hygiene (relating to dress, hair care, footwear and oral hygiene)

- ▶ using personal protective clothing such as aprons, gloves and masks appropriately

- ▶ following standard health, safety and hygiene precautions in the workplace

- ▶ washing hands regularly and thoroughly

- ▶ ensuring that equipment such as commodes and hoists are thoroughly cleaned and disinfected between uses

- ▶ disposing of waste safely in the correct bags, bins or containers.

Infection control policies and procedures

There should be a detailed set of infection control policies and procedures relating to your workplace. You should know what these say about:

- ▶ hand washing

- ▶ use of personal protective equipment

- ▶ cleaning standards and procedures

- ▶ dealing with spillages (blood, vomit, diarrhoea and other body fluids)

- ▶ handling soiled clothes and laundry

- ▶ dealing with 'sharps'

- ▶ touching and looking after animals (e.g. cats, dogs)

- ▶ coughing, sneezing and outbreaks of infectious illnesses such as chickenpox, measles, norovirus, for example

- ▶ infestations of head lice.

Your assessment criteria:

4.1 Demonstrate the recommended method for hand washing

4.2 Demonstrate ways to ensure that own health and hygiene do not pose a risk to others at work

Key terms

Bacteria: single-cell organisms that can carry disease but which can also be helpful to human beings

Immunity: resistance to disease

Virus: a disease-carrying microorganism that infects other cells in the human body

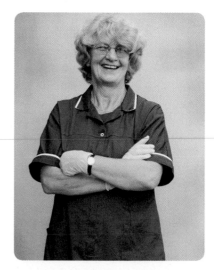

The policies and procedures used in your work setting should explain when and why personal protective equipment, such as gloves, should be used to provide care

Washing and drying your hands

Regular, effective hand hygiene is the single most important infection control measure you can undertake in a health or social care setting. Washing your hands thoroughly with a decontamination agent and drying them properly denies bacteria and viruses the conditions in which they can exist and develop. You should always wash and dry your hands before and after:

▶ helping a person to use the toilet or commode

▶ changing a person's incontinence pad, dressing or soiled clothes (remember to wear gloves)

▶ using the toilet yourself

▶ preparing or providing food for people, including yourself

▶ taking part in messy creative or outside activities.

You should encourage and demonstrate good hand hygiene to the people for whom you provide care, assistance and support, so that they develop effective hand washing habits too.

Reflect

When do you wash your hands at work? Think of the types of activities and tasks you do and reflect on the infection risks that these might involve. Are you protecting yourself and others appropriately through regular and thorough hand washing?

Investigate

Go to the Health Protection Agency website (**www.hpa.org. uk**) and find the information and guidance on infection prevention and control in hospitals and care homes. Consider how this guidance can be used in your own work setting.

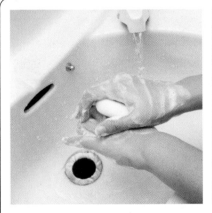

1. Lather hands with soap

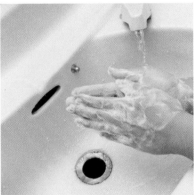

2. Rub both palms together

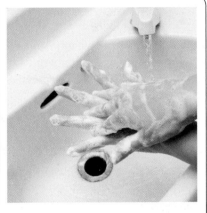

3. Rub each fingers and between fingers

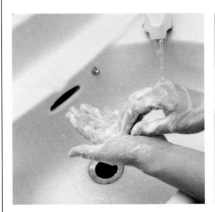

4. Rub palms with finger nails

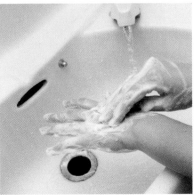

5. Rub back of hand with finger nails

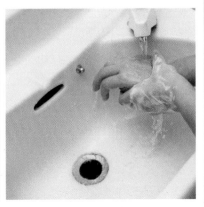

6. Wash thoroughly and towel dry

Using personal protective clothing

Personal protective clothing and equipment plays an important part in infection control because it is generally used to provide a barrier to infections being transmitted from one person to another. Using the personal protective clothing and equipment available in your workplace reduces the risk that you will contract an infection from others and the risk of you passing one on. Examples of personal protective clothing and equipment generally available in health and social care settings include:

- disposable aprons
- disposable gloves
- face masks
- eye-protector goggles.

Health and social care practitioners may need to use these items of equipment when:

- changing dressings, incontinence pads or bandages
- helping people to use the toilet
- caring for people who are unwell (bleeding or vomiting) or who have open wounds such as pressure sores
- picking up and washing soiled clothing or linen
- cleaning up body fluid spillages.

You should always dispose of personal protective equipment in the appropriate waste bin immediately after each use (do not reuse aprons, gloves or masks) and wash your hands before and after using them. Do not wander around the workplace wearing personal protective clothing or engage in any activity other than the one you are wearing them for, as this risks spreading infection.

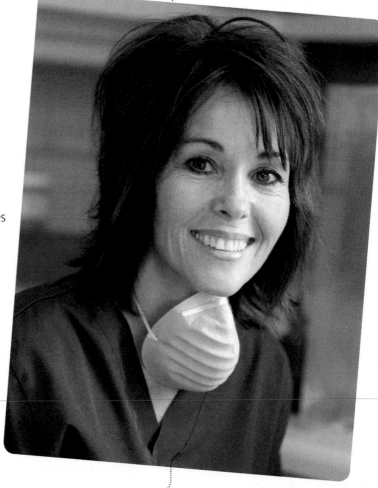

Investigate

Find out what kinds of personal protective clothing are available in your work setting and the situations in which they need to be used.

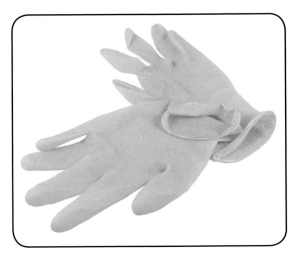

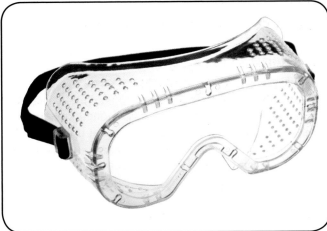

Case study

Cheryl, aged 17, is taking a BTEC First Health and Social Care course at school. She will be spending every Wednesday at your work setting on placement until the end of term. Cheryl is quite excited about working with people in a real care environment. However, she has never done any care work before, or visited your workplace. You have been asked to help with Cheryl's induction programme. Make notes, describing for Cheryl:

▶ the infection control procedures in your work setting
▶ the personal protective clothing that is used to avoid the spread of infection.

Practical Assessment Task   4.1   4.2

Your competence as a health or social care worker depends on your ability to demonstrate safe practice. For this task you need to demonstrate to your assessor that you are able to demonstrate:

▶ the recommended method for hand washing
▶ ways to ensure that your own health and hygiene do not pose a risk to others at work.

You will need to demonstrate these skills in a practical, work-based situation. One way of doing this would be to apply these basic infection control procedures when providing personal care for a service user. You may be able to identify another situation where you can demonstrate these skills but should agree on the suitability of this with your assessor.

Moving and handling in care settings

Moving and handling people, equipment and other objects is a major cause of injury at work in the United Kingdom. Health and social care practitioners are particularly at risk of back injuries unless they understand and use safe moving and handling techniques. The importance of using correct moving and handling procedures is reflected in the fact that this area of care practice is regulated by a number of laws.

Regulations relating to safe moving and handling

The moving and handling of people, equipment and objects is regulated by the Manual Handling Operations Regulations 1992. This law requires employers to avoid all manual handling activities where there is a risk of injury 'so far as is reasonably practicable'. This might involve modifying the plan for a task or using specialist lifting equipment to carry it out. However, there are situations in health and social care settings where manual handling cannot be avoided. A suitable and sufficient risk assessment must be carried out and all reasonable steps taken to minimise risks to those involved in these situations.

Provision and Use of Work Equipment Regulations (PUWER) 1998

These regulations make employers responsible for ensuring that workplace equipment is:

▶ suitable for its intended use and for the conditions in which it is used

▶ safe for use, and maintained and inspected where necessary

▶ used only by those with adequate knowledge, training and experience to use it safely

▶ fitted with suitable safety measures (e.g. safety guards, brakes, protective devices, instructions and warning labels).

Where the use of equipment involves a risk to users it must be inspected by qualified people on a regular basis.

All lifting equipment for handling objects must have an annual inspection. Lifting equipment for handling or moving people must be inspected every six months.

Your assessment criteria:

5.1 Identify legislation that relates to moving and handling

5.2 Explain principles for moving and handling equipment and other objects safely

5.3 Move and handle equipment or other objects safely

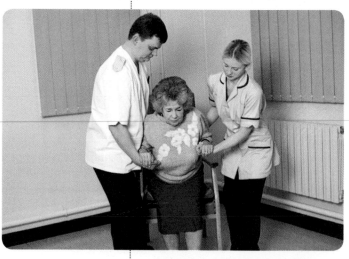

Assisting people with their mobility can present risks for care practitioners if the person requires physical support and is not weight bearing

Principles of moving and handling equipment and other objects safely

It is now rare to lift a person or object manually in a health or social care setting. Where this does happen, a risk assessment must be carried out and risk control measures followed. This may involve using a team of people to carry out a lift or using specialist equipment. The safety of the person being moved or lifted as well as those carrying out the move is the key concern.

Responsibility for ensuring that moving and handling activity is carried out safely is shared between employers and employees.

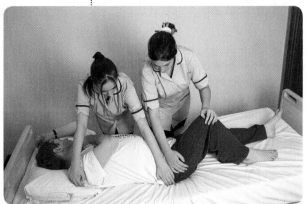

Care practitioners should have regular training and be competent in moving and handling techniques before undertaking this kind of activity

It is the *employer's* responsibility to:

▶ provide an induction and training course in current manual handling practice, with compulsory yearly updates

▶ produce and implement a manual handling policy

▶ provide equipment that meets both the specific and collective needs of the individuals concerned

▶ employ a competent person to monitor manual handling practice or seek advice from an expert, such as a back care adviser

▶ minimise risks in the workplace environment by providing adequately trained staff, clear guidelines and support and an appropriate uniform or clothing policy

▶ ensure that members of staff are fit to carry out work and that there are sufficient reporting mechanisms in place if injuries do occur

▶ investigate any injuries and aim to prevent any reoccurrence through risk assessment and clear policies and procedures.

It is the *employee's* responsibility to:

▶ be accountable for their own actions and to seek advice if unsure of safe practice

▶ undertake manual handling training and update practice at least once yearly

▶ report any manual handling concerns regarding individuals, equipment or staff to a manager or supervisor

▶ use moving and handling equipment appropriately and responsibly

▶ carry out a personal risk assessment to consider safety of self, individual and equipment.

Your assessment criteria:

5.3 Find out what kinds of personal protective clothing are available in your work setting and the situations in which they need to be used

Moving and handling policies

Your care organisation should have an organisational policy on moving and handling. It is important – and your responsibility – to find out what this says, and to follow the practices and procedures that it sets out. The moving and handling policy should incorporate all of the most recent moving and handling regulations and laws. You will not be covered by your employer's insurance policies, and may not have any legal redress, if you fail to follow the moving and handling policy and subsequently get a back injury due to unsafe practice.

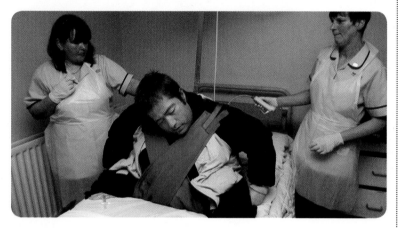

Good practice in moving and handling usually involves the use of appropriate equipment

Using moving and handling equipment

The majority of health and social care settings have a policy of no manual lifting. This ensures that individuals are assisted to move with the aid of equipment or support aids. However, it is known that when there are staff shortages and equipment is lacking or defective, many care practitioners will continue to lift or manually handle individuals. In doing so, they are putting themselves at risk of sustaining back, arm and neck injuries and may also be endangering the safety of the individuals they are caring for.

Risk assessment will determine what constitutes safe handling practice in any situation. The starting point for risk assessment should be that lifting an adult's weight is likely to be unacceptably hazardous to an individual practitioner. The Department of Health also advises that certain moves, such as the shoulder or 'Australian' lift, are now considered to be unacceptable from a risk control point of view.

Detailed advice on safe moving and handling practice in your workplace should be sought from a specialist practitioner or adviser with responsibility for this area of work. You should also consult the safe moving and handling policy and any in-house training guidance that your employer provides on these matters. Remember that no one working in a hospital, nursing home or community setting should need to manually lift patients any more. Non-weight-bearing individuals should only be moved using appropriate equipment and safe techniques.

▶ Before attempting any moving or handling, explain to the individual what you need to do and obtain their assistance where appropriate.

▶ Prepare the area first so that it is free from clutter and objects on the floor.

▶ Confirm that the equipment to be used has been checked and is safe to use. If this is not the case, do not use it.

▶ The correct sling or hoist should be used to suit the weight and size of the individual.

▶ Sufficient time and space must be allowed when carrying out the manoeuvre so that the individual does not feel rushed.

▶ The individual's dignity must be maintained throughout and they should not be unduly exposed or made to feel vulnerable.

▶ The hoist should be placed in a suitable position near to the person's bed, chair or bath, for example. At least two people should support the individual during the procedure: one person to operate the device and one to support the individual so that no injuries occur.

▶ If the individual is being transferred to another area it is advisable to transport them in a wheelchair first and then to use the hoist in the transfer area, such as a bathroom.

▶ The individual should never be left alone whilst in the hoist. To avoid this, before you begin take all of the necessary equipment, toiletries, clothing and belongings to the area where care will be provided.

▶ Provide the minimum level of manual handling required in the situation: encourage the person to do as much for themselves as they can.

Reflect

What kinds of moving and handling equipment are provided in your work setting? Do you feel competent and confident about using this equipment? If not, what could you do to develop your knowledge, skills and ability to move and handle people safely?

Practical Assessment Task   5.1   5.2   5.3

The safety of yourself and others should be your main priority when moving and handling equipment and other objects in your work setting. In this task you need to show that you are able to:

▶ identify legislation that relates to moving and handling
▶ explain the principles for moving and handling equipment and other objects safely
▶ move and handle equipment or other objects safely.

The evidence that you produce for this task must be based on your practice in a real work environment. Your assessor may want to observe you moving and handling equipment or other objects and may wish to ask you questions about this and the legislation and principles involved in this area of practice.

Handling hazardous substances and materials

The various kinds of clinical and everyday waste that are produced in health and social care settings present an infection hazard unless they are dealt with correctly. There should be a detailed waste disposal policy and a clear set of procedures relating to waste disposal in your workplace. You need to know about these policies and procedures and must follow them carefully. If you are unsure about what to do with a certain type of waste, always ask your supervisor or a senior colleague for assistance. The waste disposal policy and procedures should identify how to dispose of different types of waste (see Figure 8.5) and contain information on how the waste should be stored and removed.

Your assessment criteria:

6.1 Identify hazardous substances and materials that may be found in the work setting

6.2 Describe safe practices for: storing hazardous substances; using hazardous substances; disposing of hazardous substances and materials

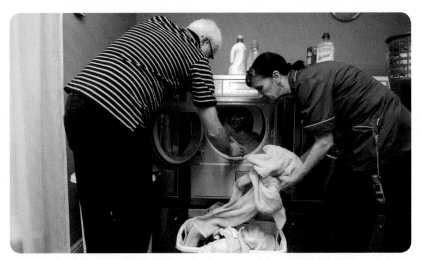

Soiled clothing and linen should be treated as hazardous materials in a care setting

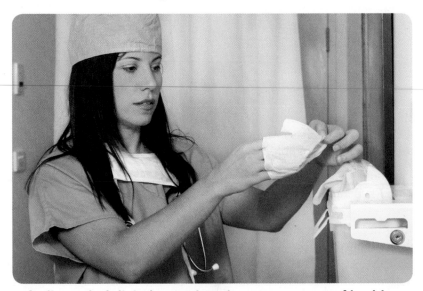

Safe disposal of clinical waste is an important aspect of health and safety practice in care settings

Figure 8.5 Methods of disposal of different types of waste

Type of waste	Method of disposal
Linen and clothing	Soiled sheets, towels and clothing should be kept and washed separately from non-soiled linen. They should be washed as soon as possible after soiling.
Sharps	Needles, blades, glass and other sharps should be disposed of in a special sharps bin. Broken glass or pottery should be carefully wrapped and disposed of in the domestic waste bin or according to the local procedure.
Body products	Blood, urine, faeces, vomit and sputum should be cleaned up using the spillage procedure and flushed down the toilet or a sink, as appropriate. All spillage areas should be disinfected following the local policy and procedures.
Clinical waste	Dressings, plasters, bandages, gloves, aprons, nappies and pads should be put in the clinical waste bags in foot-operated bins. This should be stored in a designated area and removed by a specialist waste contractor.
Recyclable waste	Place recyclable materials in the appropriate recycling bin or, for clinical equipment that will be sterilised and reused, in the special packages/bags provided.
Leftover food	Put it in the kitchen bin or food bin as soon as a meal is finished.
Household waste	Dispose in the domestic rubbish bin using the waste disposal system provided by the local authority.

Case study

Chelsey Hughes recently obtained a job as a care support worker at Redwood residential care home for frail older people. An incident occurred whilst she was working with Doreen, another experienced care support worker, and Irene Philips, the home manager. Whilst Irene was on her lunch break Chelsey realised that Charlie Roberts, a quiet 80 year-old resident with Parkinson's disease, had wet his trousers whilst watching television and needed cleaning and changing. Chelsey had never dealt with this situation before and wasn't sure what to do. Because she didn't know how to deal with the situation, Chelsey waited until Irene returned from her break and then pointed out that Charlie seemed upset about something.

1. Identify reasons why Chelsey should have got help sooner in this situation.

2. Describe the potential hazards that need to be dealt with in order to provide appropriate and safe care for Charlie.

3. What should Chelsey have done to maximise health and safety and minimise the risk of infection in the situation described?

Controlling hazardous substances

The Control of Substances Hazardous to Health (COSHH) Regulations 2002 apply to any substance that is toxic, corrosive or irritant. The regulations require every work setting to have a COSHH file that lists all of the hazardous substances used in the work setting. The file should identify:

▶ where hazardous substances are kept

▶ how they are labelled

▶ their effects

▶ the length of time a person can safely be exposed to each substance

▶ what to do in an emergency involving each hazardous substance.

Health and social care employers are now required to:

▶ find out what the health hazards are with regard to each substance used

▶ decide how to prevent harm to health via risk assessment

▶ provide control measures to reduce harm to health

▶ make sure that all control measures are used

▶ keep all control measures in good working order

▶ provide information, instruction and training for employees and others

▶ provide monitoring and health surveillance in appropriate cases

▶ plan for emergencies.

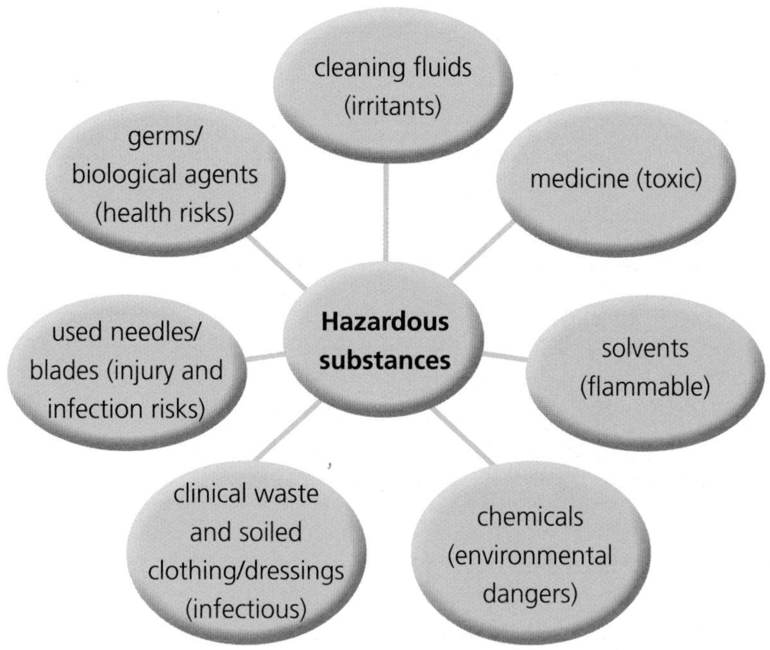

Figure 8.6 Substances hazardous to health

Health and social care workers should identify tasks or aspects of practice that expose them to, or require them to use, hazardous substances. You should know how each substance may cause harm and should also know what you can do to reduce the risk of harm occurring to you and others. It is best to try to prevent yourself being exposed to any hazardous substance. Always try to prevent exposure at source by choosing an alternative or by ensuring that you minimise the contact you have with the substance to maximise your own safety. The COSHH

Regulations 2002 outline a number of principles of good practice and require employers to:

▶ design and operate processes and activities to minimise emission, release and spread of substances hazardous to health

▶ take into account all relevant routes of exposure – inhalation, skin absorption and ingestion – when developing control measures

▶ control exposure by measures that are proportionate to the health risk

▶ choose the most effective and reliable control options that minimise the escape and spread of substances hazardous to health

▶ provide (in combination with other control measures) suitable personal protective equipment (PPE), where adequate control of exposure cannot be achieved by other means

▶ check and review regularly for their continuing effectiveness all elements of control measures

▶ inform and train all employees on the hazards and risks from the substances they work with and the use of control measures developed to minimise the risks

▶ ensure that the introduction of control measures does not increase the overall risk to health and safety.

You have a responsibility to know what the COSHH file says and to work in ways that minimise risk. It is vital to always read and understand the labels on containers and to replace lids and caps securely. You should always use personal protective equipment, such as gloves and goggles, when working directly with hazardous substances, and minimise your exposure to them.

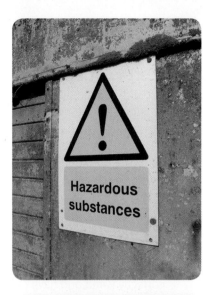

Reflect

Have you heard about the COSHH regulations before? How do you think they affect your work role? Reflect on the impact that these regulations should have on the way you practise in your work setting.

Knowledge Assessment Task   6.1   6.2

Health and social care practitioners need to know how to handle hazardous substances and materials safely. For this assessment task you are required to design a leaflet or poster which:

▶ identifies examples of hazardous substances and materials that can be found in your work setting
▶ describes safe practice in relation to:
  ▶ storing hazardous substances
  ▶ using hazardous substances
  ▶ disposing of hazardous substances and materials.

Your leaflet or poster should provide useful information for colleagues or students who join the care team in your work setting. Your assessor may also wish to ask you questions about or witness the way that you deal with hazardous substances.

Fire safety and security in the work setting

Fire prevention

Fire emergencies are frightening and can be very dangerous. There should be a detailed fire and evacuation policy for your work setting. You must be familiar with this. You should also take part in all fire drills and know what your role is in any evacuation procedure. Practices that prevent fires from starting include:

▶ being aware of the fire hazards and risks in your work place

▶ avoiding leaving cookers unattended and never leaving service users alone in the kitchen

▶ not overloading sockets and ensuring all electrical items are correctly wired and have been checked before use

▶ ensuring that people do not smoke in the work setting

▶ keeping matches and lighters in a safe, secure place that is accessible only to staff members

▶ avoiding the use of candles indoors

▶ making sure that people do not sit close to open fires and that fireguards are used in such circumstances

▶ ensuring that care practitioners and service users avoid putting clothes, towels or other objects on top of heaters or lamps that could overheat as a result

▶ fitting and regularly testing fire alarms and smoke detectors.

Health and social care employers are responsible for carrying out a fire risk assessment in the care settings they provide. The Health and Safety Executive breaks the fire risk assessment into five steps:

1. Identify the fire hazards.

2. Decide who might be harmed and how.

3. Evaluate the risks and decide on precautions.

4. Record your findings and implement them.

5. Review your assessment and update if necessary.

Your employer is also required to provide fire training for all employees each year (which you must attend) and should install a range of fire prevention and emergency systems including smoke alarms, fire blankets, fire extinguishers, sign posted fire exits and fire doors in the workplace.

Fire evacuations

In the rare event that a fire does start in your care setting, you should understand what can be done to prevent it from spreading and also what your role is in any evacuation procedure. A care

Your assessment criteria:

7.1 Describe practices that prevent fires from starting and spreading

7.2 Outline emergency procedures to be followed in the event of a fire in the work setting

7.3 Explain the importance of maintaining clear evacuation routes at all times

Key terms

Assembly point: an agreed place everyone must go to when they are evacuated away from potential danger in an emergency

practitioner's role during a fire incident is to keep themselves and others safe. If you are the person who notices a fire (or smoke), you should first raise the alarm, either activating a fire alarm, phoning 999 yourself or instructing someone else to do this. Other actions to take include:

▶ closing doors and windows to prevent draughts from fanning the flames and allowing the fire to spread

▶ tackling the fire if it is very small and manageable and you have the correct equipment

▶ ensuring that all service users are moved away from the area and are supervised by care practitioners

▶ reassuring people by staying calm and providing information about what is happening and what they need to do

▶ evacuating the building and going to the agreed **assembly point** with the people you are taking care of.

A successful fire evacuation depends on there being a clear set of fire procedures; good understanding of what to do developed through regular fire drills; and, very importantly, clear evacuation routes within the building. All corridors, fire exits, stairways and the usual entrance and exit doors to your workplace should be kept free of obstructions at all times. If you notice that any of the fire evacuation routes are blocked, you should inform the person in charge of your work setting at that point and have the items obstructing the evacuation route removed.

The person in charge of an evacuation during a fire incident needs to keep a register of all people in the building to check that everyone is present at the assembly point. No one should return to the building unless authorised by the person in charge and/or the emergency services personnel. You should also remain at the assembly point until you are directed to go somewhere else or are allowed back into the building.

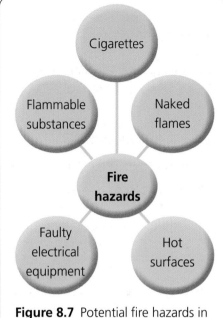

Figure 8.7 Potential fire hazards in the workplace

Reflect

Have you taken part in a fire drill at your workplace in the past three months? Can you remember where the assembly point outside of the building is?

Knowledge Assessment Task   7.1   7.2   7.3

Health and social care practitioners should attend a fire safety session to update their knowledge about fire prevention each year. For this assessment task, produce a handout for a fire safety briefing that:

▶ describes practices that prevent fires from starting and spreading in your workplace

▶ outlines emergency procedures to be followed in the event of a fire

▶ explains the importance of maintaining clear evacuation routes in your workplace at all times.

Keep any written work that you produce for this activity as evidence towards your assessment.

Security in health and social care settings

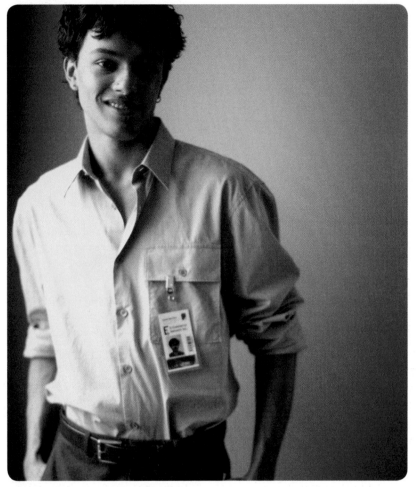

Wearing an identity badge is an important part of the security procedures in many care settings

Reflect

Would you feel confident about approaching an apparently unauthorised person present in your workplace? What could you say that was both polite but also assertive to find out what they were doing there?

Security procedures

It is important to consider the security of the setting where you work as this affects the safety of the service users, visitors and care practitioners who use it. Security incidents can occur as a result of:

▶ intruders or unauthorised people entering the building

▶ service users leaving the building unexpectedly through unlocked doors or windows

▶ care practitioners giving confidential information to people who are not authorised to have access to it.

Care settings can minimise the risk of security incidents by:

▶ having a single entry and exit point that is controlled by staff

▶ using a security system, such as a keypad or locked door, to control entry and exit to the setting

▶ ensuring that identity badges are worn by staff and visitors and that only authorised visitors accompanied by a member of staff are allowed entry

▶ training staff members to approach and politely challenge visitors who are not wearing appropriate visitor badges or who appear in the setting (including the outside areas) unexpectedly

▶ ensuring that service users only leave the setting with the knowledge of a senior member of staff.

You should know and understand what the security procedures are relating to your work setting. You must always follow the procedures, which are designed to protect you and others in the work setting. There may be occasions where you have to leave the work setting to carry out a work-related task somewhere else, to escort visitors or service users to another part of the building or to visit a person in their own home. In all of these cases, your supervisor or the person in charge of the workplace should know where you are going, who you are with or will be seeing and what time you are expected to return. If you do have to visit a service user at home, your organisation should have a lone-working policy and must train you in ways of managing your own safety when working alone.

You should never lend your identity badge to anyone else nor reveal the keypad code to non-staff members. If you are asked to check ground-floor windows and doors, you should do this thoroughly to ensure that they are safe and secure. You should always report any concerns that you have about visitors and about any apparent attempts to break into the building or inappropriately enter your workplace. The personal safety of people in the workplace is always a high priority in a care setting so if you have any serious suspicions, or become aware of an intruder, it is advisable to seek help quickly and to call onsite security staff and/or the police. Care organisations generally discourage staff from approaching or directly restraining intruders in order to minimise the risk of violence occurring.

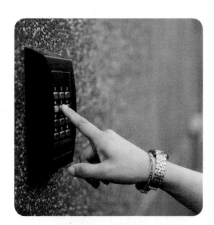

> **Investigate**
>
> What does the security policy of your work setting say about the agreed way of dealing with intruders or people who you are suspicious of in your workplace? Find out what the procedure is for dealing with this kind of situation.

Practical Assessment Task   8.1 8.2 8.3

Protecting the security of yourself and others is a key part of your role as a care practitioner. Health and social care organisations must always have security-related policies and procedures that safeguard members of staff and other people who use the care setting. In this activity you are required to produce evidence that shows you are able to:

▶ use agreed ways of working for checking the identity of anyone requesting access to your work setting or to information relating to service users or care practice

▶ implement measures to protect your own security and the security of others in the work setting

▶ explain the importance of ensuring that others are aware of your whereabouts when you are working.

Your evidence for this task must be based on your practice and experience in a real work environment. Keep any written work that you produce for this activity as evidence towards your assessment. Your assessor may also want to observe or ask you questions about the way you implement security measures in the work setting.

Managing stress

What is 'stress'?

'Stress' is the feeling of emotional tension, worry or pressure that a person feels when they face a demanding or challenging situation. It has both psychological and physical symptoms.

A person who is experiencing high levels of stress may display this through their behaviour, perhaps by being irritable, argumentative and quick to lose their temper or by smoking or drinking more heavily to cope with the anxiety that stress causes. Prolonged or extreme stress can lead to health problems. It can trigger mental health problems such as depression and anxiety-based illnesses. Stress is also associated with high blood pressure and heart disease, and leads some people to misuse drugs and alcohol as a way of coping with their symptoms.

Exercise, recreation and leisure activities provide effective ways of reducing stress levels. Having supportive relationships and satisfying work also helps. Increasingly, people use sports activities to help them to relax and 'de-stress'. Massage, talking to others about problems and feelings, thinking positively and being assertive (saying 'no' to extra work!) are all good ways of reducing stress levels.

Health problems associated with stress include:

▶ anxiety

▶ stomach ulcers

▶ high blood pressure

▶ angina

▶ depression

▶ migraine

▶ eczema

▶ heart attack.

Your assessment criteria:

9.1 Identify common signs and indicators of stress

9.2 Identify circumstances that tend to trigger own stress

9.3 Describe ways to manage own stress

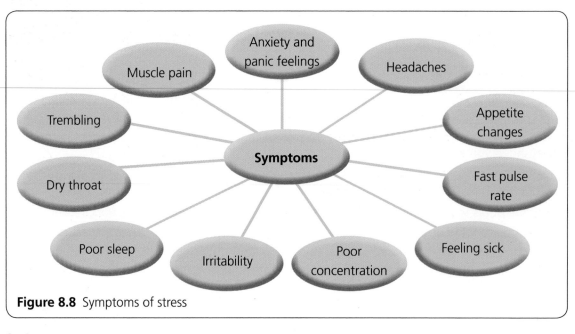

Figure 8.8 Symptoms of stress

Identifying stress triggers

Stress can be triggered by a wide variety of factors that affect different people in different ways. Common causes of stress include:

- ▶ debt and other money worries
- ▶ work pressures and long hours
- ▶ relationship difficulties or breakdown
- ▶ lack of rest, sleep and relaxation
- ▶ bereavement or other forms of loss
- ▶ exam and study pressures
- ▶ physical and mental ill health
- ▶ poor working relationships and lack of job satisfaction
- ▶ unemployment and redundancy worries.

Health and social care practitioners have diverse social and cultural backgrounds as well as differing lifestyles and personal circumstances. Your main sources of stress, or the work-related factors that trigger off your feelings of stress, may be different to those of your colleagues as a result.

Reflect

Identify three occasions when you've felt very stressed. What were your symptoms? What caused your stress? Make a note of these points or discuss them with a colleague in your class.

Reflect

What are the three main stress triggers in your work life? If you could remove or at least control one of these sources of stress, which one would you choose?

Case study

Neville is a 37 year-old plumber. He wants to retire as a rich, happy man when he is 50. Neville runs his own plumbing company, working between 60 and 80 hours every week. He is feeling under a lot of pressure at the moment. Neville has complained to his wife that he has had a headache for a week, feels faint at times and is having trouble sleeping. Neville will not go and see his GP as he says he is too busy. His wife is trying to persuade him to take a holiday but he is reluctant to do so because of the amount of work he has to do.

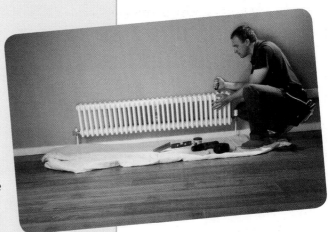

1. What symptoms of stress does Neville have?
2. What might be causing Neville's current stress problems?
3. Explain what might happen to Neville's health and wellbeing if he continues to experience high stress levels.

Managing stress

Awareness of the symptoms, causes and triggers of your stress is the first step to managing it. There are a variety of ways of managing stress, though to be effective any strategy must respond appropriately to the underlying causes. For example, if your stress is triggered by working excessively long hours or by the emotionally draining nature of your work, an appropriate response would be to take some time off work and to ensure that you have a clear work life balance. Exercise is an effective way of reducing stress as it quickly releases tension and 'nervous energy' from the body. Drinking alcohol, smoking and over- or under-eating are strategies that people sometimes use to make themselves feel better or to try to regain a sense of control when life becomes very stressful. However, these kinds of responses tend to make people feel worse rather than better and may have negative health consequences. They are likely to do little to address the causes or triggers of an individual's stress.

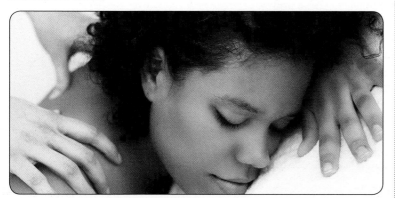

Your assessment criteria:

9.3 Describe ways to manage own stress

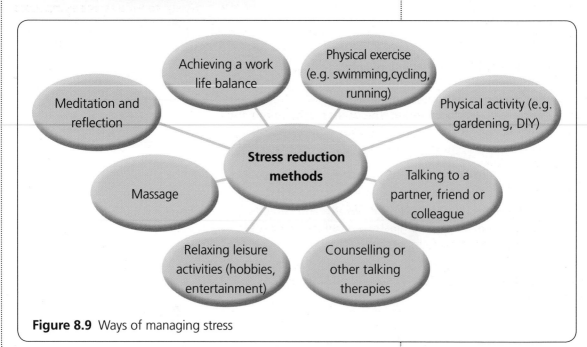

Figure 8.9 Ways of managing stress

(Diagram: Stress reduction methods)
- Achieving a work life balance
- Physical exercise (e.g. swimming, cycling, running)
- Meditation and reflection
- Physical activity (e.g. gardening, DIY)
- Massage
- Talking to a partner, friend or colleague
- Relaxing leisure activities (hobbies, entertainment)
- Counselling or other talking therapies

Using advice, guidance and support services

Persistent stress can cause physical and mental health problems to develop. It is worth trying a variety of different strategies to deal with the causes and symptoms of your stress. Being able to confide in somebody and talk through the issue and your feelings with them can be a very helpful way of managing stress. A common strategy is to talk to a partner or close friend informally to express feelings and receive some support. Similarly, you should use the advice, guidance and support services provided by your employer to seek help for and manage work-related stress.

Your supervisor or a trusted colleague may be the first person to approach. They may be able to help or may refer you to the occupational health and support services provided by your employer. Talking through and learning about time management, assertiveness and basic task management strategies with colleagues or stress counsellors can be very helpful and may lead to new skills and understanding that prevent a repetition of stressful situations in the future. Where stress symptoms are persistent and unresponsive to informal or workplace support, you may need to see your GP (family doctor) for assessment and treatment of your physical and psychological symptoms.

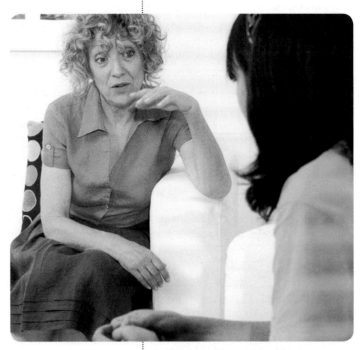

Talking about stressful situations and the triggers to your stress reactions can often help to relieve the symptoms you feel

Knowledge Assessment Task   9.1   9.2   9.3

Health and social care practitioners spend the majority of their time caring for and supporting others. This focus on the needs and wellbeing of other people can sometimes lead to practitioners failing to look after themselves! Produce a personal health and wellbeing plan as follows:

1. Identify common signs and indicators of stress.
2. Identify circumstances that tend to trigger your own stress.
3. Describe ways in which you manage your own stress, or could do so if you became stressed in the future.

Your written work for this task should relate to your health or social care role. Keep a copy of the work you produce as evidence for your assessment.

Are you ready for assessment?

AC	What do you know now?	Assessment task	✓
1.1	How to identify legislation relating to general health and safety in a health or social care work setting	Page 193	
1.2	The main points of the health and safety policies and procedures agreed with the employer	Page 193	
1.3	The main health and safety responsibilities of: • self • the employer or manager • others in the work setting	Page 193	
1.4	How to identify tasks relating to health and safety that should not be carried out without special training	Page 193	
1.5	How to access additional support and information relating to health and safety	Page 193	
2.1	Why it is important to assess health and safety hazards posed by the work setting or by particular activities	Page 197	
2.2	How and when to report potential health and safety risks that have been identified	Page 197	
2.3	How risk assessment can help address dilemmas between rights and health and safety concerns	Page 197	
3.1	Different types of accidents and sudden illness that may occur in own work setting	Page 201	
3.2	The procedures to be followed if an accident or sudden illness should occur	Page 201	
6.1	Identify hazardous substances and materials that may be found in the work setting	Page 213	
6.2	Describe safe practices for: • storing hazardous substances • using hazardous substances • disposing of hazardous substances and materials	Page 213	
7.1	Practices that prevent fires from: • starting • spreading	Page 215	
7.2	Emergency procedures to be followed in the event of a fire in the work setting	Page 215	
7.3	The importance of maintaining clear evacuation routes at all times	Page 215	
9.1	Common signs and indicators of stress	Page 221	
9.2	Circumstances that tend to trigger own stress	Page 221	
9.3	Ways to manage own stress	Page 221	

AC	What can you do now?	Assessment task	✓
4.1	Demonstrate the recommended method for hand washing	Page 205	
4.2	Demonstrate ways to ensure that own health and hygiene do not pose a risk to others at work	Page 205	
5.1	Identify legislation that relates to moving and handling	Page 209	
5.2	Explain principles for moving and handling equipment and other objects safely	Page 209	
5.3	Move and handle equipment or other objects safely	Page 209	
8.1	Use agreed ways of working for checking the identity of anyone requesting access to: • premises • information	Page 217	
8.2	Implement measures to protect own security and the security of others in the work setting	Page 217	
8.3	Explain the importance of ensuring that others are aware of own whereabouts	Page 217	

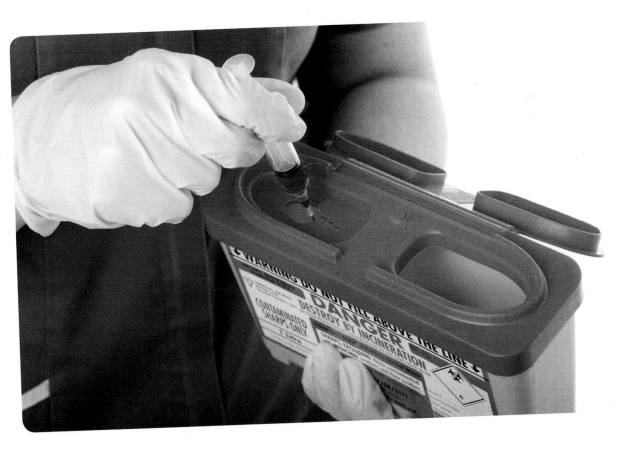

9 | Handle information in health and social care settings (HSC 028)

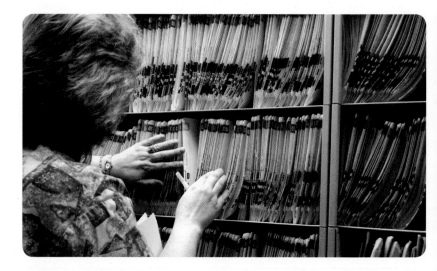

Assessment of this unit

This unit introduces you to the process of recording, storing and sharing information in health and social care settings. It focuses on the need for sensitive handling of information relating to service users and care practice and to the legal and organisational issues that affect this area of your work. You will need to:

▶ understand the need for secure handling of information in health and social care settings

▶ know how to access support for handling information

▶ be able to handle information in accordance with agreed ways of working.

The assessment of this unit is partly knowledge-based and partly competence-based. Knowledge-based assessments test the things you need to know. Competence-based assessments test the things you need to do in the real work environment. To successfully complete this unit, you will need to produce evidence of both your knowledge and your competence as a care worker. The tables opposite outline what you need to know and do to meet each of the assessment criteria for the unit.

Your tutor or assessor will help you to prepare for your assessment, and the tasks suggested in the unit will help you to create the evidence that you need.

CHAPTER 9

AC   What you need to know

1.1	Identify the legislation that relates to the recording, storage and sharing of information in health and social care
1.2	Explain why it is important to have secure systems for recording and storing information in a health and social care setting
2.1	Describe how to access guidance, information and advice about handling information
2.2	Explain what actions to take when there are concerns over the recording, storing or sharing of information

AC   What you need to do

3.1	Keep records that are up-to-date, complete, accurate and legible
3.2	Follow agreed ways of working for: • recording information • storing information • sharing information

AC 3.1 and 3.2 must be assessed in a real work environment.

This unit also links to some other units:

SHC 21	Introduction to communication in health and social care
HSC 026	Implement person-centred approaches in health and social care
HSC 2013	Support care plan activities

Some of your learning will be repeated in these units, and will give you the chance to review your knowledge and understanding.

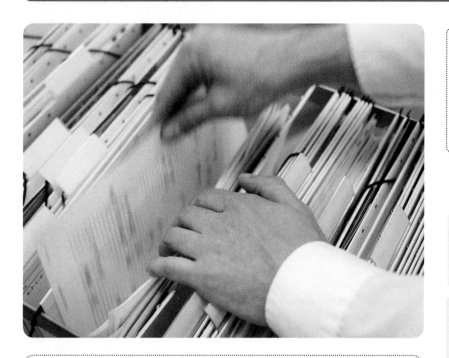

Your assessment criteria:

1.1 Identify the legislation that relates to the recording, storage and sharing of information in health and social care

Key terms

Legislation: written laws, in this case governing the use of information

Secure: applies to information that is not just physically safe, e.g. secure in a locked cabinet, but also protected from people who do not need to know about it

What do you need to know about the law?

The main legislation affecting the recording, storage and sharing of information is outlined in Figure 9.1 below. You should know the main points of each law as described in the table. The law affects all kinds of uses of information, and not just written information.

Figure 9.1 Legislation affecting information recording, storage and handling

Legislation	What does it say?
Data Protection Act 1998	This includes the principles that as well as being kept secure, information should be accurate, be adequate for its purpose, observe a person's rights and be kept no longer than is necessary. It must be used for limited purposes, in a fair and legal manner, and not be transferred to or shared with others without proper safeguards.
Human Rights Act 1998	Even if a person is in care, or can no longer give their own consent for information about them to be shared, they have a legal right to have their privacy respected.
Freedom of Information Act 2000	Most public authorities are obliged to provide information about their policies and services to people requesting that information through the agreed channels. You should know whom to ask in case someone approaches you with a request for certain kinds of information.
Equality Act 2010	This includes measures in the previous Disability Discrimination Act and Race Relations Act. It requires employers and carers to take all reasonable steps to treat all people equally well. This applies whether or not an individual has the capacity to understand the issues themselves.

The Caldicott principles

In addition to the laws above, you may come across the Caldicott principles. These apply to the release of information that identifies individuals either by name or in some other way. There will be one or more senior people in your organisation who can give advice on this, but the principles apply broadly to all the work you are likely to do. For example, if you need to share information on someone with a doctor or social worker these principles will affect what you do and how you do it. All the people you care for have the same rights as you to have their information recorded correctly, stored safely and only shared with those people who really need to know – usually with the person's consent.

Figure 9.2 The Caldicott principles

- You must be able to justify the purpose of every proposed use or transfer of information.
- You should not use or share personal information unless it is absolutely necessary.
- You should use the minimum amount of personal information necessary to do a particular task.
- Access to personal information should be on a strict need-to-know basis.
- Everyone with access to personal information must be aware of their responsibilities.
- Everyone must understand and comply with the law.

Reflect

Who has private records or confidential information about you? Identify an example, either related to health, or income, or to a family matter. Think about the reasons why you want to keep this information private. What could happen if the information recorded was not correct or up-to-date? What could happen, and how would you feel, if this information were given to someone who didn't need to know it?

Investigate

Think of a recent task you were asked to carry out with an individual who uses your care setting. What information did you need to know to carry out that task? Were you allowed to see all the information held about the individual? If not, why not?

Knowledge Assessment Task   1.1

Case study

You are working in a care home. You are caring for an elderly woman, Mrs Ahmed. As with all residents of the care home, Mrs Ahmed's case notes have to be kept securely and written up accurately. Someone from the local council wants to know how many people like Mrs Ahmed are in your home. You refer this person to your manager, who will have to decide whether to give out this information. Mrs Ahmed has dementia, so you can no longer ask her if she is happy or not to share information about herself with others. However, her privacy must still be respected. Mrs Ahmed's dementia is a type of disability; this means she still has rights about the correct handling of her information.

1. Identify the four pieces of legislation that protect Mrs Ahmed's rights.
2. Identify when and why each piece of legislation applies to Mrs Ahmed's situation.

Keep the work that you produce for this activity as evidence towards your assessment.

How can information be recorded and stored securely?

There are many different ways of recording information, and this information may be stored on paper or electronically on computers or portable memory devices. Whichever way information is recorded and stored, you must ensure that it is done securely. If information about people is not stored or disposed of securely, it can get lost, stolen or damaged. Confidential information about an individual may also get mixed up with someone else's, or be seen or heard by a person not privy to such information if it is recorded or stored incorrectly.

Ways of dealing with confidential information

There are different ways of dealing with confidential information. Many of these ways of dealing with confidential information will depend on the source of the information presented. Figure 9.3 on the page opposite, details the main ways of dealing with a variety of information sources.

Your assessment criteria:

1.2 Explain why it is important to have secure systems for recording and storing information in a health and social care setting

Key terms

Legible: refers to writing that is easy to read, especially handwriting

Encrypted files: electronic files protected by a code; they can only be accessed by means of a password

Case study

Several nurses and carers work in a small dementia unit in a nursing home. As they go in and out of the office many times a day, they have got into the habit of leaving the office door closed but unlocked, as they find it annoying to keep using the numbered keypad. One morning when most of them are helping residents in their rooms, a mobile resident wanders into the office unnoticed. By the time he is discovered, he has pulled several residents' files out of the open cupboard, there is paper all over the floor and he is busily covering some file pages with black marker pen.

1. What was the basic mistake that the nurses and carers made as regards storing information?
2. How could they have made the file cupboard more secure?
3. What do you think they might do about the pages of information which are now unreadable because they have been drawn over?

Figure 9.3 Recording and storing information

Source of information	Recording and storage issues
Handwritten records	• Handwriting must be legible. • Only write what's most important, so things are easy to find. • Sign and date everything you write. • Make sure there is a tidy place for different kinds of paper, including test results and messages on slips of paper. • Don't erase or white-out mistakes. Instead, score through, initial and rewrite. • Only record factual information, and not opinions or hearsay.
Personal files	• Each name should be clear, easy to read and obviously different from all the other names. • Files should be kept in a locked cabinet, with access restricted to named staff. • Files should, ideally, not be taken out of their storage place – the office, for example – so write notes or take photocopies if information from the files needs to be taken away from their storage place; if notes need to be taken to a meeting, check with senior staff what the procedure is; make sure a note is put in the file or cabinet as to what has been taken. • Write up notes as soon as possible after the event – you may not remember all the details later on; and they may be required in court, as evidence and as an aide memoire.
Computer files and emails	• Normally, people's initials, rather than names, are used in emails or other 'public' communications, and only if absolutely necessary. • You may have to use encrypted files/emails or passwords to get in to the work computer. *Never* give anyone else your password(s).
Telephone calls	There will usually be a procedure for recording calls – if you jot something down on a pad before writing in someone's notes, those jottings need to be disposed of securely.
Face-to-face communication	• Make sure you are the correct person to receive this information. If not, ask for the minimum information in order to successfully pass it on to a person who can deal with it. Often this person will be a senior colleague. Decide whether any information needs to be recorded as well as passed on verbally. • If you receive face-to-face information from individuals outside your organisation, make sure you record names, the reasons why the information is being given, and remember to take contact details.

Confidentiality

Confidentiality does not mean keeping things secret. It means making sure that only *appropriate* individuals are privy to **confidential information**. These people will usually need to access confidential information in order to support the individual(s) concerned. Health and social care organisations will have written procedures as to how confidential information is handled. Occasionally, the normal rules on confidentiality can be broken. This occurs when other people in positions of legal authority – the police or courts, for example – need to access specific information in order to protect someone, or to prevent a crime. For example, confidentiality may be broken in the following circumstances:

▶ to protect a person at risk of harm

▶ to protect a person's health

▶ if the person appears to be about to commit a crime

▶ to protect the health or safety of others

▶ to help an investigation into suspected child abuse

▶ if a court or tribunal orders certain information to be disclosed.

It is part of your duty of care to make sure that you know the rules in your workplace for sharing information about the people you care for. It is never acceptable to share information about the people you care for – named or unnamed – outside the workplace.

Your assessment criteria:

1.2 Explain why it is important to have secure systems for recording and storing information in a health and social care setting

Key terms

Confidential information: information that can only be accessed by individuals who have the authority or permission to access it

Investigate

How many ways is information about individuals recorded in your workplace? See if your workplace uses any or all of the examples below:

▶ handwritten daily records

▶ care plans

▶ computer files

▶ hospital/GP letters

▶ medical charts and test results

▶ professional reports

▶ records of phone calls

▶ family/personal correspondence.

Discuss

With your supervisor or a colleague talk about who you might need to share information with about people in your care. What procedures does your workplace have for sharing information with outside agencies, such as doctors or social workers?

Case study

Mr Green lives alone and is supported by various people. He can walk with difficulty, takes many different medications and has memory problems. Members of his family have employed a carer, who comes every morning, and recently a volunteer has been visiting once a week from the local befriending scheme.

The family tell the carer that the volunteer is going to pick up Mr Green's test results and new medication for him once a week on the day she visits. This has previously been the carer's job.

After discussion with her boss, the carer decides first to approach the befriending scheme, and enquires whether their volunteers have the same duty of confidentiality that she has. She learns that they do; this reassures her that Mr Green's medical information will be treated confidentially by the volunteer. She then contacts the volunteer to discuss Mr Green's taking of his medication, and they agree together on how to mark the doses on the drug boxes to help Mr Green do this. Everyone, including Mr Green, then knows what he has taken or has not taken on any day by looking at the box. This proves very useful a week later when Mr Green has a fall and is attended by a paramedic. Neither the carer nor the volunteer is present. The paramedic needs to know about Mr Green's medicines in order to decide on appropriate first aid.

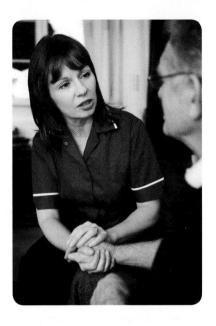

1. Why did the carer have concerns about *sharing* information with the volunteer?

2. Why was it important for the carer and the volunteer to discuss together how to *record* the doses on the drug boxes?

3. Why was it important that, in this case, the secure *storage* of the drug boxes had to include them being easily accessed by others?

Reflect

For how long does information of different kinds have to be kept in your workplace? How is information disposed of securely (by shredding, for example) and who is allowed to do this?

Knowledge Assessment Task   1.2

1. Read the following scenarios. Make a note of what is wrong in relation to the information referred to in each scenario, how it relates to the importance of having secure systems, and what should have happened.

   a. Mr Ali's medication notes are in badly written handwriting.

   b. The manager takes her computer memory stick home but it gets left on the bus.

   c. There are files on several people called Smith in the office.

   d. A phone message from the district nurse is written on a scrap of paper.

   e. A carer discusses all the clients with the home cleaner over coffee every day.

   f. Mrs McGregor's case notes are left in an unlocked cabinet.

2. Think of three individuals in your workplace and explain what might go wrong if information on each one was not recorded or stored properly, or shared inappropriately, using a different example each time. Remember to protect confidentiality by disguising each person's true identity in your written work.

Keep a copy of the work that you produce for this activity as evidence towards your assessment.

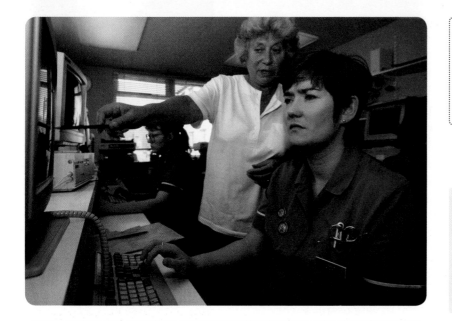

Your assessment criteria:

2.1 Describe how to access guidance, information and advice about handling information

Key terms

Appraisal: a formal meeting, between a care practitioner and a senior staff member, to monitor the practitioner's progress and discuss any concerns

Information governance rules: these are written systems of procedures and checks designed to ensure that information is properly recorded, stored and shared

How to access guidance and support about handling information

Every health and social care workplace should have written policies and procedures relating to the way information should be handled. You should know:

▶ where to find this information

▶ what it says about information handling procedures

▶ how this affects your work role.

If the policies and procedures are very detailed or technical, it is best to ask someone senior to help you identify which parts are relevant for your work role. You may also be told about procedures and issues related to safe handling of information during staff meetings and appraisals. Whether it is a regular topic for a meeting or not, you should never feel reluctant to ask or check what the correct procedure is in any particular case. Your workplace should offer training in handling information – it is important that you attend these sessions, as they will help you understand in more detail how information governance rules determine access to and use of information.

Case study

Ann is a fairly new care practitioner working in a mental health unit. She reports to a senior nurse practitioner, and they share a manager. She has been shown where the patients' paper files are kept, and has been given a computer password so she can send emails within the organisation. Ann can also fill in assessment forms on the computer.

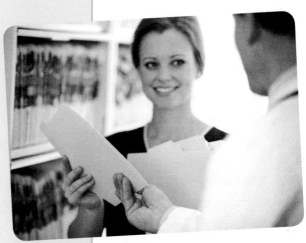

1. What questions does Ann need to ask, as a new employee, regarding information handling?
2. Whom could she ask to help her decide what she needs to look at?
3. When could Ann bring up any questions or concerns about handling information in her unit?

Knowledge Assessment Task 2.1

Information handling is a key part of all health and social care work roles. There are always situations where care practitioners are unsure about the correct procedures or what they should do in response to a request for information about a person they provide care for. Accessing guidance and support is the key to dealing with these situations appropriately. In this activity you are required to produce evidence that:

▶ describes how to access guidance, information and advice about handling information in your work setting
▶ identifies the names and contact details of people in your workplace who can give you guidance and support around handling information and confidentiality issues on an everyday basis.

You should keep the written work that you produce as evidence for your assessment.

Discuss

To whom do you report on a day-to-day basis? To whom do you report if that person is not around? Are these people senior enough to give you advice about using people's information? If not, whom should you ask?

Dealing with concerns about recording, storing or sharing of information

Preventing and dealing with bad practice in information handling

There are normally various measures in place in health and social care settings to prevent bad practice in information handling. For example:

▶ employees and volunteers are expected to go through a set of vetting procedures when beginning a job; they are legally required to have a CRB (Criminal Records Bureau) check

▶ staff should be properly supervised, particularly during their training period, but also afterwards

▶ agreed ways of working should be outlined in the workplace's policies and procedures, and clear rules established on reporting questions or concerns to senior managers

▶ there should be physical and electronic measures in the workplace for the purpose of safely storing information (see page 237).

Your assessment criteria:

2.2 Explain what actions to take when there are concerns over the recording, storing or sharing of information

Key terms

Vetting: a formal procedure to check out an individual's past record and qualifications, and particularly any police record

Figure 9.4 Some typical concerns and what you might do about them

Concern	What you might do
Confidentiality of records written by yourself on home visits	• Keep electronic notes in a secure folder on a password-protected laptop. • File the notes securely back at the office as soon as possible. • Discuss with your manager and any other appropriate persons whether you need to leave some kind of record at the home, and if so, the most secure method in that particular instance.
Confidentiality of a patient's personal and medical information when recorded by professionals other than yourself	• Discuss privately with other professionals involved, with regards to your organisation's rules. • Involve your and their manager if unsure.
Concern that many different people are recording information about a patient or client in different places, and that this is not all being shared with everyone involved, and may in some cases be inaccurate	• Consult your manager about the policy in your workplace: there may need to be an overview of that person's information; for example, at a regular case conference.

continued...

Concern	What you might do
Concern that paper or electronic information in your workplace is not being stored as securely as possible	• Discuss with your manager why this appears to be so – there may be some good reason. • If s/he can give no good reason then correct procedures may need to be discussed at a staff meeting. • In the event of security lapses continuing, you may need to consider contacting someone more senior in the organisation.
Concerns about confidential information being overheard when other care workers have telephone conversations	• Discuss with your managers – they may need to remind all staff of the correct procedures.
Confidentiality of information shared with you by a patient or client which gives you concerns	• Never promise to keep information secret. • Tell the patient or client that you may need to share that information with some appropriate person, their GP for example. *You must share the information if you suspect neglect or abuse.* • Make an official note of what you were told, and to whom you passed on that information.
Information shared with you by family or friends of a patient or client that appears to conflict with what you are told by the patient or client	• Do not make assumptions or take sides. Your duty of care to the person you care for means that their needs and wishes are your priority, so try to establish these first. • You or your manager may need to use a third party – for example, an advocate – in order to make sure all views are heard, and that the person's needs and wishes are respected and fulfilled as far as possible.

Knowledge Assessment Task   2.2

Health and social care practitioners have a duty of care towards the people they provide care or support for. This includes protecting confidentiality and ensuring that information relating to the individual is recorded, stored and shared appropriately. This task requires you to explain how you would deal with a number of different information-handling concerns.

1. Explain whom you would speak to if you had concerns about a professional visiting your care home whose writing in people's notes was not legible.

2. Explain what you would do if you kept finding people's notes or records lying around in public areas of your workplace.

3. Explain what you would do if a person for whom you provided care or support told you that a family member was abusing them.

You should keep the written work that you produce as evidence for your assessment.

Handling information in accordance with agreed ways of working

Keeping, storing and sharing records

As well as knowing the procedures in your workplace, you will need to make sure that you follow them when dealing with people's confidential records. To show that you have effective and competent information-handling skills, you will need to make sure that service users' records are:

▶ up-to-date

▶ complete

▶ accurate

▶ legible

▶ stored safely

▶ shared appropriately.

Ensuring records are up-to-date

Tasks such as writing in someone's care file, recording medication given and making notes about conversations, should be done as soon as possible after you have carried them out. Any entry you make, in writing or on computer files, should be signed and dated. In addition, some records, such as medication charts, will require you to record the time of day you carried out an action (such as giving a particular medication). Also, make sure that any information coming from outside the workplace, such as professional reports, are filed in accordance with your organisation's filing system, making them easy to find. If necessary, check with the people you provide care for (or their relatives), and senior staff, that any recorded postal addresses, email addresses and telephone numbers you have for them are up-to-date.

Ensuring records are complete

Make sure you know the rules in your workplace about when, and how often, you need to record something in a person's file. Get into the habit of recording information as you go; only recording information at the end of a shift results in incomplete records. In the event that a record is incomplete, *never* make up information to fill the gap. Instead, inform a senior member of staff immediately. You may then be asked to contact an outside professional, or talk with others who were present, and so complete the record.

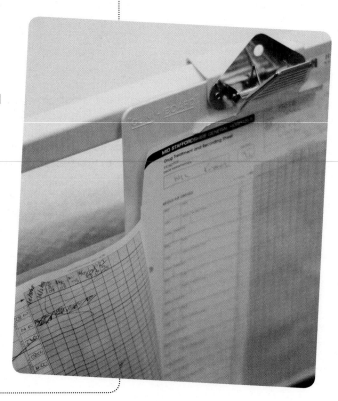

Ensuring records are accurate

Accurate records are those which are up-to-date and complete. However, the individual entries that you make in someone's records must also be correct in the details, especially with regards to *who* said or did what. Only record what you have done yourself, and sign only for yourself. If a senior staff member asks you to record something, make it clear that that senior manager has asked you to make the record. Similarly, always record the name of a source of information for which you cannot personally vouch. For example, if a family member asks you to put something in an individual's record, then you should record their name and make it clear that you are quoting information supplied by someone other than yourself. Finally, be extra careful with the recording of numbers and quantities – this is particularly important when it comes to administering prescribed drugs.

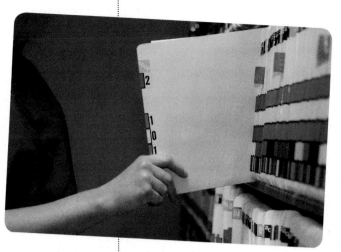

Ensuring records are legible and easy to understand

Your own handwriting must be clear and easy to read, neither too large nor too small. Write in clear, simple sentences. Avoid flowery descriptions. Make sure your words are evenly spaced. You may be required to leave a blank or scored line between entries. Try not to use abbreviations unless the information is so confidential that you are required by your organisation's procedures to use abbreviations for people's names. However, be aware that some workplaces accept common abbreviations, and insert a sheet into people's files for recording common abbreviations and their meaning. Whether using a typed or a cursive (handwritten) script, make sure you check that your spellings are correct. Do not over-rely on computer spell-checkers; they will not always know the correct spelling of surnames or words particular to your practice.

Ensuring records are stored safely

Always put files or other paperwork back as soon as you have used it. Don't leave files or other information lying about, even in the office. Check that files are filed in accordance with your organisation's filing system. If you are allowed to unlock a locked cabinet, lock it again as soon as possible, and immediately return the key to its rightful place. Don't allow members of the public (including relatives) to be in record storage rooms unsupervised. If using files or records on the computer, change your password as often as you can, and don't let anyone else use it. When working on a computer, make sure that you regularly save the document, and ask senior staff about the facilities for backing up information on the computer.

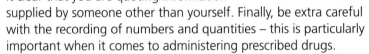

> **Key terms**
>
> **Abbreviations:** shortened forms of words or phrases; for example, 'meds' for 'medicines', or ENT for 'Ear, Nose and Throat'

Sharing information appropriately

Information must only be given to those who really need to know it. It is equally important to make sure that this information is passed on when it is needed. This includes passing on information you have gained from someone you provide care for about their expressed needs or preferences, especially if these have changed. Staff or visitors who do not know individuals as well as you do may need brief information about their likes and dislikes. Any change in an individual that worries you should be reported, in as private a way as possible. In the same way, any new information about a person – provided, for example, by a district nurse – should be recorded and shared with a senior member of staff. Avoid merely filing a report: make the information available to whosoever needs it *before* filing it. In particular, any apparent problems with an individual's behaviour must be shared and recorded in a manner that is **objective**, and neither criticises nor demeans that individual.

Your assessment criteria:

3.2 Follow agreed ways of working for:
- recording information
- storing information
- sharing information

Key terms

Objective: describing something in a purely factual, non-emotional way

Case study

Jon works in a home for young adults with learning disabilities. He is the main carer for one young man, but also does activities with another two. One day, when he is helping the three clients make a meal in the kitchen, they begin arguing and fighting. After Jon and another carer calm the clients down, they all sit down to eat. During the meal, Jon and the other carer discuss what happened, with the clients present, and share opinions about which of the clients is easiest or most difficult to work with. After the meal, Jon records the incident in the home's incident book. He records whose fault he thought the incident was. At the end of his shift, he also leaves a note for his manager in the kitchen. The note details the incident.

1. Why should Jon not have discussed the incident with the clients present during lunch?

2. What was wrong about the way Jon recorded the incident in the book?

3. Why was the kitchen the wrong place to leave the note for his manager?

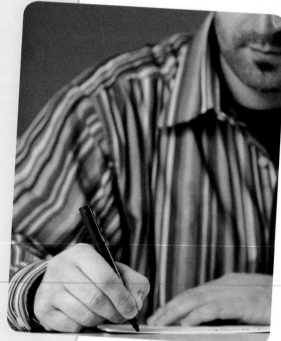

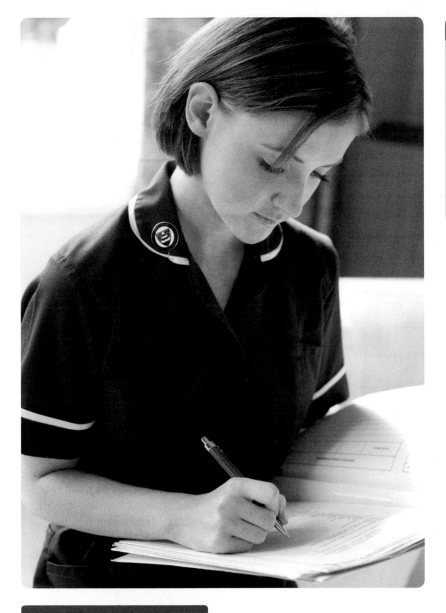

Investigate

Find out what procedures are used in your workplace for recording certain incidents, for example someone having a minor accident or a carer being threatened by a member of an individual's family. How do the rules on accurate and objective recording, and appropriate information sharing, apply in this kind of case?

Practical Assessment Task

3.1 **3.2**

Health and social care practitioners must follow agreed ways of working when recording, storing or sharing information in their work setting. To complete this activity you need to show that you are able to follow agreed ways of working:

1. for recording information: to do this you could make entries in a person's written or electronic records during or just after a working shift. These should be up-to-date and legible, and follow the guidelines of your work setting.

2. for storing information: to do this you could show how you stored the records completed in task 1 above.

3. for sharing information in your work setting: to do this you could participate appropriately in a team meeting where individuals' needs or care issues are discussed.

The evidence for this assessment task must be assessed in a real work environment and should relate to your practice as a health or social care practitioner. Your assessor may want to observe or ask questions about your practice.

Are you ready for assessment?

AC	What do you know now?	Assessment task	✓
1.1	Identify the legislation that relates to the recording, storage and sharing of information in health and social care	Page 227	
1.2	Explain why it is important to have secure systems for recording and storing information in a health and social care setting	Page 231	
2.1	Describe how to access guidance, information and advice about handling information	Page 233	
2.2	Explain what actions to take when there are concerns over the recording, storing or sharing of information	Page 236	

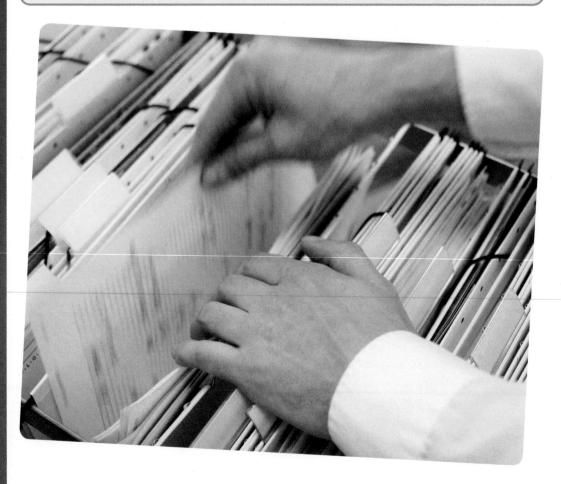

AC	What can you do now?	Assessment task	✓
3.1	Keep records that are up-to-date, complete, accurate and legible	Page 239	
3.2	Follow agreed ways of working for: • recording information • storing information • sharing information	Page 239	

10 | Dementia awareness (DEM 201)

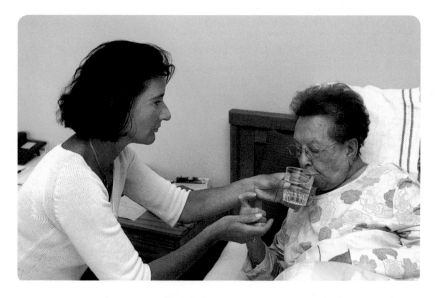

Assessment of this unit

Developing an awareness of dementia is very important. It ensures that people with this condition and their carers get the support that they need; and it helps dispel various myths and misconceptions about the condition. Crucially, it shines a light on the fact that many individuals diagnosed with dementia go on to live satisfying lives for several years after diagnosis.

The aim of this unit is to enable you to gain knowledge about dementia. It clarifies the meaning of dementia, outlines different forms of dementia and examines the reasons why people develop the condition. The unit also looks at the various factors that affect an individual's experience of dementia, and considers the impact carers can have on that experience.

The assessment of this unit is entirely knowledge-based (things that you need to know). You will need to:

▶ understand what dementia is

▶ understand key features of the theoretical models of dementia

▶ know the most common types of dementia and their causes

▶ understand factors relating to an individual's experience of dementia.

In order to successfully complete the unit, you will be required to produce evidence of your knowledge of dementia, as shown in the tables opposite. Your tutor or assessor will help you to prepare for your assessment; the tasks suggested in the unit will help you to create the evidence that you need.

AC	What you need to know
1.1	Explain what is meant by the term 'dementia'
1.2	Describe the key functions of the brain that are affected by dementia
1.3	Explain why depression, delirium and age-related memory impairment may be mistaken for dementia
2.1	Outline the medical model of dementia
2.2	Outline the social model of dementia
2.3	Explain why dementia should be viewed as a disability
3.1	List the most common causes of dementia
3.2	Describe the likely signs and symptoms of the most common causes of dementia
3.3	Outline the risk factors for the most common causes of dementia
3.4	Identify prevalence rates for different types of dementia
4.1	Describe how different individuals may experience living with dementia, depending on age, type of dementia and level of ability and disability
4.2	Outline the impact that the attitudes and behaviours of others may have on an individual with dementia.

There is no practical assessment for this unit. However, it is important that can apply your knowledge of dementia in the work setting.

This unit also links to some other units:

DEM 204	Understand and implement a person-centred approach to the care and support of individuals with dementia
DEM 210	Understand and enable interaction and communication with individuals with dementia

Some of your learning will be repeated in these units, and will give you the chance to review your knowledge and understanding.

What is dementia?

Dementia is a long-term condition that normally affects older people aged 65 and over; however, younger people can also be affected. The condition is predicted to become more common as a result of ageing populations.

Dementia covers a range of symptoms, which interfere with an individual's ability to function normally. These include:

▶ loss of memory

▶ confusion

▶ speech and language problems

▶ changes in personality and behaviour.

Generally, an individual will need to exhibit the above symptoms for at least six months before positive diagnoses of dementia can be made. Initially, the person may seem grumpy, appear withdrawn, and will tend to opt out of social activities. As the condition progresses, they may experience difficulties with time, with not knowing the day of the week, the date of the month or even what year it is. Gradually, a person with dementia may go on to develop problems identifying friends, key family members and eventually themselves. They can become disorientated, and frequently fail to recognise their surroundings. They may also experience difficulties communicating emotions, remembering how to do everyday things and recalling specific events. Dementia is progressive: the person's ability to function deteriorates over a period of time.

Your assessment criteria:

1.1 Explain what is meant by the term 'dementia'

Key terms

Dementia: a progressive long-term condition that affects the function of brain, leading to memory loss

Investigate

Using the internet, your local library and other resources, conduct further research into the symptoms of dementia.

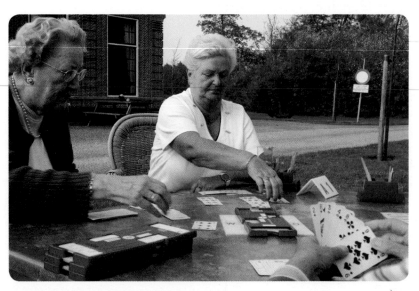

A dementia related condition in someone who appears to be participating in normal activities can be difficult to identify

Case study

George is 70 years old. He lives with his daughter and grandson in Scotland. He is an active man who plays bowls three times a week and belongs to a group of ramblers. His daughter has noticed that George is becoming forgetful and gets very frustrated when he cannot remember simply things like how to boil an egg. He also becomes quite aggressive when she tries to help.

Make notes on the following three questions about George.

1. What symptoms is George exhibiting?
2. What would you do in order to find out more about George's problem?
3. How can you help his daughter understand George's problem?

Reflect

Think about a recent conversation you have had with an individual with a dementia related condition in your work or placement setting. What symptoms did this individual exhibit that made you consider that the cause was dementia?

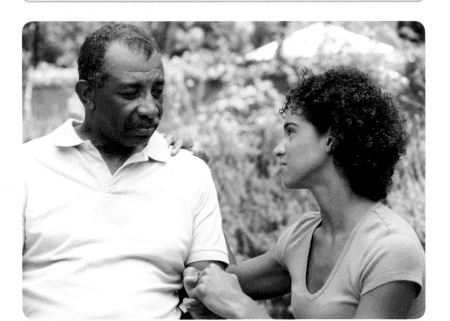

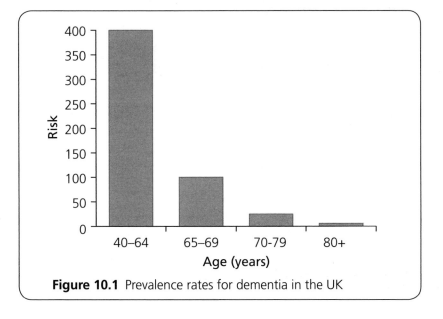

Figure 10.1 Prevalence rates for dementia in the UK

How dementia affects the brain

The Alzheimer's Society (2010) states that the brain consists of three main sections: the **hindbrain**, **midbrain** and the **forebrain**. Each section of the brain is responsible for controlling specific physical or mental functions. The hindbrain and midbrain are concerned with basic life support functions such as blood pressure and respiration. The forebrain is concerned with memory and language, and is further divided into four sections: the frontal, parietal, occipital and temporal lobes (see Figure 10.2).

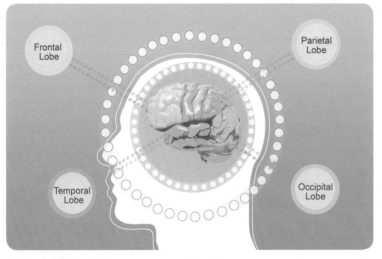

Figure 10.2 The four sections of the forebrain

The forebrain is the section of the brain affected by dementia. The Alzheimer's Society is very clear as to how each lobe is affected by the onset of dementia:

▶ The frontal lobe enables the individual to plan actions and learn new tasks. If there are problems with this lobe, the individual has to relearn certain routine tasks affected by dementia. These tasks may include shopping or cooking.

Your assessment criteria:

1.2 Describe the key functions of the brain that are affected by dementia

Key terms

Hindbrain: this part of the brain regulates essential functions such as breathing, swallowing, blood circulation and maintaining balance

Midbrain: regulates vision, hearing and body movement

Forebrain: the part of the brain concerned with receiving and processing information

Spatial: refers to general awareness of your immediate surroundings

Perception: a process by which a person detects and interprets information from within the environment

▶ The parietal lobe provides the individual with information about **spatial** relationships and **perception**. If the parietal lobe is damaged, the individual's ability to recognise objects, people or surroundings can be severely affected. This is why a person with dementia may sometimes fail to recognise a familiar face.

▶ The occipital lobe deals with visual information. An individual affected by dementia may consequently have difficulty *seeing* what an object is, despite having reasonable eyesight or wearing a visual aid such as spectacles.

▶ The temporal lobe is focused on memory and language. Short-term memory, or memory for recent events, is often impaired in individuals with dementia. Recalling the day's events, therefore, is much more difficult than remembering childhood or distant memories, which are more deeply stored, and thus less affected by dementia. The ability to describe, explain, sequence thoughts and to think logically is also affected by damage to the temporal lobe.

Reflect

Can you think of anybody you know well who has experienced the symptoms of a dementia-related disease? Which aspects of their functioning were affected? Can you link their symptoms to changes in one of the four lobes of the forebrain?

Case study

Victor is a 79 year-old man who lives on his own. He has lived an active life; since his retirement he has looked after his personal needs, prepared his own meals and most days had a cup of tea with his neighbour Miriam. About six months ago she noticed a change in his behaviour. Victor no longer goes shopping like he used to and seems to have lost his cooking skills. He mainly eats meat pies and biscuits. On occasions Victor seems to forget where he is or doesn't recognise Miriam. He has also complained of not seeing very well when trying to read his newspapers even though he has recently had his eyes tested and has been using his new glasses.

1. What signs or symptoms suggest that Victor has a dementia-related disease?

2. Which sections of Victor's brain are likely to be affected by the dementia-related disease?

3. How is dementia affecting Victor's everyday living skills?

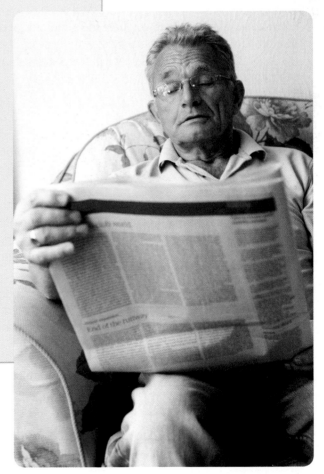

Depression, delirium and age-related memory impairment

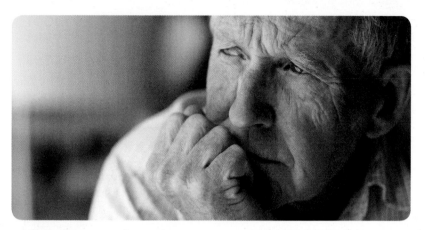

Feeling intense sadness does not necessarily mean you have dementia; you could be experiencing depression

Depression, delirium and age-related memory impairment are sometimes mistaken for dementia. This is because these conditions can have a similar effect on a person's behaviour and communication skills as a dementia-related condition. As a result, it is important to know about and be able to compare the symptoms of depression, delirium and age-related memory loss with those of dementia. This makes understanding the difference between dementia and these other conditions much easier.

Depression

Depression and dementia share a number of symptoms including:

- ▶ low motivation
- ▶ apathy
- ▶ memory problems
- ▶ slow speech
- ▶ slow movements.

Similarities between the symptoms of dementia and depression can make a diagnosis of dementia difficult. However, there are some key differences between the symptoms of the two conditions. The symptoms of depression, for example, include:

- ▶ rapid mental decline
- ▶ slow speech or movement
- ▶ a negative view on life.

These symptoms are not a feature of dementia but may co-exist with the symptoms of dementia if the person has dementia and is also depressed. Symptoms of dementia that are not a feature of depression include:

Key terms

Depression: a mood disorder characterised by intense sadness that disrupts an individual's daily life

248

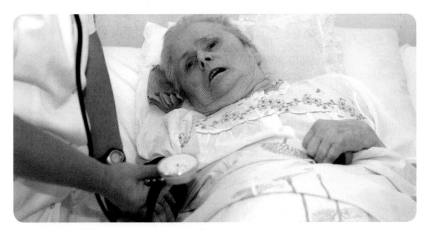

Delirium is a serious condition requiring hospitalisation that can sometimes be mistaken for dementia

- ▶ slow mental decline
- ▶ loss of touch with familiar surroundings
- ▶ progressive confusion and disorientation
- ▶ impaired motor skills, and loss of the ability to write, read and even speak
- ▶ short-term memory loss
- ▶ problems with time.

A person with dementia may try to cover up their memory loss, either by making excuses for their forgetfulness, confusion or other symptoms or by hiding their difficulties from acquaintances, friends and family. The condition tends to be progressive: it worsens rather than improves over time. In contrast, depression is treatable with medication, responds well to talking therapies like counselling, and will often improve even without the help of drugs or talking therapies.

Delirium

A person with delirium can suffer a form of cognitive impairment similar to that affecting someone with dementia. Delirium is also known as acute confusion, and is caused by illness or drug toxicity. Delirium is diagnosed by the following symptoms:

- ▶ mental incoherence
- ▶ difficulty in maintaining concentration and attention
- ▶ unconsciousness.

In dementia, a person's concentration may be severely reduced and there is a great deal of mental confusion but they are not unconscious. Another difference between the two conditions is that delirium is often reversible because it can be treated and cured. Dementia, however, is irreversible and cannot be cured.

Key terms

Delirium: sudden, severe confusion and rapid changes in brain function that occur with physical or mental illness. Delirium is also described as an acute toxic confusional state

Cognitive impairment: loss of ability to think, concentrate and remember information

Age-related memory impairment

Age-related memory impairment is not easy to distinguish from dementia. This causes a lot of anxiety for some older people who are fearful of developing dementia. As we have seen, memory loss is a significant aspect of dementia. However, memory impairment is also an accepted result of the ageing process. A naturally occurring, age-related decline in the brain's cognitive function means that as people age they will inevitably find remembering things more difficult. The naming of people, places and things is especially affected by age-related memory impairment.

However, intellectual brain function remains intact, and while unable to name them, a person with age-related memory impairment will continue to recognise people, places and objects, and will not experience the depth of memory loss experienced by a person with dementia.

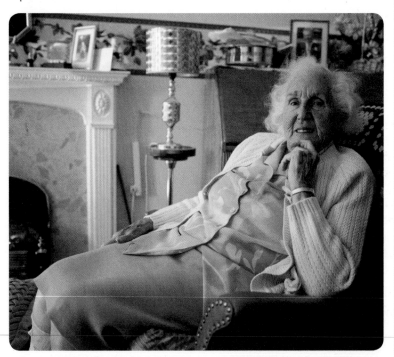

Slower recall of memories and knowledge is a normal part of human ageing

Key terms

Memory impairment: a part of the normal ageing process characterised by episodes of forgetfulness

Case study

Mimi is an 85 year-old woman who has been admitted to a ward in a hospital trust. On admission, Mimi was tearful but she couldn't explain why. Her clothes were dirty and she just wanted to lie in bed and sleep. In the two days since her admission, Mimi's appetite has been poor, even though, according to her son, she normally eats well. Mimi does not seem to know where she is at the moment, even though members of staff have told her on several occasions that she is in hospital. Mimi's admission notes say that she did not recognise her son when he visited her at home and found her in this tearful, dirty and confused state. It was her son who called her GP. The GP then referred her to hospital for admission and assessment.

1. Identify three signs or symptoms that suggest Mimi may be mentally unwell.

2. Why might a relative or neighbour think that Mimi has a dementia-related illness?

3. What do you think could be wrong with Mimi?

Reflect

What do you see as the main differences between age related memory impairment and dementia?

Discuss

Discuss with colleagues why depression and age-related memory impairment are mistaken for dementia.

Knowledge Assessment Task   **1.1** **1.2** **1.3**

Case study

Maureen Jacobs is 78. She is in good physical health and lives an active lifestyle. Maureen's daughter, Jenny, has noticed that her mum has started to become forgetful and sometimes gets confused when she takes her shopping to the local supermarket. Maureen has laughed this off as 'having a senior moment' but Jenny thinks there may be more to it. Maureen doesn't want to go to see her GP (family doctor) about her forgetfulness and Jenny accepts this. However, Jenny is keen to find out more about mental health conditions that can affect people in later life. You have been asked to produce information for Jenny that:

▶ explains what the term 'dementia' means

▶ describes the key functions of the brain that are affected by dementia

▶ explains why depression, delirium and age-related memory impairment are sometimes mistaken for dementia.

Keep the work that you produce as evidence towards your assessment.

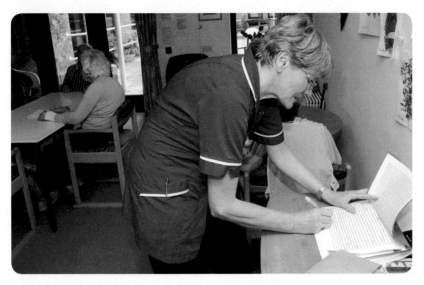

Care practitioners may use one particular model of dementia or elements from different models in their care practice

In the context of health and social care, **models** are ways of thinking about, understanding and responding to health and care-related issues. Models of health and illness also enable practitioners to develop practical ways of caring for people. In this section, we will examine three theoretical models considered suitable for working with individuals with dementia. These are known as the:

▶ medical model

▶ social model

▶ dementia as a disability model.

Medical model of dementia

Practitioners who use a medical model view dementia as an incurable physical illness. The priorities of practitioners who use a medical model approach are to:

▶ identify signs and symptoms of brain disease so that a diagnosis can be given

▶ prescribe drugs considered appropriate for treating the symptoms of dementia.

The medical model approach to dementia focuses on the physical changes in the person's brain and on finding treatments that slow these changes down and improve a person's ability to function. However, many in health and social care see limitations in the medical model of dementia. They argue that focusing on prescribing drugs as the main form of treatment devalues the individual,

Key terms

Models: ways of thinking about, describing or explaining something

and that people are disempowered and further disabled by the process of becoming 'dementia patients'. Some health and social care practitioners also claim that those who use a medical model approach tend to dismiss the effectiveness of other models of care for people living with dementia.

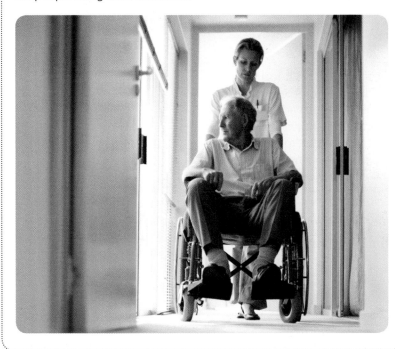

Social model of dementia

The social model of dementia encourages care practitioners to focus on understanding the individual's experiences of living with dementia and on ways of enabling people to maintain their daily living skills. The social model places an emphasis on carers building a relationship with the individual and on maintaining a positive, supportive social environment for the person living with dementia. This is because a well-structured social network and an appropriate living environment, supported by carers with an understanding of dementia, can help individuals with dementia to help themselves in many ways. The social model of dementia attempts to provide individuals with the necessary tools with which to manage the effects of their condition for as long as possible.

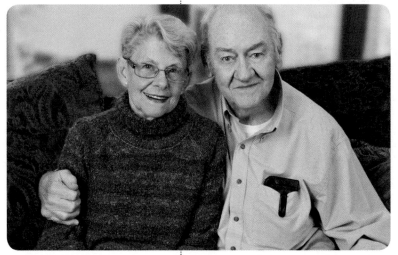

Carer support is a key part of the social model of dementia

Dementia as a disability

The dementia as a disability model uses the concept of **disability** to help people:

▶ understand the disabling impact of dementia

▶ identify how they can learn to cope with their condition as 'disabled people'.

The dementia as a disability model is person-centred, as it focuses on the particular effects of an individual's dementia on their ability to function, and on developing ways in which they can adapt to and overcome the problems they face within their own life. The model helps individuals to manage their dementia from the start and continues to help them adapt to new problems as the condition develops. Health and social care practitioners who use this model suggest it:

▶ gives dignity back to the individual with dementia

▶ promotes and protects the rights of individuals with dementia

▶ ensures that a **needs-led assessment** is carried out when an individual is first diagnosed with dementia.

A needs-led assessment that identifies and takes into account an individual's strengths and abilities is an important part of this approach. This type of assessment enables an individual and their carers to make decisions about the kinds of care and support that are required and which are best suited to the individual. Health and social care practitioners who adopt a dementia as disability approach would argue that where a person can manage their own daily living needs, perhaps with a suitable level of community care support, they should remain living in their own home for as long as possible. Inpatient care is only considered when a person can no longer be supported at home and requires safeguarding against risks associated with later stages of dementia (see Figure 10.3).

Key terms

Disability: a limitation that prevents an individual from carrying out a certain task or action

Needs-led assessment: an assessment of an individual that focuses on their health and social care needs

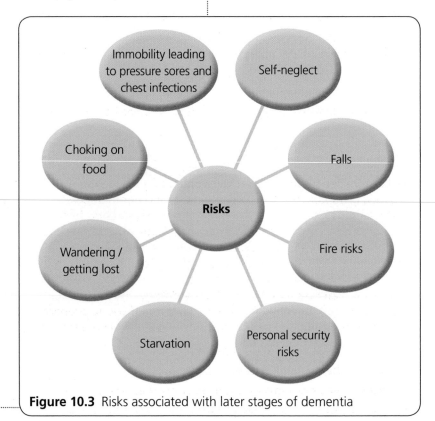

Figure 10.3 Risks associated with later stages of dementia

- Immobility leading to pressure sores and chest infections
- Self-neglect
- Choking on food
- Falls
- Risks
- Fire risks
- Wandering / getting lost
- Personal security risks
- Starvation

A person's care needs will increase as their dementia progresses. As this happens, a person's mental capacity is affected to the point where they may require the assistance of an advocate and protection from the Mental Capacity Act 2005. Among other things, the Mental Capacity Act ensures that the incapacitated individual is provided with an advocate, who is legally bound to act on their behalf. For example, an advocate may have to make a decision about where the person they represent is cared for and what type of care services they receive. These are difficult decisions to make and an advocate must keep the person with dementia informed throughout the process.

Key terms

Mental Capacity Act 2005: a law that protects the rights of people who cannot make decisions for themselves due to a learning disability or mental health condition, or for any other reason.

Case study

Beryl is now in the advanced stages of dementia. She was managing well at home with the help of two professional carers who visited twice a day and her niece Marion who lived nearby and often visited during the day. However, Marion recently noticed that her aunt had started to become aggressive and abusive towards her and was refusing to eat. Marion has withdrawn her services and now refuses to visit Beryl. The carers have also became concerned about the situation and following discussion with Beryl contacted Social Services. A care manager suggested that Beryl will need protection from the Mental Capacity Act and an advocate to represent her interests as she does not have any other surviving relatives.

1. How could Beryl's care be managed using the medical model?
2. How would the social model improve the relationship between Beryl and her niece Marion?
3. How does the disability model enhance the care that is delivered to Beryl?
4. What would the advocate do for Beryl in this particular situation?

Reflect

What do you see as the strengths and weaknesses of the dementia as a disability model? Jot down some of your ideas, particularly relating to the value of a needs-led approach to assessment.

Knowledge Assessment Task | 2.1 | 2.2 | 2.3

Barbara Davies-Hughes is the chairwoman of a Women in Business group in your local area. Barbara and her members meet every other Thursday to discuss business issues and find out about services in the local community. Your work setting has received a letter from Barbara asking whether somebody would be able to attend one of their meetings in a few weeks time to tell them about different approaches to dementia and dementia care. Your manager is aware that you are studying for the Adult Diploma in Health and Social Care and has asked you to prepare some information for a talk on this. You have been asked to:

▶ outline the medical model of dementia
▶ outline the social model of dementia
▶ explain why dementia should be viewed as a disability.

Keep a copy of the work that you produce for this activity as evidence towards your assessment.

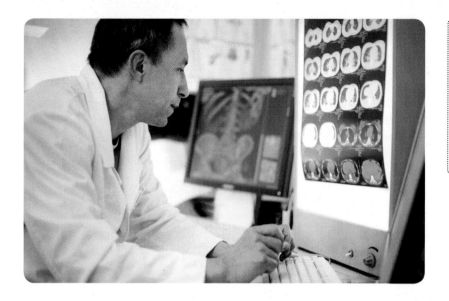

Your assessment criteria:

3.1 List the most common causes of dementia

3.2 Describe the likely signs and symptoms of the most common causes of dementia

Common causes, signs and symptoms of dementia-based conditions

The term 'dementia' is used to describe a range of conditions that affect the brain and cognitive functioning. In reality, there are many causes of dementia. The most common forms are:

▶ **Alzheimer's disease**

▶ **Lewy body dementia**

▶ **vascular dementia**

▶ **fronto-temporal dementia.**

Alzheimer's disease

Alzheimer's disease is one of the most common causes of dementia. It kills brain cells and nerves, causing changes in the chemistry and structure of the brain. Gaps develop in the temporal lobe and in the hippocampus, both of which are responsible for storing and retrieving new information. These gaps affect the individual's ability to remember, speak, think and make decisions. The Alzheimer's Society lists the following as signs and symptoms of Alzheimer's disease:

▶ lapses in memory, especially for recent events

▶ mood swings – busting into tears for no reason, for example

▶ forgetfulness of recent events

▶ personality changes

▶ wandering, particularly in the middle of the night

Key terms

Alzheimer's disease: a disease that causes changes in the brain, affecting a person's speech, thoughts and communication

Hippocampus: stores long-term memories of personal events

Lewy body dementia: a form of dementia caused by Lewy bodies, which have been likened to clumps of protein in the brain. The presence of these bodies damages brain cells, giving rise to dementia

▶ getting lost

▶ loss of inhibitions –inappropriate sexual advances

▶ neglect of personal hygiene.

Alzheimer's disease accounts for between 50% and 60% of all cases of dementia (Alzheimer's Society, 2010).

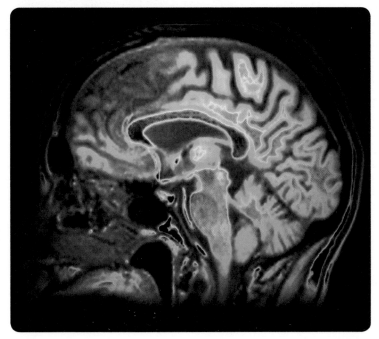

Lewy body dementia

Lewy body dementia is caused by the development of Lewy bodies inside the nerve cells. These disrupt the brain's capacity to function normally, leading to degeneration of brain tissue. This then gives rise to dementia. The signs and symptoms of Lewy body dementia are:

▶ memory loss

▶ persistent visual hallucinations – seeing things or people or animals that are not there

▶ problems with attention and alertness

▶ decline in problem-solving skills – for example, finding it difficult to plan ahead

▶ loss of facial expression

▶ confusion and delirium with nightmares

▶ propensity to faint or fall.

Investigate

Using the internet, your library and other resources, find out the common causes of dementia based conditions and identify which part of the brain is affected for each cause.

Reflect

Think about a conversation you have had with an individual who has had either Alzheimer's disease or Lewy body dementia. What were the signs and symptoms of that particular condition?

Vascular dementia

Vascular dementia occurs when the blood vessels in the brain are damaged, causing oxygen supply to be diminished. This can result in a series of mini strokes (infarcts), causing the brain cells to die. Initially, the strokes will have either no symptoms, or simply leave the individual feeling confused. However, over a period of time, the cumulative effect of these mini strokes leads to vascular dementia. The signs and symptoms of vascular dementia are:

- problems with communication and concentration
- stroke symptoms; for example, leg or arm weakness
- stepped progression – symptoms level off then condition deteriorates
- acute confusion
- memory loss
- dizziness
- slurred speech
- rapid shuffling steps
- loss of bladder and bowel control.

Fronto-temporal dementia

Fronto-temporal dementia consists of a range of conditions, including Pick's disease, frontal lobe degeneration and a type of dementia associated with motor neurone disease. Fronto-temporal dementia occurs as a result of damage to the frontal lobe or temporal parts of the brain, where there is an abnormal accumulation of proteins between the spaces of the cells. In the case of Pick's disease, these proteins are called Pick's bodies. The signs and symptoms of fronto-temporal dementia are:

- lack of insight
- an inability to empathise
- changing or inappropriate behaviour
- loss of inhibitions
- development of compulsive rituals
- increased interest in sex
- agitated or blunted emotions
- a decline in personal hygiene
- language difficulties – not understanding the spoken word or failure to speak.

Your assessment criteria:

3.1 List the most common causes of dementia

3.2 Describe the likely signs and symptoms of the most common causes of dementia

Key terms

Vascular dementia: a form of dementia resulting from the accumulative effect of a series of mini strokes, causing the brain cells to die

Fronto-temporal dementia: also known as Pick's disease, it is caused by damage to the temporal lobe of the brain

Case study

Isobel is a 65-year-old lady who lives with her husband, Gavin. She has led a very sociable and active life until a year ago when Gavin became increasingly concerned with his wife's short term memory loss. Isobel had a fall eight months ago and following the fall, Gavin noticed a change in his wife's behaviour. She became confused, started to ask the same questions over and over again and lost interest in her daily activities of cooking and cleaning the house. She also started hoarding things.

A few weeks later, she complained of feeling dizzy and sustained another fall that resulted in her having slurred speech and walking with rapid shuffling steps. Isobel has a history of hypertension and heart problems.

1. Identify what you think might be cause of Isobel's problems?

2. What are the signs and symptoms of this condition?

3. Which part of the brain do you think is affected?

Investigate

Using online and library sources, investigate one of the four common forms of dementia further. Try to find out about ways of assessing and diagnosing your chosen form of dementia, its specific causes, the impact it has on an individual's behaviour and functioning as the disease progresses.

Knowledge Assessment Task   3.1   3.2

The manager of your work setting has looked through the information you produced about dementia for the Women in Business group in a previous task (see page 255). She has suggested that the information could be extended a little to broaden the understanding of people attending the meeting. You have been asked to:

▶ list the most common causes of dementia

▶ describe the likely signs and symptoms of the most common causes of dementia.

You could add this information to the information leaflet or presentation notes that you have prepared for the previous task. Remember to keep your work so that you can use it as evidence towards your assessment.

Risk factors

It is not understood exactly why some people develop dementia-related conditions, but there are certain **risk** factors that are associated with the condition. These are:

- ▶ age – people aged 65 years and older are at much higher risk of dementia

- ▶ family history – you are more likely to develop the illness if a close relative has been affected

- ▶ environmental and lifestyle factors – these include excess intake of alcohol, lack of exercise, exposure to aluminium and other metals, inappropriate diet

- ▶ head injury – a connection has been found between head injuries and dementia

- ▶ physical conditions – risk factors include hypertension, heart disease, HIV and multiple sclerosis

- ▶ genetics – risk factors include Down's syndrome

- ▶ learning disabilities.

Your assessment criteria:

3.3 Outline the risk factors for the most common causes of dementia

3.4 Identify prevalence rates for different types of dementia

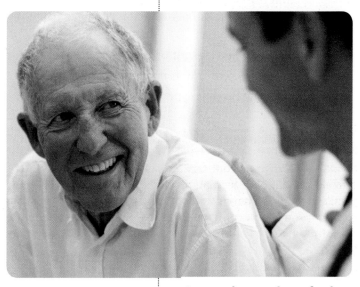

Age and a number of other physical and environmental factors raise an individual's risk of experiencing a dementia-related condition

Case study

Tom, aged 65, lives on his own and is due to retire from his job as a postman soon. Tom has an active social life and hates the thought of getting old. He plays darts every weekend with his mates, drinks heavily and does not exercise. As a result, Tom is overweight and has hypertension but he rarely visits his GP. Tom's mother lived until she was 80 years old, but died of a dementia-related disease. Tom is worried that he might get dementia too, but is not doing anything to address the possibility. He has decided to take each day as it comes.

1. What factors increase Tom's risk of developing a dementia-related disease?

2. What advice or guidance would you give to Tom about his lifestyle?

3. Whom should Tom contact regarding his weight and hypertension?

Key terms

Risk: the likelihood or chance of something happening

Prevalence: the number of cases

Prevalence rates

The **prevalence** rate for dementia is the frequency with which the condition occurs in a population. It has been estimated that by 2021 there will be about 940,000 people living with dementia in the UK. This is expected to rise to 1.7 million by 2051. The relative frequency of different forms of dementia is as follows:

▶ Alzheimer's disease (AD): 62%

▶ vascular dementia (VaD): 17%

▶ mixed dementia (AD and VaD): 10%

▶ Lewy body dementia: 4%

▶ fronto-temporal dementia: 2%

▶ Parkinson's dementia: 2%

▶ Other dementias: 3%

Source: Alzheimer's Society (2010)

It is estimated that there are about 15,000 people from black and minority ethnic (BME) communities with dementia in England. This estimate is based on the 2001 census. The proportion of older people from black and minority ethnic groups in the UK is small but is projected to rise as this population grow older. There is limited published research or statistical information regarding dementia in BME communities.

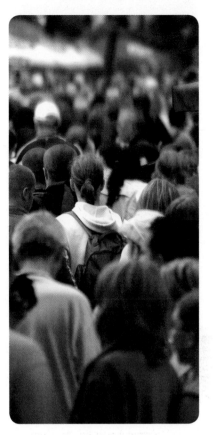

Dementia can be experienced by anyone regardless of their age, social status or ethnicity

Knowledge Assessment Task   3.3   3.4

The manager of your care setting has asked you to produce an information leaflet for other care professionals and students who visit your workplace to find out about care and services for people living with dementia-related conditions. Many visitors ask about the causes and prevalence of dementia. You have been asked to produce an information leaflet that:

▶ outlines the risk factors for most common causes of dementia
▶ identifies the prevalence rates for different types of dementia.

Your leaflet should provide the information clearly, using words, graphs or other images, and should state the source of any data or statistical information you use. You should keep a copy of the work that you produce as evidence towards your assessment.

An individual's experience of dementia

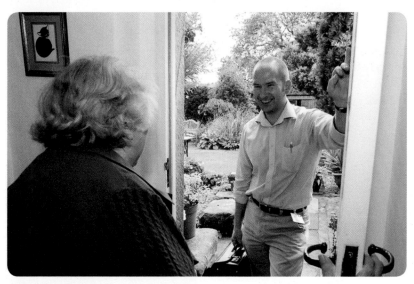

Many individuals with dementia live at home and receive support from community-based health and social care practitioners

Investigate

When you are next at your work or placement setting, find out as much as you can from colleagues and members of the multidisciplinary team about the support offered by the statutory services for people with dementia related conditions.

Reflect

Write a brief reflective account of about 100 words of how you would help an individual with a dementia related condition in your care setting to recognise their symptoms and manage their condition.

Living with dementia

This section highlights some of the issues that people living with dementia may face and describes how health and social care practitioners working in statutory and voluntary services can provide them with help and support.

Recognising the symptoms

Living with dementia is not easy. A person with dementia is constantly trying to manage a worsening condition. It may be that in the early stages an individual has decided to keep the condition private, and has not told anyone. It may be that the person does not recognise the signs and symptoms they are experiencing as being the onset of dementia, or has failed to accept the possibility of having developed dementia. In the early stages of dementia, an individual may experience some or all of the following symptoms:

▶ memory loss

▶ problems with recalling names and words

▶ language difficulty

▶ loss of hearing

▶ effects on visual acuity

▶ changes in behaviour from being a cheerful and responsive person to someone who has become hostile and aggressive with significant mood swings.

Statutory support

In the early stages of dementia an individual experiencing the symptoms described above may be assessed by their local general practitioner (GP) and referred on to a multidisciplinary services team for older people. These teams usually consist of:

▶ nurses

▶ speech and language therapists

▶ occupational therapists

▶ physiotherapists

▶ psychologists

▶ psychiatrists.

Each member of the multidisciplinary team can carry out further assessments of a person's skills, abilities, problems and care needs. These may include a needs-led assessment, which helps determine the individual's strengths and abilities. A member of the team may act as the individual's advocate if the person goes on to lose the ability to make decisions independently or to live safely at home, for example. The outcome of a series of assessments is usually an individualised outreach programme of care, designed specifically to support and empower the person and to maximise their quality of life.

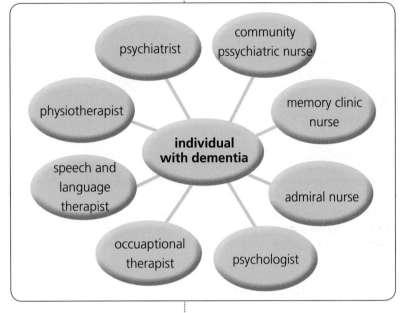

The role of statutory services is vital for people with dementia-related conditions. Increasingly, health and social care practitioners also provide support for the families and carers of people affected by dementia. This is important as it helps to maintain the individual's social and support networks and can be the factor that enables them to remain living in their own home. For those in the early stages of Alzheimer's disease, or with undiagnosed memory impairment, a new range of drugs administered by **memory clinic nurses** may be prescribed. These drugs are proving relatively effective: the rate of their success improves the earlier a diagnosis is made. **Admiral nurses** and **community psychiatric nurses** also work with people with dementia (and their families and carers) as outreach workers in the community. These specialist health and social care practitioners offer a range of support, education and counselling services that can be specially tailored to individual needs. Their introduction has also had the effect of increasing the wider community's awareness of dementia, and thus improving the quality of life of those with dementia.

Key terms

Memory clinic nurses: health care practitioners who provide drug and other treatments in specialist clinics for people showing early signs and symptoms of memory impairment, particularly Alzheimer's disease

Admiral nurses: specialists providing care for people with all forms of dementia and support for their carers in the community

Community psychiatric nurses: mental health nurses who work in the community, often with people who have dementia-related conditions

Case study

Enid and Martin have been married for 50 years and enjoyed a happy married life. About ten years ago Enid noticed a change in Martin's behaviour. He was a fairly patient and mild-mannered man who gradually became very hostile and aggressive, with rapid changes in his mood. One moment he would be happy and laughing and the next very tearful. He seemed confused at times, finding it difficult to hold a conversation and not remembering his wife's name or those of his two sons. Eventually, Martin agreed to see his GP. While conducting the assessment, Dr White noticed significant memory loss

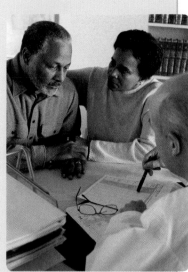

and language difficulties. He informed Martin that he was going to refer him to the multidisciplinary team for older people for a specialist assessment.

1. Identify the symptoms of dementia that Martin is experiencing.

2. Describe who will perform the assessment and what help and treatment you think statutory services should be able to offer Martin and Enid.

3. How can the community psychiatric nurse support Martin in living at home with his wife in the community?

Voluntary support

The voluntary sector has a key role in supporting people with dementia and their families. The Alzheimer's Society **(www.alzheimers.org.uk)** and Dementia UK **(www.dementiauk.org)** provide a useful range of information about dementia issues through their websites. Both organisations work with and on behalf of people with dementia to raise awareness of the common types of dementia, their causes, symptoms and treatments. In addition to these national bodies, there are many local community-based support groups working with people with dementia, their carers and families throughout the UK. These groups are flexible, generally easy to access and use and resourceful. They provide day-to-day support for individuals with dementia, as well as for the family members of individuals with dementia. Their services typically include the provision of practical help, advice on benefits, treatment and local services, and support

Dementia UK
Improving quality of life

A number of organisations exist to help individuals, carers and their families.

to alleviate carers' and sufferers' feelings of isolation. Voluntary groups are important because they are able to act as links between individuals with dementia and the statutory services.

Inpatient care

Dementia is a progressive illness. This means that every individual's dementia will get worse over time. This often results in people needing inpatient care in a hospital or specialist care home setting. When a person is admitted for inpatient care, tensions can arise because the individual has been placed in an unfamiliar environment. Consequently, the person can present a number of challenges that may require careful handling by the healthcare practitioner. These challenges can include the person exhibiting violent, argumentative or unresponsive behaviour. This can upset the other patients or residents within an inpatient setting. The individual exhibiting this behaviour could be experiencing a sense of loss or fear in leaving a known environment for another that is alien to them. An individualised person-centred approach is needed to put the individual at ease, monitor their concerns and promote a sense of wellbeing and harmony. This will subsequently improve the quality of care they receive.

Reflect

Reflect on the skills you need in order to manage the tensions that may arise when an individual with a dementia related condition is admitted to an unfamiliar environment. What would you do to promote a sense of wellbeing and harmony for that individual? Write down these thoughts in your journal.

Case study

Margaret Lawrence is a retired 60 year-old woman who had a successful career as a journalist. She is married with three grown-up children and five grandchildren. Margaret lives in the outer suburbs of the city and until recently was a relaxed and pleasant woman who socialised with friends at work and at home. However, since retirement Margaret has found it difficult to engage with her local community or to pursue any of her former social activities, such as yoga and gardening. She is aware that she has not been herself for sometime, but has hidden these feelings from her husband and children. Margaret has become forgetful, bursting into tears for no apparent reason, has developed volatile moods and can suddenly become very angry with others. She forgets the time of day and sometimes fails to recognise where she is. Margaret does not know how to cope with the present situation.

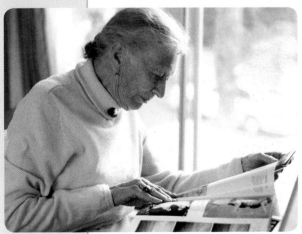

1. What signs, symptoms or changes in behaviour suggest that Margaret may have a dementia-related condition?

2. What type of dementia do you think Margaret has?

3. What support services are available for Margaret and for her husband?

Keep your notes you make in response to this activity as evidence for your assessment.

Behaviour of others

In the past, some health and social care practitioners may have felt that nothing could be done for people diagnosed with dementia. Attitudes like this may have had a negative impact on the quality and standard of care that some practitioners provided for people with dementia. As a result, some people with dementia have been left vulnerable to neglect and abuse by carers, practitioners and others. Negative attitudes and unscrupulous, uncaring behaviour by carers and care practitioners fails to recognise the capabilities and needs of people with dementia or the safeguarding responsibilities of those who are supposed to provide care. However, there has been a shift in attitudes in recent years. Dementia is now recognised as a serious and disabling condition requiring the care practitioner's understanding of the individual's lived experience. The shift has been linked to the development and use of the person-centred approach (see page.154). This approach values each individual as a unique person regardless of the way they act or communicate. It asks that practitioners tailor their approaches to the needs of the individual who also happens to be a patient, resident or service user. Tom Kitwood, a pioneer of the person-centred approach, recommends that those providing care for people with dementia should:

▶ encourage individuals to tell their life stories because this helps carers to understand a person with dementia as a distinct individual rather than just as someone with a long-term condition

▶ use pictures and photographs to communicate with and maintain an individual's dignity, particularly in the less personal surroundings of an inpatient facility

▶ protect dignity and seek to reduce embarrassment when providing personal and intimate care for people with dementia

▶ respect each person's privacy and continually promote a person's sense of self through the way care is provided.

Your assessment criteria:

4.2 Outline the impact that the attitudes and behaviours of others may have on an individual with dementia

Discuss

Discuss with colleagues, fellow students and your tutor the knowledge and skills that care practitioners require in order to promote a more positive attitude to individuals with dementia related conditions in the caring setting.

Reflect

Think about how you can protect a person's privacy when providing personal and intimate care in order to reduce their embarrassment. Write down your thoughts in your journal.

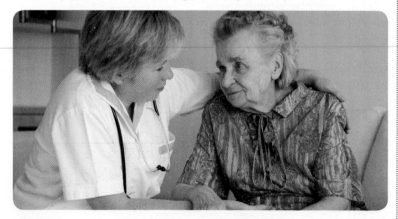

Compassionate care that respects individuality and promotes each person's sense of self is a key part of care practice in dementia care settings

Knowledge Assessment Task   4.1   4.2

Identify two people with dementia-related conditions from your workplace environment or placement area to focus this activity on. If the people you have chosen are able to communicate verbally, ask each of them to tell you their life story. Alternatively, you could talk to the person's carers, relatives or members of staff in your workplace who know them well. You could also review each person's records for background information. Focus your research, questions and the conversation on:

▶ how the person experiences living with dementia

▶ what impact the person's dementia has had on their daily living skills

▶ how the attitudes and behaviours of others have affected the person since they developed the condition.

Using the information you obtain, create two profiles that:

▶ describe how each person experiences living with dementia

▶ outline the impact that the attitudes and behaviours of others have had on the individual with dementia.

Keep the work you produce for this activity as evidence for your assessment.

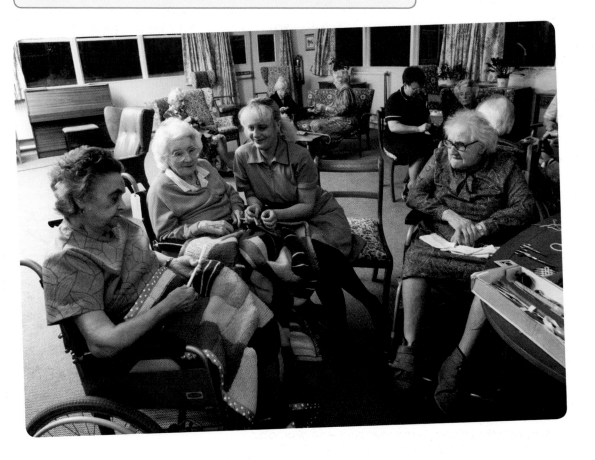

Are you ready for assessment?

AC	What do you know now?	Assessment task	✓
1.1	Explain what is meant by the term 'dementia'	Page 251	
1.2	Describe the key functions of the brain that are affected by dementia	Page 251	
1.3	Explain why depression, delirium and age-related memory impairment may be mistaken for dementia	Page 251	
2.1	Outline the medical model of dementia	Page 255	
2.2	Outline the social model of dementia	Page 255	
2.3	Explain why dementia should be viewed as a disability	Page 255	
3.1	List the most common causes of dementia	Page 259	
3.2	Describe the likely signs and symptoms of the most common causes of dementia	Page 259	
3.3	Outline the risk factors for the most common causes of dementia	Page 261	
3.4	Identify prevalence rates for different types of dementia	Page 261	
4.1	Describe how different individuals may experience living with dementia, depending on age, type of dementia and level of ability and disability	Page 267	
4.2	Outline the impact that the attitudes and behaviours of others may have on an individual with dementia	Page 267	

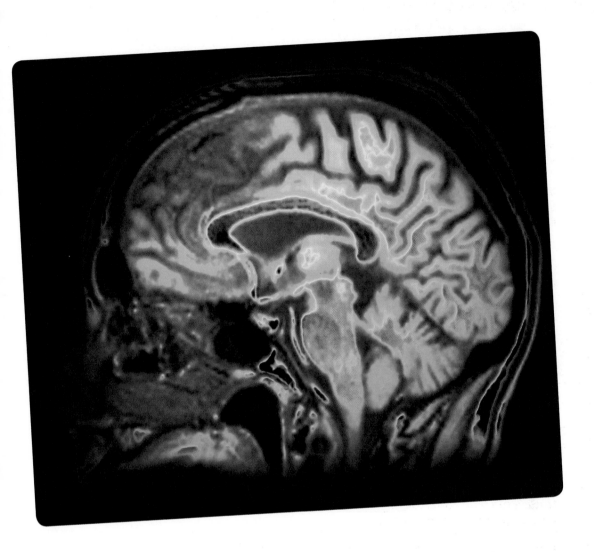

11 | The principles of infection prevention and control (ICO 1)

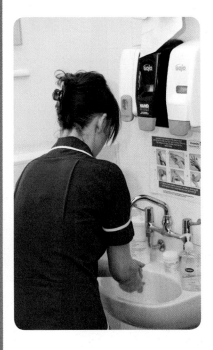

AC	What you need to know
1.1	Explain employees' roles and responsibilities in relation to the prevention and control of infection
1.2	Explain employers' responsibilities in relation to the prevention and control of infection
2.1	Outline current legislation and regulatory body standards which are relevant to the prevention and control of infection
2.2	Describe local and organisational policies relevant to the prevention and control of infection
3.1	Describe procedures and systems relevant to the prevention and control of infection
3.2	Explain the potential impact of an outbreak of infection on the individual and the organisation
4.1	Define the term 'risk'

4.2	Outline potential risks of infection within the workplace
4.3	Describe the process of carrying out a risk assessment
4.4	Explain the importance of carrying out a risk assessment
5.1	Demonstrate correct use of personal protective equipment (PPE)
5.2	Describe different types of PPE
5.3	Explain the reasons for use of PPE
5.4	State current relevant regulations and legislation relating to PPE
5.5	Describe employees' responsibilities regarding the use of PPE
5.6	Describe employers' responsibilities regarding the use of PPE
5.7	Describe the correct practice in the application and removal of PPE
5.8	Describe the correct procedure for disposal of used PPE
6.1	Describe the key principles of good personal hygiene
6.2	Demonstrate good hand washing technique
6.3	Describe the correct sequence for hand washing
6.4	Explain when and why hand washing should be carried out
6.5	Describe the types of products that should be used for hand washing
6.6	Describe correct procedures that relate to skincare

This unit also links to some of the other units:

HSC 027	Contribute to health and safety in health and social care
HSC 2014	Support individuals to eat and drink
HSC 2015	Support individuals to meet personal care needs

Some of your learning will be repeated in these units and will give you the chance to review your knowledge and understanding.

Roles and responsibilities

Everyone working in a health and social care setting is responsible for preventing **infection**. Health and social care practitioners must avoid getting and passing on **pathogens**, such as **bacteria** and **viruses** that cause illness. Employees and employers working in health and social care settings have particular roles and responsibilities for preventing infection.

Employees' roles and responsibilities

As a health or social care practitioners you should:

- ▶ maintain high standards of personal health and hygiene
- ▶ be aware of the infection control policies and procedures that are used in your workplace
- ▶ follow best practice in infection prevention and control
- ▶ maintain a clean and hygienic environment
- ▶ report infection risks to your employer
- ▶ attend training days relating to infection prevention and control.

Roles and responsibilities of the employer

Your employer must make sure all laws and legal regulations concerning infection prevention and control are followed in the workplace and should:

- ▶ undertake risk assessment and management to identify and minimise the impact of infection hazards
- ▶ produce infection prevention and control policies and procedure
- ▶ provide relevant equipment to enable you to prevent and control infection
- ▶ identify and distribute relevant information about infection hazards and prevention and control methods
- ▶ provide training and supervision in aspects of infection and control relevant to your work setting
- ▶ keep records relating to infection prevention and control in your workplace.

Your assessment criteria:

1.1 Explain employees' roles and responsibilities in relation to the prevention and control of infection

1.2 Explain employers' roles and responsibilities in relation to the prevention and control of infection

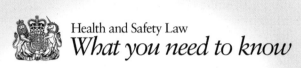

Health and Safety Law
What you need to know

All workers have a right to work in places where risks to their health and safety are properly controlled. Health and safety is about stopping you getting hurt at work or ill through work. Your employer is responsible for health and safety, but you must help.

What employers must do for you

1 Decide what could harm you in your job and the precautions to stop it. This is part of risk assessment.

2 In a way you can understand, explain how risks will be controlled and tell you who is responsible for this.

3 Consult and work with you and your health and safety representatives in protecting everyone from harm in the workplace.

4 Free of charge, give you the health and safety training you need to do your job.

5 Free of charge, provide you with any equipment and protective clothing you need, and ensure it is properly looked after.

6 Provide toilets, washing facilities and drinking water.

7 Provide adequate first-aid facilities.

8 Report injuries, diseases and dangerous incidents at work to our Incident Contact Centre: **0845 300 9923**

9 Have insurance that covers you in case you get hurt at work or ill through work. Display a hard copy or electronic copy of the current insurance certificate where you can easily read it.

10 Work with any other employers or contractors sharing the workplace or providing employees (such as agency workers), so that everyone's health and safety is protected.

Your health and safety representatives:

Other health and safety contacts:

What you must do

1 Follow the training you have received when using any work items your employer has given you.

2 Take reasonable care of your own and other people's health and safety.

3 Co-operate with your employer on health and safety.

4 Tell someone (your employer, supervisor, or health and safety representative) if you think the work or inadequate precautions are putting anyone's health and safety at serious risk.

If there's a problem

1 If you are worried about health and safety in your workplace, talk to your employer, supervisor, or health and safety representative.

2 You can also look at our website for general information about health and safety at work.

3 If, after talking with your employer, you are still worried, phone our Infoline. We can put you in touch with the local enforcing authority for health and safety and the Employment Medical Advisory Service. You don't have to give your name.

HSE Infoline: **0845 345 0055**

HSE website: **www.hse.gov.uk**

Fire safety
You can get advice on fire safety from the Fire and Rescue Services or your workplace fire officer.

Employment rights
Find out more about your employment rights at
www.direct.gov.uk

 HSE **Health and Safety Executive**

Employers must display this poster outlining British health and safety law in the workplace, or provide it in pocket card format to workforce

Case study

Fatimah, a community support worker, visited Mrs Yates at home to help her wash and dress this morning. During today's visit, Fatimah used the last of the plastic aprons and also noticed there was only one pair of disposable gloves left. Mrs Yates's husband, who is also her main carer, said he thought that throwing these items away after one use seemed wasteful. He also suggested that he and Fatimah should use (and share) cloth aprons and washing up gloves to provide personal care for Mrs Yates in future.

1. Who is responsible for ensuring that aprons and gloves are provided and replenished in this kind of care situation?
2. What role and responsibilities does Fatimah have regarding infection prevention and control in this situation?
3. What could Fatimah say to Mr Yates to explain why disposable rather than reusable aprons and gloves are used to provide care for his wife?

Knowledge Assessment Task   1.1   1.2

Infection prevention and control should be a high priority in all health and social care settings. Health and social care practitioners should receive clear information about their own and their employer's role and responsibilities for preventing and controlling infection.

You have been asked to produce a concise and clear information leaflet for your workplace that:

▶ explains the employee's role and responsibilities in relation to the prevention and control of infection
▶ explains the employer's role and responsibilities in relation to the prevention and control of infection.

Keep the written work that you produce for this activity as evidence towards your assessment.

Discuss

With a colleague or your supervisor, talk about how you could respond to a colleague who failed to keep to guidelines about infection prevention and control in your workplace. How could you draw this to their attention and what would you tell them about their infection prevention and control role and responsibilities?

Reflect

What do you do to prevent infection (to yourself and others) while at work? Do you remember to wash your hands, wipe surfaces and use gloves when delivering care?

Key terms

Infection: an invasion of disease-causing micro organisms that multiply in the body and cause illness

Pathogen: a micro organism such as bacterium or a virus that causes disease

Bacterium: types of micro-organism that can carry disease

Virus: a micro-organism containing genetic material that replicates within a host's cell causing illness

Legislation, standards and policies for infection prevention and control

In the UK, laws, legal regulations and standards relating to infection prevention and control cover a number of different issues that are relevant to health and social care practice. These include health and safety at work, public health issues, environmental safety and food safety.

Figure 11.1 Laws relating to infection prevention and control

Law	How does it affect care practice?
Health and Safety at Work Act 1974	Sets standards to prevent infection occurring and spreading
Public Health (Control of Disease) Act 1984	Sets standards for sanitation, water supply and disposal of rubbish
Food Safety Act 1990	Concerns food production and consumption
Environmental Protection Act 1990	Ensures the safe management (handling, transfer, disposal) of controlled waste
Management of Health and Safety at Work Act 1999	Introduced risk assessment

Your assessment criteria:

2.1 Outline current legislation and regulatory body standards which are relevant to the prevention and control of infection

2.2 Describe local and organisational policies relevant to the prevention and control of infection

GUIDANCE TO THE FOOD SAFETY ACT 1995

ALL STAFF PLEASE NOTE:

Always wash your hands before handling food and after using the toilet.

Tell your boss at once of any skin, nose, throat or bowel trouble.

Ensure cuts and sores are covered with waterproof dressings.

Keep yourself clean and wear clean clothing.

Do not smoke in a food room it is illegal and dangerous. Never cough or sneeze over food.

Clean as you go. Keep all equipment and surfaces clean.

Prepare raw and cooked food in separate areas. USE COLOUR CODED CHOPPING BOARDS AND KNIVES to avoid cross contamination.

Ensure food is at correct temperature at all times. READ COOK CHILL GUIDELINES.

Keep your hands off food as far as possible.

Ensure waste food is disposed of properly. Keep the lid on the dustbin and wash your hands after putting waste in it.

Deliveries of food to your premises should be checked to ensure they are at correct temperature on receipt. IF IN DOUBT ADVISE YOUR SUPERVISOR.

Tell your supervisor if you cannot follw the rules. Do not break the law.

This notice gives guidance only and should not be treated as a complete and authoritative statement of law. For more information contact the environmental health officer at your local council.

Figure 11.2 Regulations relating to infection prevention and control

Legal regulations	How does it affect care practice?
Personal Protective Equipment (PPE) at Work Regulations 1992	Employers must supply and employees must use appropriate protective clothes and equipment (see page 292)
Food Safety (General Food Hygiene) Regulations 1995	Introduced safe hygiene practices to prevent pathogen contamination during handling and storage of food
Reporting of Injuries, Diseases and Dangerous Occurrences (RIDDOR) 1995	Ensures that work-related infection from handling body fluids and highly infectious diseases are reported
The Control of Substances Hazardous to Health (COSHH) 2002	Regulates storage and use of chemicals (e.g. cleaning solutions) that pose a danger. All workplaces must have a COSHH information file available for workers
Hazardous Waste Regulations 2005	Concerns the disposal of sharps and clinical waste, which pose a particular infection hazard
Code of Practice for the Prevention and Control of Healthcare Associated Infection (HCAI); Regulation 12; 2010	Provides guidance on ways to reduce the incidence of HCAI

Key terms

Controlled waste: household, industrial and commercial waste

Risk assessment: the process of identifying likelihood of harm from hazards

Contamination: the pollution or infection of an object or person

Body fluid: any fluid that circulates around or is expelled from the body, such as blood, sputum or urine

Clinical waste: waste produced from healthcare premises, such as hospitals and care homes

Health Care Associated Infection (HCAI): an infection that originates from a healthcare setting

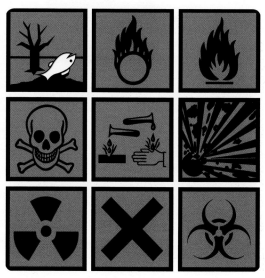

COSHH warning symbols

Reflect

Which of the laws and regulations relating to infection control are you already aware of? Are there any that you haven't heard of or which you could investigate further as a way of developing your knowledge and care practice?

Regulatory body standards

Health and social care professions produce standards which describe the skills, knowledge and understanding needed by a practitioner in order to demonstrate competence and protect the public from harm. Some examples of regulatory body standards which concern infection prevention and control include:

▶ National Occupational Standards (NOS) for health workers produced by Skills for Health.

▶ guidance for NHS and local authorities produced by the National Institute for Health and Clinical Excellence (NICE).

▶ *Essential Standards of Quality and Safety*, 2010, including eight cleanliness and infection control measures, produced by The Care Quality Commission (CQC).

Health and social care practitioners should also be aware of other sources of guidance about standards, such as those provided by the Department of Health and the Royal College of Nursing (RCN).

Infection control policies

The infection control policies developed for your workplace should incorporate all of the current laws, regulations and standards relating to infection prevention and control. If you put these policies into practice through the way you provide care, you should always stay within the law, uphold the conditions of your work contract and protect yourself and others from the risk of infection. The infection prevention and control policies used in your work setting must:

▶ be seen and read by all members of the care team (you may be asked to sign to show that you have done this)

▶ provide enough information for care workers to practice safely

▶ set out step-by-step guidance for using the infection prevention and control systems and procedures that operate in your work setting

▶ be available to visitors or family members of people receiving care.

Reflect

How do you use the infection prevention and control policies written for your workplace?

Which elements are most relevant to your work role?

Investigate

Think about ways to improve the information about infection control issues given to visitors to your workplace. Talk with your manager about the possibility of developing a simple questionnaire to check visitors' understanding about such issues as washing hands, use of hand gel and not visiting when feeling unwell.

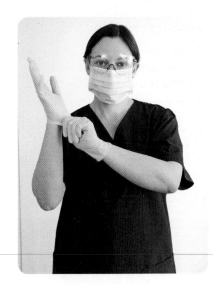

Case study

Davina has just started working at a care home and has been given the infection prevention and control policy to read over. This isn't what Davina hoped to be doing on her first day at work. Shortly after starting to read through the infection prevention and control policy and procedures file, Davina gives up and starts playing a game on her mobile phone instead.

1. Why should Davina read the infection prevention and control policy?

2. What risks does Davina take by not reading the policy?

3. What could you say to Davina to help her recognise the benefits of knowing how to work within policy guidelines?

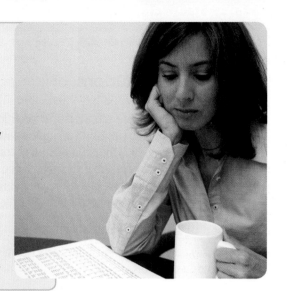

Knowledge Assessment Task   2.1   2.2

Infection prevention and control is a very important issue for all health and social care practitioners. However, the legal and regulatory framework relating to this issue can seem complex and isn't always well understood by practitioners. Consequently, the manager of your work setting has asked you to produce a summary, ideally in an easy to read table format, of:

▶ current legislation and regulatory body standards that are relevant to the prevention and control of infection in health and social care settings

▶ the local and organisational policies and procedures relating to the prevention and control of infection in your work setting.

The work that you produce should be factually correct, concise and useful to your colleagues. Keep a copy of your written work to use as evidence for your assessment.

Discuss

Talk together with colleagues, other learners and your manager or tutor about ideas to make and improve links between infection control policy and working practice. Perhaps there are issues which could be addressed by a training session for staff which you could help to run?

Standard precautions

Standard precautions or 'universal' precautions, as they are sometimes called, recognise that all individuals pose a potential infection risk to you and that you pose a potential infection risk to others. It is not always possible to know when a person is infectious, so it is best to treat everyone as if they are contaminated, including yourself. To apply standard precautions in practice you should:

- risk-assess all potential infection hazards in your day-to-day work
- wash your hands using correct procedure (see page 301) at appropriate times
- use personal protective equipment (see page 292) to create a barrier against pathogens
- clean and disinfect items and areas at appropriate times and with appropriate chemicals for the job
- dispose of waste, including sharps, safely.

Procedures and systems

A range of infection prevention and control systems and procedures are used in health and social care settings. These relate to food hygiene, disposal of waste, cleaning and laundry.

Food hygiene

Food hygiene is an important focus for infection prevention and control because food provides an environment suitable for pathogens to multiply and eating provides a route for infection to enter the body. Food poisoning causes vomiting and diarrhoea. This can lead to dehydration and, in severe cases, is sometimes fatal. Contamination of food can occur during the preparation, cooking, serving or storage of food. To avoid **cross-contamination** and **cross-infection** when dealing with food, pay particular attention to:

- personal hygiene – keep hands clean, wear PPE, and do not work if unwel
- kitchen and dining environment – keep surfaces and cooking equipment clean
- safe food practices – including thorough thawing, heating and cooking of food; correct food storage; preparing meat and fish separately to avoid contaminating foods that are eaten raw.

Disposal of waste

Rubbish and other waste products provide a perfect environment for harbouring pathogens and spreading infection. If left lying

Key terms

Standard precautions: a set of guidelines to minimise the spread of infection between individuals

Cross-infection: the spread of infection from one person to another

Cross-contamination: the transfer of pathogens from one person, object or area to another

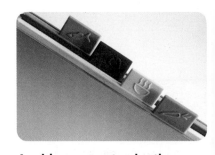

Avoid cross contamination by using different coloured chopping boards to prepare different food types

around rubbish also attracts vermin, such as rats, which carry disease. The way waste is disposed on depends on the:

▶ type of waste involved

▶ risk the waste poses to people

▶ risk the waste poses to the environment.

You need to understand the waste disposal arrangements and procedures for your work area. Figure 11.3 outlines methods for disposing of healthcare waste. You should also be aware that different local authorities have different waste disposal arrangements for other forms of waste.

Key terms

Healthcare waste: any waste produced as a result of healthcare activities in hospital or community settings

Reflect

How many times in a day do you take measures to reduce or remove the potential for infection? Could (or should) you do this more frequently?

Figure 11.3 Disposal of healthcare waste

Category of waste	Example	Colour-coded waste stream	Method of disposal
Hazardous waste: infectious, dangerous or toxic			
1. Clinical waste: items soiled with infected body fluids, such as blood	• catheter bags • dressings	Yellow or orange bag	Incineration
2. Sharps: used to take blood, perform surgery, give injections	• needles, razors, scalpels	Rigid yellow receptacle, marked with a fill-to line – different coloured lids indicate content	Incineration
Drugs: medicines and tablets	• discarded medicines • toxic chemicals	Yellow receptacle with blue lid	Specialist disposal
Non-hazardous: also called domestic waste, which can be safely recycled or will compost	• packaging • food waste • vacuum cleaner dust	Black or clear bags	Recycle: (paper, glass, tin, cardboard, plastic) Compost: (vegetable and fruit peelings) Landfill: the rest
Offensive hygiene waste: non-infectious and non-hazardous, but may be unpleasant if individuals come into contact with it	• nappies • incontinence pads • sanitary wear	Yellow bag with a black stripe to alert handlers to content Picked up by arrangement with local authority	Landfill

Disposal of sharps

'Sharps' include needles, razors and scalpels. These pose a serious risk, because they may be contaminated with infected blood and can cause a penetrating wound, taking infection into the body.

Seriously harmful pathogens, such as HIV and Hepatitis B and C, can be transmitted directly into a person's blood stream through a sharps injury. When dealing with sharps you should:

▶ bring the disposal box to the used sharps, not the other way round

▶ never fill the disposal box beyond the mark indicated (approximately two thirds)

▶ keep handling of sharps to a minimum

▶ avoid passing items directly from hand to hand

▶ never recap, bend or break sharps or separate a needle from its syringe

▶ report all sharps incidents, in line with RIDDOR.

Investigate

Find out about the ways different types of healthcare waste are managed in your work setting. Include hazardous waste (clinical waste and sharps), offensive hygiene (incontinence products) and check how the colour-coded waste streams operate in your workplace.

Case study

Tilak is a personal care assistant visiting Mr Jenkins for the first time. While Mr Jenkins is in the toilet, Tilak finds used incontinence pads tied up in carrier bags under the bed. When asked about this Mr Jenkins explains that he is embarrassed to tell his daughter about his incontinence. He orders pads over the internet, but she sorts his rubbish on bin collection day, so getting rid of them has been a problem. Every few weeks Mr Jenkins removes the bags of pads from beneath his bed and burns them in the lounge fireplace.

1. What category of waste do incontinence pads fall into?

2. How is Mr Jenkins's behaviour increasing his risk of infection?

3. Explain how Mr Jenkins's incontinence pads should be disposed of to minimise infection risks.

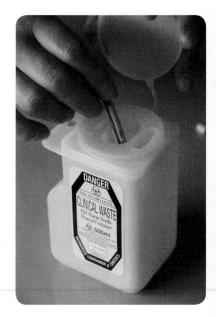

Decontamination procedures

There are three levels of **decontamination**:

1. Cleaning: using soap-based products to remove surface dirt and odour. This must take place before disinfection or sterilisation takes place.

2. Disinfection: using chemicals to kill pathogens.

3. Sterilisation: removing all pathogens and the conditions in which they survive. This is used for high risk items, such as surgical instruments.

Regular cleaning with appropriate cleaning products is necessary to create hygienic surroundings.

Key terms

Decontamination: the process of making a person, object or environment free from pathogens

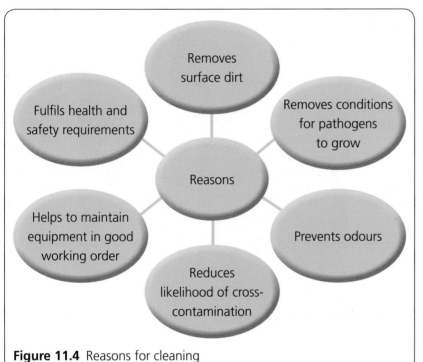

Figure 11.4 Reasons for cleaning

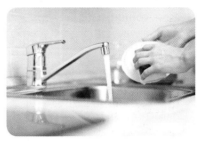

Cleaning

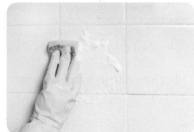

Disinfection

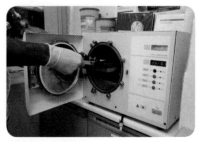

Sterilisation

Cleaning policy

Healthcare settings must have an environmental cleaning policy which provides guidance about the use of cleaning equipment and chemicals, and cleaning regimes. Chemicals must be handled with care, used in the correct concentrations, and stored and disposed of safely in accordance with COSHH. Equipment such as mops and cloths should be colour-coded to indicate the area they are intended for. This prevents cross-contamination. Mops and cloths must always be cleaned after use, left to dry in the air and replaced as necessary. A cleaning timetable ensures all areas are cleaned regularly. For example, in a healthcare setting, floors will be cleaned daily, but windows less frequently.

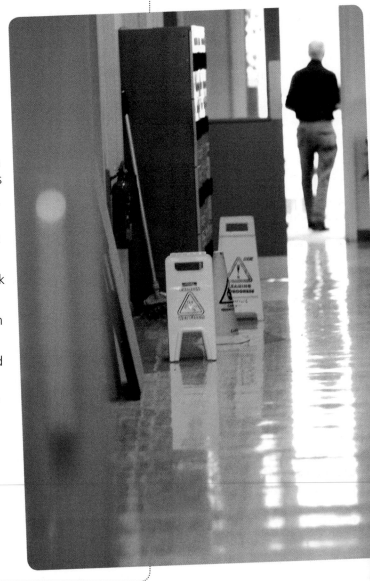

Due to the risk of body fluids carrying infection, healthcare settings usually have a specific procedure for dealing with spillages of blood, vomit, urine or faeces:

▶ the person on the spot should deal with the spillage immediately and must *never* leave it for a cleaner

▶ do an immediate risk assessment to check if the area needs to be cordoned off

▶ use appropriate equipment to deal with the spillage

▶ use appropriate PPE, such as gloves and aprons

▶ sanitiser granules can be sprinkled over the spillage to absorb the fluid and prevent it spreading

▶ use paper towels to absorb spillage

▶ dispose of using correct clinical waste stream

▶ clean area with disinfectant

▶ wash your hands thoroughly after all cleaning tasks.

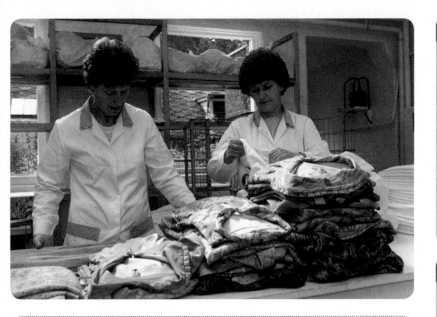

Laundry procedures

Soiled laundry is a potential source of infection when it has been contaminated with body fluids. For this reason, you should:

▶ always wear personal protective equipment (PPE) when dealing with soiled laundry

▶ place soiled items directly in the correct type of laundry bag. In some work settings specific bags for soiled laundry which dissolve on contact with hot water are used.

▶ bring the laundry bag to the bedside to minimise cross-infection risks – don't carry soiled laundry around!

▶ remove and flush any solid faeces down the toilet.

Knowledge Assessment Task   3.1

Procedures and systems to prevent and control infection when dealing with food, disposal of waste, cleaning and laundry must be followed in your working practice. Think about one task associated with each of these areas which you carry out regularly, and describe the ways in which your actions follow the infection control procedures and systems at your place of work.

Keep your notes as evidence towards your assessment.

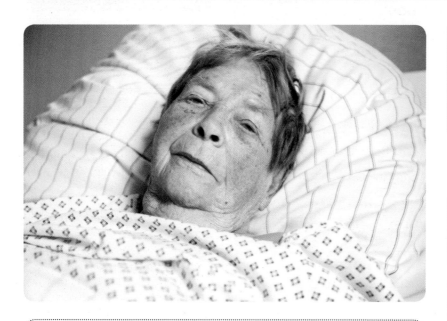

Key terms

Localised infection: an infection that is limited to a particular part of the body

Systemic infection: an infection that affects the whole body

Signs and symptoms: evidence indicating that a person is unwell

Impact of infection on the individual

Infections range from mild to very serious, and can be fatal. They can be **localised** or **systemic** and are identified by **signs and symptoms**. An infection can have a significant impact on an individual's life (see Figure 11.5).

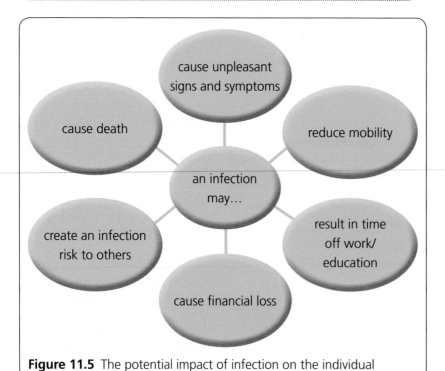

Figure 11.5 The potential impact of infection on the individual

Signs and symptoms of infection

The signs and symptoms of an infection will differ according to whether it is **localised** or **systemic**. Localised infections can spread to become systemic.

Figure 11.6 Signs and symptoms of infection

Localised infection	Systemic infection
Inflammation causing redness	Raised body temperature
Heat	Aching joints
Pain	Enlarged lymph glands
Swelling	Loss of appetite
Formation of pus	Listlessness and apathy

Adults vulnerable to infection

A number of adult groups are more vulnerable to infection than the average person. These include:

▶ older people

▶ people with chronic illnesses or disabilities

▶ people who have had surgery

▶ people who are being looked after in a hospital.

Older people and those with medical conditions may have reduced immunity. If this is the case, then it is easier for an infection to be picked up, and it is harder to fight the infection. Immobility due to frailty or illness means the lungs don't breathe as deeply and body systems are more sluggish, giving pathogens greater opportunity to invade. Surgical operations provide additional routes for infection to get into the body, such as through a wound, or at the site of an intravenous infusion or catheter.

Reflect

What signs and symptoms did you have the last time you were ill with an infection?

Investigate

Using internet or library sources find out about septicaemia (blood poisoning) which is one of the most serious affects of systemic infection.

Discuss

With colleagues, talk together about service users you have looked after who were more vulnerable to infection. Identify the reasons for this and the ways in which it impacted on their life.

Key terms

Immunity: the body's natural defence against infection provided by the immune system

Localised infection of the thumb causes swelling, inflammation and pus formation, but without treatment this could spread via the blood stream to cause potentially fatal systemic infection.

Impact of infection on the organisation

Healthcare settings are particularly vulnerable to outbreaks of infection because sick people frequently carry pathogens. With many older, less mobile and vulnerable people gathered in one place the potential for cross-infection increases dramatically.

Health Care Associated Infection (HCAI)

Health Care Associated Infections (HCAI) are infections that originate from a healthcare environment. If a person develops an infection during their stay in a healthcare setting, or within three days of their arrival or discharge, it is classed as an HCAI. One complication of HCAI is that many of the infections do not get better with common antibiotics. This antibiotic resistance has given these pathogens the nickname 'superbugs'. One common HCAI is caused by Methicillan Resistant Staphlococco Aureus (MRSA). Many people carry MRSA in or on their bodies without it causing infection. However, carriers can also transfer pathogens to others, who do develop infection. Without testing, it is not possible to know who carries MRSA.

Your assessment criteria:

3.2 Explain the potential impact of an outbreak of infection on the individual and the organisation

Key terms

Antibiotics: treatments used for infections caused by bacteria

Antibiotic resistance: the ability of some bacteria to thrive despite antibiotics

Methicillin Resistant Staphylococcus Aureus (MRSA): a staphylococcus bacterium that has developed resistance to the usual antibiotics and is a widespread HCAI

Carrier: a person who carries pathogens on or in their body without becoming ill

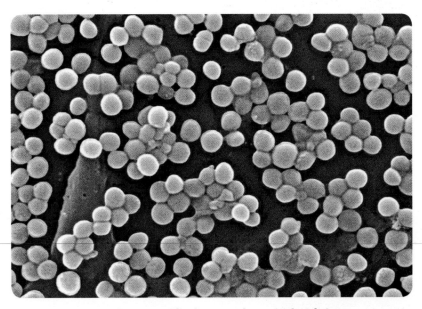

MRSA bacteria cells, magnified many thousands of times.

Case study

Mr Renfrew has dementia and attends a day hospital. This gives his wife respite and provides Mr Renfrew with a hot meal, interest and company. Before this, Mr Renfrew used to wander outside whenever his wife moved into another room. He continuously asked the same questions, and had episodes of frustration sometimes resulting in aggression towards his wife. However, Mr Renfrew has not been able to attend the day hospital since developing a chest infection, is now more confused, and has a cough which wakes him at night.

1. What factors make Mr Renfrew vulnerable to acquiring an infection?
2. What are the negative effects of acquiring an infection for Mr Renfrew?
3. How might this impact on him and his wife?

Investigate

Using newspapers, the internet and the library, find out about a recent epidemic of infection (swine flu, for example), or the increasing incidence of an infectious disease (measles, for example) in the population. What has to happen for an infection to be classed as an epidemic, or even a pandemic? What procedures are put in place in the event of an epidemic?

Key terms

Pandemic: an epidemic spread over a wide geographical area and affecting a high percentage of the population

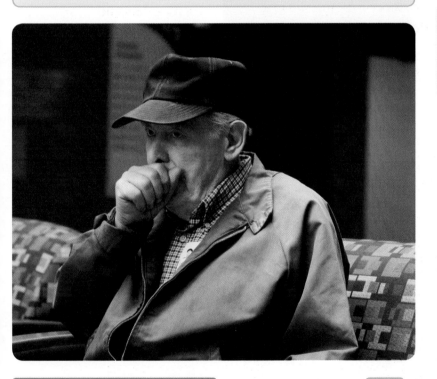

Knowledge Assessment Task   3.2

When you work in health and safety settings there is always a risk of an outbreak of infection. Make an information poster that explains how infection can affect individuals and impact on an organisation.

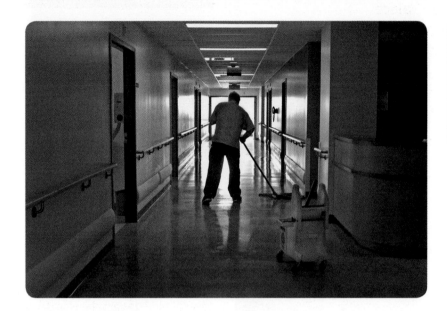

Key terms

Infection hazard: any situation that could spread pathogens

Host body: the person or animal which accommodates a virus or parasite

Cell division: the way in which bacteria reproduce and multiply

Managing the risk of infection in the workplace

In every work setting there will be potential infection hazards that pose a risk to those you care for, their families, your colleagues and yourself. Some of these risks can be removed, whilst others can be reduced to an acceptable level.

The meaning of 'risk'

Pathogens can be present anywhere. Being microscopic, it is impossible to know which area, objects or people are contaminated. Risk, or the chance of infection developing, is higher where the conditions are suitable for pathogens to multiply and be transmitted to others. A virus, for example, needs a host body in order to multiply, and cannot survive for long outside the body it invades. Similarly, bacteria need the following conditions to flourish:

▶ nutrients (broken down from deceased animals, plants, excreta, soil)

▶ moist conditions

▶ warmth

▶ oxygen, or no oxygen – depending on type of bacteria

▶ time – for cell division to take place

Infection hazards in the workplace

Infection hazards can be found in the work environment as well as being associated with the activities that commonly take place in a care setting.

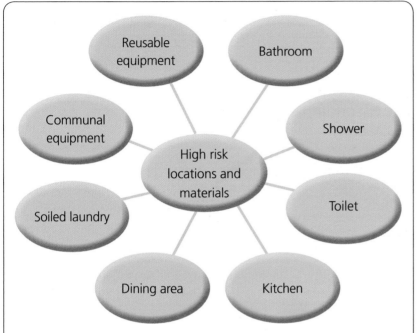

Figure 11.7 Work environment infection risks

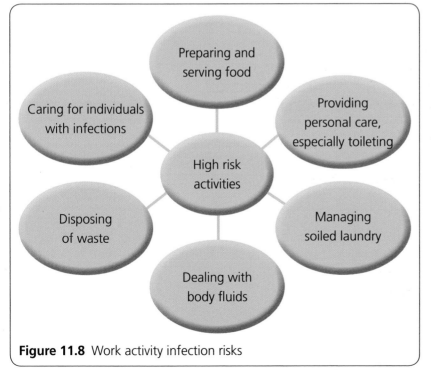

Figure 11.8 Work activity infection risks

Investigate

Using local resources and the internet, research MRSA, finding out when it was first identified, the conditions in which it develops and how it is treated and managed.

Reflect

What environmental and work-related infection hazards do you face in your work setting?

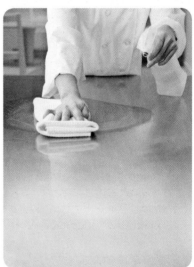

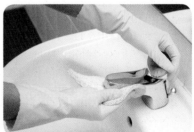

Why is risk assessment important and how is it done?

The risk assessment process

Risk assessment is a legal requirement and is central to providing infection-free work environments and working practices in health and social care settings. The steps involved in a risk assessment process relating to infection control are outlined in figure 11.9.

Your assessment criteria:

4.3 Describe the process of carrying out a risk assessment

4.4 Explain the importance of carrying out a risk assessment

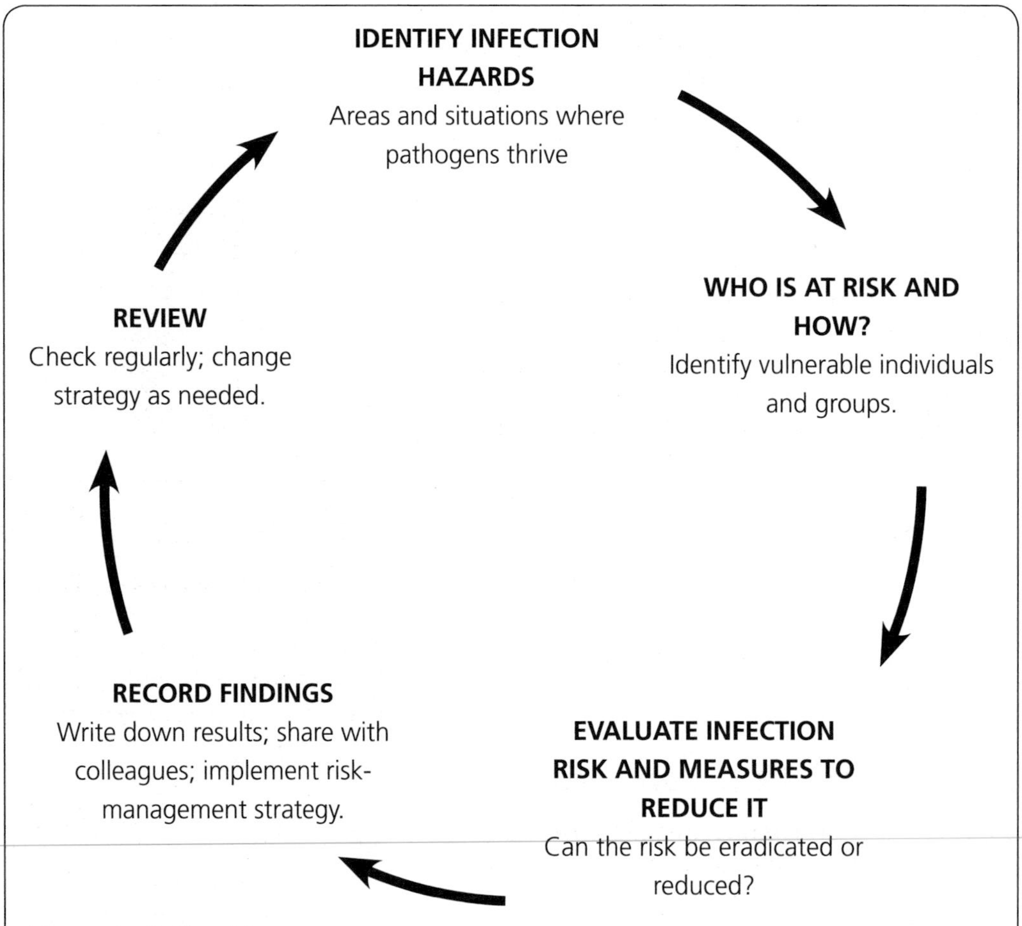

IDENTIFY INFECTION HAZARDS
Areas and situations where pathogens thrive
WHO IS AT RISK AND HOW?
Identify vulnerable individuals and groups.
EVALUATE INFECTION RISK AND MEASURES TO REDUCE IT
Can the risk be eradicated or reduced?
RECORD FINDINGS
Write down results; share with colleagues; implement risk-management strategy.
REVIEW
Check regularly; change strategy as needed.

Figure 11.9 The risk assessment process

Monitoring and reviewing risk assessments

Risk assessment is an on-going process that needs continuous review until the hazard has been eliminated or reduced to an acceptable level. Risk assessment reviews should consider:

▶ any changes in conditions that have occurred in the work setting since the last risk assessment

▶ whether the different individuals present different infection risks

▶ whether there are any new potential hazards arising.

Infection risk assessments are important because they provide an audit of infection hazards, draw attention to high risk activities and behaviours, indicate measures to reduce or remove risk, identify areas for staff training, and can be used to inform policy.

Key terms

Risk assessment: the process of identifying hazards and taking measures to reduce risk to an acceptable level

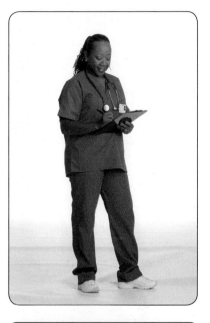

Case study

Enid Wright, aged 85, is an insulin-dependent diabetic and Precious is her carer. When helping Enid have a bath Precious notices one of Enid's toes looks red. Enid thinks it is just a mark from her shoes, as it doesn't hurt. Precious is concerned because she knows diabetics are more susceptible to infection and that diabetes can affect blood flow and cause nerve damage to the feet. She tells her manager, who advises her to carry out a risk assessment for infection.

1. What are the risks for Enid?
2. Why is it important for Precious to carry out a risk assessment on Enid?
3. What should Precious do at each stage of the risk assessment process?

Reflect

Do you think your colleagues and service users are aware of common infection hazards that exist in your work setting? Could anything be done to improve this situation?

Investigate

Talk to your manager and relevant staff members about ways to improve your understanding of infection prevention and control. Are there any local training courses or sources of information you could use to develop your knowledge further?

Knowledge Assessment Task   4.1   4.2   4.3   4.4

There are likely to be a number of potential infection risks related to your workplace and the activities that take place there. Plan a teaching session to inform staff about the importance of the risk assessment process. You must include:

▶ a definition of risk

▶ an outline of the potential risks of infection within your workplace

▶ an example that describes the process of carrying out a risk assessment for infection

▶ an explanation of why risk assessment is important.

Keep the work that you produce as evidence towards your assessment.

Using personal protective clothing (PPE) in the prevention and control of infection

What are the correct ways to use personal protective equipment?

In adult health and social care settings **personal protective clothing (PPE)** creates a barrier between care practitioners and service users, protecting both parties from acquiring and transmitting pathogens.

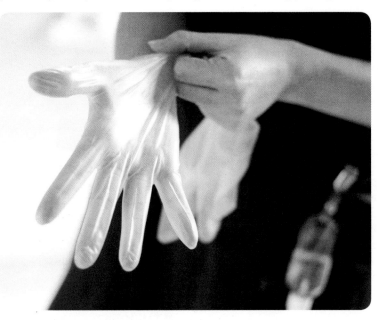

PPE only remains an effective barrier when it is used correctly. Most items are disposable and designed for single use. If you repeatedly use the same item of PPE, it will become an infection hazard, and cease to protect against infection. PPE is used to cover areas of the body that can be both routes for pathogens to enter the body and cause infection, as well as routes for pathogens to exit the body to spread infection to others. PPE also protects against pathogens that are present in the air, on skin, on objects and in fluids, and which can be passed from person to person and from person to objects.

These are the main steps for correct use of PPE:

▶ wash your hands before using PPE

▶ select the appropriate type of PPE for the task

▶ make sure PPE is intact and undamaged

▶ make sure PPE fully covers the area intended

▶ remove PPE immediately following use

▶ dispose of PPE into the appropriate waste stream

▶ wash your hands after disposing of PPE.

Your assessment criteria:

5.1 Demonstrate correct use of personal protective equipment (PPE)

5.2 Describe different types of PPE

5.3 Explain the reasons for use of PPE

Key terms

Personal Protective Equipment (PPE): equipment and clothing, such as disposable gloves and aprons, that are used to create a barrier against pathogens that cause disease

Mucosa: skin that lines areas inside of the body, such as inside the mouth

Sterile: free from pathogens

Reflect

Consider the types of PPE that you use at work on a regular basis. Do you know the occasions when these should be worn? Do you know how to dispose of them correctly?

Using different types of personal protective equipment

A range of PPE items is commonly used in health and social care settings. These are set out in Figure 11.10, along with the reasons for their use.

Figure 11.10 Types of PPE and their uses

Type of PPE	Reason for use	Occasions to use
Plastic aprons	Cover clothes or uniform. Made from slippery plastic, it is harder for pathogens to stick. Suitable to protect from body fluids and to be worn during other tasks that hold a risk of bringing you into contact with pathogens	**1.** Helping service users with: • toileting • washing **2.** Contact with **mucosa**: • giving oral care • administering suppositories • doing dressings **3.** Preparing and serving food **4.** Dealing with body fluids: • cleaning spillages • obtaining specimens • emptying catheter bags **5.** Disposing of rubbish
Plastic or latex gloves	Protection for hands and nails, which are the main way pathogens are transmitted	
Paper masks	To cover mouth and nose, which are key sources of pathogens, as well as routes for pathogens to gain entry into the body	**1.** Tasks bringing you in close proximity to a source of infection, such as a wound
Cloth or paper gowns (sometimes fluid repellent)	Provide a complete covering for the body and can be used with plastic aprons on top	**2.** In areas where there is a need for **sterile** conditions, such as operating theatres
Plastic over-shoes	Worn over normal shoes to prevent pathogens from outside being brought into clean areas	**3.** Where there is the likelihood of splashing with body fluids, such as when assisting with childbirth
Paper hair-cover	Covers head to prevent stray hairs escaping	Handling, preparing, cooking and serving food
Plastic goggles	Completely cover eyes, including fitting over glasses	Used where there is particular risk of body fluid splashes, such as to protect dentists and hygienists

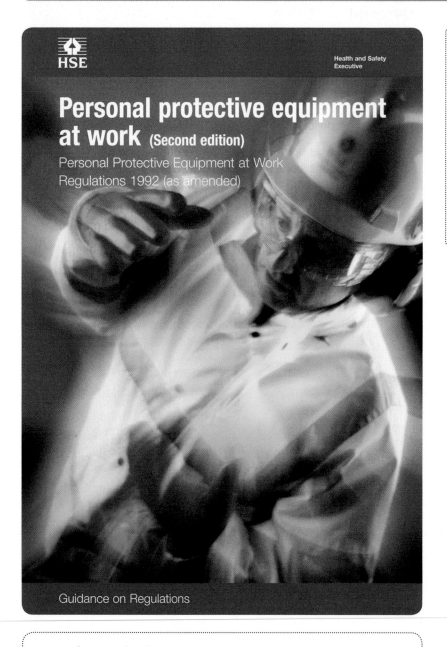

HSE

Health and Safety Executive

Personal protective equipment at work (Second edition)

Personal Protective Equipment at Work Regulations 1992 (as amended)

Guidance on Regulations

Your assessment criteria:

5.4 State current relevant regulations and legislation relating to PPE

5.5 Describe employees' responsibilities regarding the use of PPE

5.6 Describe employers' responsibilities regarding the use of PPE

Legal regulations

Employers must manage the workplace and their workforce to satisfy the law regarding PPE, and employees must follow the guidance set out in organisational policy and procedures. The Personal Protective Equipment (PPE) at Work Regulations set out these responsibilities; European legislation means PPE must carry the CE marking.

Key terms

CE marking: the marking on an item of equipment that shows the product conforms to European standards to do with consumer safety, health or environmental requirements

Figure 11.11 Employer and employee roles and responsibilities

Your manager must:	You must:
• supply appropriate PPE • maintain and store PPE correctly • provide training, instruction and notices about PPE • carry out risk assessments to inform decisions about appropriate PPE • ensure PPE is being used and used properly	• use PPE at appropriate times • report if PPE is faulty or stocks are low • attend training and follow instructions about using PPE • carry out and follow risk assessments about appropriate PPE for task • use PPE on all appropriate occasions, and never cut corners. • dispose of PPE appropriately

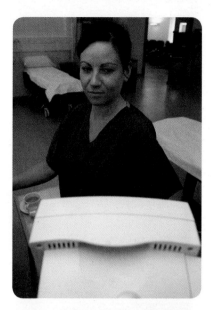

Knowledge Assessment Task · 5.4 · 5.5 · 5.6

Case study

Maria is a new healthcare assistant working in an orthopaedic rehabilitation ward. She has recently returned to work after having a family and remarks that a lot has changed in the last ten years, especially the frequent use of plastic aprons and gloves. She feels the aprons look cheap and spoil the look of her uniform and the gloves get in the way when she is doing tasks. She says she cannot understand why their employer bothers.

1. Which current legislation and regulations relating to PPE does Maria need to know about?
2. Describe employee responsibilities regarding the use of PPE that Maria needs to be aware of.
3. What does Maria need to know about her employer's responsibilities regarding the use of PPE?

Keep the work that you produce as evidence towards your assessment.

Reflect

Do you or your colleagues ever 'cut corners' or avoid using PPE when providing care? Do you think stocks of PPE, such as aprons and gloves, are placed in the right places to remind practitioners in your setting to use and change equipment at the appropriate times?

Investigate

Using your local library, the internet and work sources, find out about training materials regarding PPE, and look at ways of adapting these to create an information poster relevant to your place of work.

Applying and removing personal protective equipment and disposing of used PPE

How to apply, remove and dispose of PPE correctly

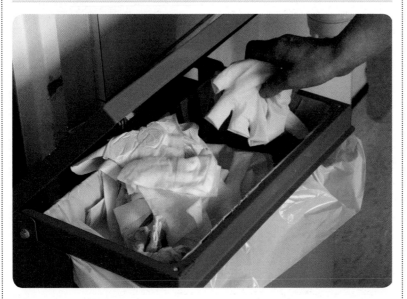

PPE must be applied, removed, and disposed of correctly, or it will become an infection control hazard rather than a means of protecting individuals from infection.

Reflect

Are there ever occasions when you may need to use PPE other than gloves and aprons? Perhaps paper masks, goggles, over-shoes. If this is the case, find out from your manager or other colleagues the correct ways to use these.

Figure 11.12 Correct application, removal, and disposal of PPE

PPE items	How to apply	How to remove	How to dispose of
Gloves and aprons	1. Wash hands before use. 2. Put on gloves and apron before starting the procedure. 3. Change gloves and aprons between caring for different service users and between different care tasks for the same service user.	1. Remove as soon as the procedure is complete. 2. Take off carefully and in such a way that your hands and clothes/uniform do not have contact with any substances contaminating the glove or apron surface.	1. Gloves are for single use only and must be disposed of after removing. 2. Dispose of as clinical waste. 3. Do not touch the bin with contaminated gloves or hands – where possible operate with a foot pedal. 4. Wash hands with soap as soon as gloves/aprons are disposed of.

Knowledge Assessment Task   5.1 5.2 5.3 5.7 5.8

Personal Protective Equipment is an important element of infection prevention and control. Complete a table like the one below with an overview of each different item of PPE used in your work environment.

Description of type of PPE	Explanation of why it is used	How to apply, use, remove and dispose of

Keep the work that you produce for this activity as evidence towards your assessment.

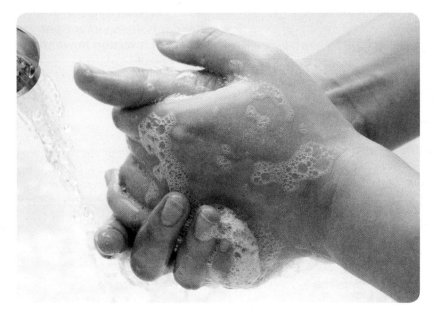

The key principles of good hygiene

Personal hygiene is a private matter, but when you work in a care setting you have a professional responsibility to maintain a *regulated* standard of personal hygiene which is set out in a personal hygiene or infection control policy.

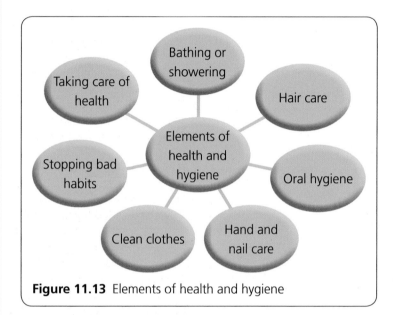

Figure 11.13 Elements of health and hygiene

Bathing and showering

Regular bathing or showering prevents the spread of bacteria, and reduces body odour.

Hair care

Regular hair washing prevents the spread of bacteria. Long hair will need to be tied back. Some care environments bring you into contact with head lice which infest clean hair as readily as dirty hair. Regular combing with a fine-toothed comb will help prevent this, but in the event of an infestation, ask your pharmacist for advice about treatment.

Oral hygiene

Good oral hygiene and six monthly visits to the dentist will prevent the build-up of bacteria and reduce halitosis (bad breath). It is especially important to brush following meals or after smoking.

Hand and nail care

Hand and nail care is vital in preventing and controlling the spread of infection. It is discussed in detail on page 300.

It is discussed in detail on page 300.

Your assessment criteria:

6.1 Describe the key principles of good personal hygiene

Key terms

Hygiene: a set of practices to achieve cleanliness and maintain health

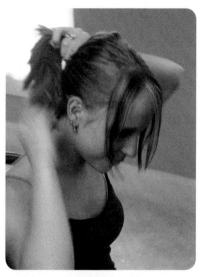

Good personal hygiene standards are an important aspect of infection prevention and control

Clean clothes

Clean work clothes are an important aspect of personal hygiene, and should be changed daily, even when covered by plastic aprons while working. Uniforms are made of hard-wearing materials that launder at high temperatures to remove most pathogens.

Cutting out certain habits

Some habits that affect personal hygiene include:

▶ smoking, which involves putting your hand to your mouth and increases the likelihood of coughing

▶ touching the face, especially nose, mouth and ears, which are routes for infection

▶ nail biting, which can produce sores and risks spreading infection

▶ sneezing and coughing without covering the mouth; not disposing of tissues properly; and not washing hands afterwards.

Taking care of health

Good personal hygiene practice is bolstered by a healthy lifestyle, which helps both avoid and fight off infection. Sleep refreshes and renews your body. Good nutrition keeps your body and brain processes working well. Fluids help to rid you of toxic waste products. If unwell stay away from work to prevent spreading infection.

Reflect

Think about the standards you keep regarding your personal health and hygiene. Do you think you do enough?

Investigate

Using a library and the internet, look up information about a number of different infection epidemics within care services – such as outbreaks of winter vomiting in care homes. What procedures are put in place when outbreaks occur? What are the effects and the outcome of outbreaks of infection?

Reflect

Staff members going off sick can pose a difficult problem for managers in a care environment. Many care workers report feeling pressurised to go into work when unwell because of staff shortages. Talk about ways to deal with this problem and improve the health of staff.

Case study

Anya works at a forensic day centre for adults who have committed serious crimes while mentally unwell. She notices most of the patients and staff smoke and have a high sickness rate, with frequent colds and chest infections.

1. How does smoking impact on standards of personal hygiene?
2. What is the connection between other bad habits and reduced standards of personal hygiene?
3. Why is it important to maintain a high standard of personal hygiene at work?

Knowledge Assessment Task   6.1

For this activity you need to produce a set of personal hygiene guidelines aimed at new staff coming to work, volunteer or undertake work experience in your workplace. You can decide how you present this, as a poster, a leaflet or a booklet, but it must include a description of the key principles of good personal hygiene and the ways this relates to infection prevention and control.

Keep your notes as evidence towards your assessment.

Good hand washing technique

Hands are the most common means of transmitting pathogens and spreading infection. Hand washing following correct procedure and carried out in the right sequence at appropriate times is the single most effective way of preventing and controlling infection. There are three stages to a good hand washing technique: preparation; washing and rinsing; drying.

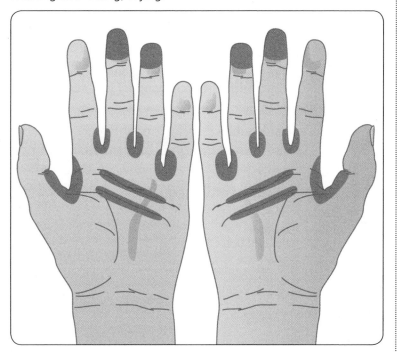

Most frequently missed areas in hand washing

Preparation

You need to carry out a number of preparations before washing your hands:

1. Check sink and taps to ensure these are clean before use.

2. Check equipment to ensure there is soap, towels or a hand drier available.

3. Remove jewellery, which harbours pathogens and may prevent you washing thoroughly for fear of damaging them.

4. Roll sleeves up to expose wrists and forearms.

5. Run water to a warm temperature as uncomfortable temperatures reduces time spent washing hands.

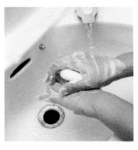
. Lather hands with soap

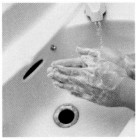
2. Rub both palms together

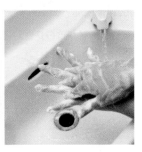
3. Rub each fingers and between fingers

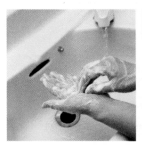
. Rub palms with finger nails

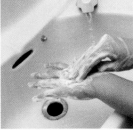
5. Rub back of hand with finger nails

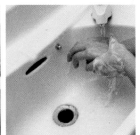
6. Wash thoroughly and towel dry

The stages of hand washing

Washing and rinsing

There are a number of important factors to consider when washing and rinsing your hands:

1. Preferably use running water.

2. Wet hands thoroughly before using soap.

3. Soap hands, making sure the solution comes into contact with all areas.

4. Rub hands together vigorously for a minimum of 10–15 seconds, paying particular attention to the tips of the fingers, the thumbs and the areas between the fingers.

5. Rinse hands thoroughly.

Drying

It is vital that hands are dried thoroughly. Ideally use a hot air drier, and continue using until your hands are totally dry. Alternatively, use paper towels, discarding them without touching the bin with your hands.

Knowledge Assessment Task   6.2   6.3

You have been asked to demonstrate the proper technique for thorough hand washing to Shilpa, a student on placement. Provide a detailed description of good hand-washing technique, including the correct sequence for each stage of the process. This will provide Shilpa with a written reminder of your demonstration.

Keep your notes as evidence towards your assessment.

When and why should hand washing be carried out?

Your assessment criteria:

6.4 Explain when and why hand washing should be carried out

Sometimes it is obvious when your hands need washing, because there is visible dirt, but at other times you must wash your hands even if they do not look dirty.

Figure 11.14 When and why to wash your hands

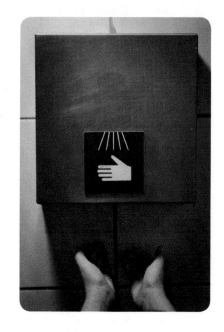

When	Why
Whenever hands are sticky or soiled with visible dirt	To remove surface dirt
After going to the toilet, touching mouth or nose	To remove pathogens present in body fluids and so remove possible contamination
Before and after direct contact with service users	To protect the service users from your pathogens and you from theirs
Between different care activities for the same service user	Some activities are cleaner than others and cross-contamination can take place between different areas of a person's body
Before putting on and after removing disposable gloves	You do not wear gloves as an alternative to washing your hands – gloves are just for higher risk activities
After any contact with body fluids	Body fluids provide a suitable environment for pathogens to multiply
Before and after handling, cooking, serving and eating food	Food is an environment where pathogens multiply; eating provides a route into the body, where infection can occur
After all cleaning tasks	To remove contamination transferred to your hands after cleaning dirty areas
After dealing with rubbish and soiled laundry	Waste and soiled laundry are environments where pathogens can multiply
After feeding and handling pets	Animals harbour pathogens that can spread to humans

Investigate

Use the internet, library or your workplace to find out as much as you can about the 'Cleanyourhands' campaign and the World Health Organization's (WHO) *Five Moments for Hand Hygiene*.

Discuss

Share ideas with colleagues for running a local hand hygiene campaign. Use the information you researched from the 'Cleanyourhands' campaign to make the campaign relevant to your workplace.

Knowledge Assessment Task   6.4

Read through the list, below, of Esther's duties, and indicate the occasions when she should wash her hands. Give reasons for your decisions.

Esther's first job of the day is to serve breakfast to all the residents. Part way through his porridge, Mr Lassiter needs to go to the toilet so Esther assists him and then helps him finish his breakfast. She makes three beds, one of which is soiled. She dispenses the medications, runs the newspaper group and goes to a supervision session with the deputy manager before going for lunch.

Keep your notes as evidence towards your assessment.

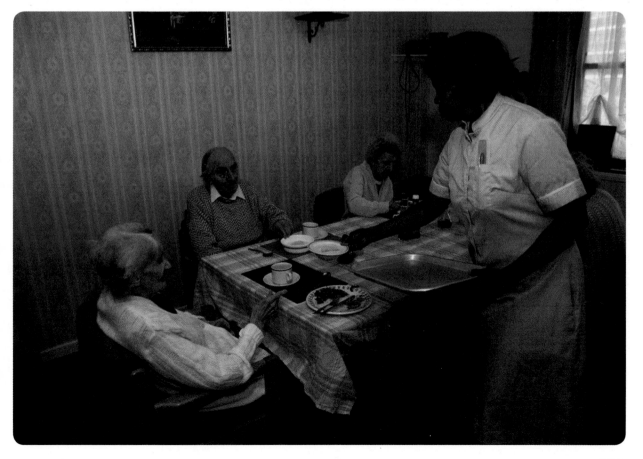

What hand washing products and skin care procedures should be used?

Hand washing products

There are two main types of hand washing products:

▶ soap-based for areas where there is a lower risk of infection

▶ **antimicrobial** products for use in high risk areas.

Ideally, soap dispensers should be used because these are more hygienic than bar soap. Bar soap is handled by a number of people and pathogens can survive on it, plus soap that has dried out to cracking point is not effective. If you are working in a service user's own home and using their facilities, it may be appropriate to request soap in a dispenser. However, there is less chance of cross-infection in a private home than in a healthcare environment.

Alcohol based hand-rub

If it is difficult to get access to running water and soap, and hands are not visibly soiled, it is acceptable to use alcohol hand-rub (gel or foam) instead. The solution must come into contact with all surfaces of the hand, and hands rubbed together vigorously, paying particular attention to the frequently missed areas (see page 300). Many care workers carry a bottle of hand-rub gel around with them.

(see page 300)

Your assessment criteria:

6.5 Describe the types of products that should be used for hand washing

6.6 Describe correct procedures that relate to skincare

> **Key terms**

Antimicrobial: a substance to kill or inhibit the growth of microorganisms, including bacteria and fungi

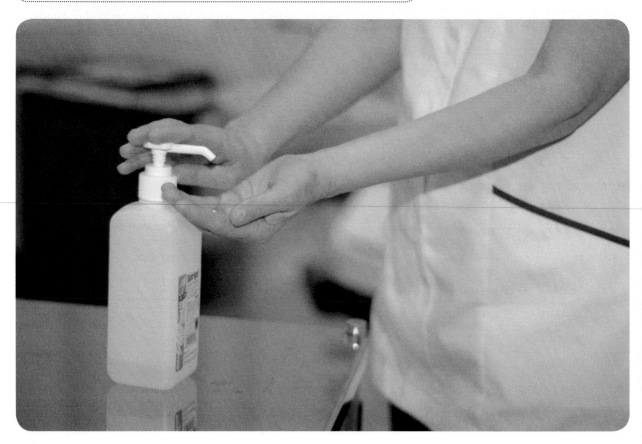

Skincare

Prevent your hands from becoming dry and sore, where abrasions can provide both a route and source of infection. Cleansing products that are gentle on the skin are recommended, also **hypo-allergenic** disposable gloves. If allergy problems arise see your doctor or ask to be referred to occupational health services.

Case study

Maxine works as a healthcare assistant and her hands are in and out of water all day. She carries a miniature bottle of alcohol hand-rub and hand cream, both of which she uses frequently. In the past couple of days Maxine has noticed a red rash on both hands made up of tiny raised pimples. It is inflamed, sore and itchy.

1. What might be happening to Maxine?
2. What implications does Maxine's skin condition have for carrying out her role as a healthcare assistant?
3. What would you do if you were Maxine?

Knowledge Assessment Task   6.5   6.6

Micah is on work experience and you have been asked to work alongside him. He is very keen and asks lots of questions. Read through these and give your answers, which must include full descriptions.

1. Why is soap from a dispenser used, rather than bar soap?
2. Why are visitors to the area asked to apply antiseptic hand gel?
3. Why do some of the care practitioners carry antiseptic hand gel in their pocket?
4. What are the correct procedures to care for skin when you work in a care environment?

Keep your notes as evidence towards your assessment.

Key terms

Hypo-allergenic: describes materials/chemicals free of substances that commonly cause allergies

Reflect

Think about the number of times you are required to wash your hands. It is no wonder they can become chapped and sore. How do you look after your hands to prevent the skin becoming damaged from hand washing?

Investigate

Find out if it is possible to hire a hand contamination box. This might be available through the infection prevention and control team based at your local hospital. This uses a particular light to show up areas of contamination – even after hands have been washed.

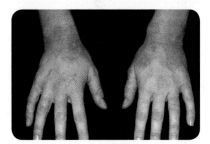

Hands affected by dermatitis, inflammation of the outer layer of skin

Are you ready for assessment?

AC	What do you know now?	Assessment task	✓
1.1	Explain employees' roles and responsibilities in relation to the prevention and control of infection	Page 273	
1.2	Explain employers' responsibilities in relation to the prevention and control of infection	Page 273	
2.1	Outline current legislation and regulatory body standards which are relevant to the prevention and control of infection	Page 277	
2.2	Describe local and organisational policies relevant to the prevention and control of infection	Page 277	
3.1	Describe procedures and systems relevant to the prevention and control of infection	Page 283	
3.2	Explain the potential impact of an outbreak of infection on the individual and the organisation	Page 287	
4.1	Define the term 'risk'	Page 291	
4.2	Outline potential risks of infection within the workplace	Page 291	
4.3	Describe the process of carrying out a risk assessment	Page 291	
4.4	Explain the importance of carrying out a risk assessment	Page 291	
5.1	Demonstrate correct use of personal protective equipment (PPE)	Page 297	
5.2	Describe different types of PPE	Page 297	
5.3	Explain the reasons for use of PPE	Page 297	
5.4	State current relevant regulations and legislation relating to PPE	Page 295	
5.5	Describe employees' responsibilities regarding the use of PPE	Page 295	
5.6	Describe employers' responsibilities regarding the use of PPE	Page 295	
5.7	Describe the correct practice in the application and removal of PPE	Page 297	
5.8	Describe the correct procedure for disposal of used PPE	Page 297	
6.1	Describe the key principles of good personal hygiene	Page 299	
6.2	Demonstrate good hand washing technique	Page 301	
6.3	Describe the correct sequence for hand washing	Page 301	
6.4	Explain when and why hand washing should be carried out	Page 303	
6.5	Describe the types of products that should be used for hand washing	Page 305	
6.6	Describe correct procedures that relate to skincare	Page 305	

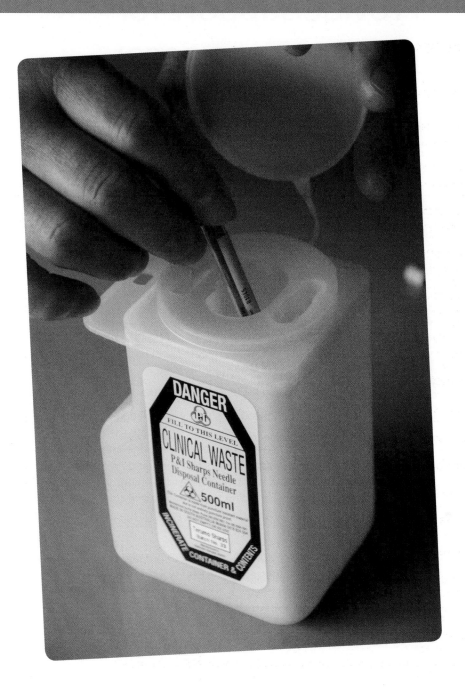

12 | Provide support for mobility (HSC 2002)

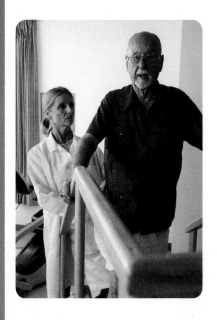

Assessment of this unit

This unit describes the importance of providing support for mobility to people who have problems moving safely by themselves. People who use health and social care services often have problems with their mobility. This can be for a wide range of reasons, including weakness in their muscles, the effects of a disease or following an accident. The unit focuses on your role in preparing for mobility activities, and in supporting individuals in keeping mobile. It provides you with the knowledge and skills needed to:

▶ understand the importance of mobility

▶ prepare for mobility activities

▶ support individuals to keep mobile

▶ observe, record and report on activities to support mobility.

The assessment of this unit is partly knowledge-based and partly competence-based. To successfully complete the unit, you will need to produce evidence of both your knowledge and your competence. Knowledge-based assessments test the things you need to know. Competence-based assessments test the things you need to do in the work environment. The tables below and opposite outline what you need to know and do to meet each of the assessment criteria for the unit.

Your tutor or assessor will help you to prepare for your assessment and the tasks suggested in the unit will help you to create the evidence that you need.

AC	What you need to know
1.1	Define mobility
1.2	Explain how different health conditions may affect and be affected by mobility
1.3	Outline the effects that reduced mobility may have on an individual's wellbeing
1.4	Describe the benefits of maintaining and improving mobility

AC	What you need to do
2.1	Agree mobility activities with the individual and others
2.2	Remove or minimise hazards in the environment before a mobility activity
2.3	Check the suitability of an individual's clothing and footwear for safety and mobility
2.4	Check the safety and cleanliness of mobility equipment and appliances
3.1	Promote active participation during a mobility activity
3.2	Assist an individual to use mobility appliances correctly and safely
3.3	Give feedback and encouragement to the individual during mobility activities
4.1	Observe an individual to monitor changes and responses during a mobility activity
4.2	Record observations of mobility activity
4.3	Report on progress and/or problems relating to the mobility activity including: choice of activities, equipment, appliances and the support provided

AC 2.1–4.3 must be assessed in a real work environment.

This unit also links to some of the other units:

HSC 2013	Support care plan activities
HSC 2015	Support individuals to meet personal care needs
HSC 2028	Move and position individuals

Some of your learning will be repeated in these units and will give you the chance to review your knowledge and understanding.

Understanding the importance of mobility for the individual's wellbeing

What is mobility?

Mobility is the ability to move, independently or with the support and assistance of others. It is about individuals moving themselves or being helped to move by others who provide support, equipment or appliances to make movement possible.

Why is mobility important?

Mobility is important because it allows people to socialise, to work, play and keep fit. Without mobility people would soon become ill and unfit. Not being able to move can also be frightening and this must be understood when communicating with people you are helping.

Figure 12.1 Challenges and problems of mobility

Challenge	Problem
Independence	Mobility is a key aspect of an individual's independence. Most people are used to moving where they want when they want. Losing this ability to move unaided seriously affects an individual's independence and makes them more dependent on other people. People should be encouraged to move independently, even if it involves using equipment. The less mobile a person is during or shortly after an episode of ill health, the less likely they are to regain their mobility.
Time	This is a key factor. The longer a person is immobile the more difficult it will be to regain the ability to move, with or without equipment or mobility appliances.
Safety	There is a risk that an individual will come to harm if they try to move when they have a health condition that prevents them moving freely.

Your assessment criteria:

1.1 Define mobility

Key terms

Mobility: the ability to move, independently or with support

Reflect

Can you think of ways in which limited or impaired mobility can affect a person's independence?

Investigate

What adaptations or procedures are there at your place of work to ensure that individuals with limited or impaired mobility can access the services and move around freely?

Case study

Peter and his friend Paul usually walk together to school and get a lift home in the afternoon with one of their parents. There is a busy road to cross which often means they have to run. One morning on the way to school they stopped to knock horse chestnuts out of a tree to play conkers later. Peter climbed a tree, but lost his footing and fell. At first he thought he had broken his ankle, but managed to walk the rest of the way to school. By the afternoon, though, his ankle was swollen and painful, and he wasn't able to walk. In the evening he was taken to the accident and emergency department where his ankle was bandaged. The doctor told him about the risks of not being treated straightaway, and that he should not have tried to put any weight on his damaged ankle. He was supplied with a crutch and told not to bear weight on his foot for a week.

1. How is Peter's independence affected by his *mobility* problem?
2. What are the potential risks for Peter?
3. Reflect on what it is like to have your mobility impeded.

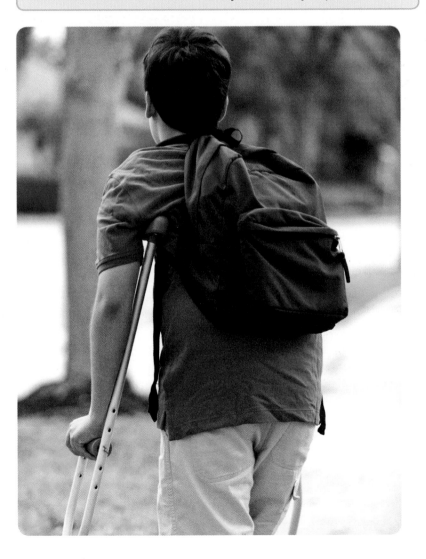

Health conditions that affect mobility

Different health conditions may affect and be affected by mobility. Any disease or condition that requires **bed rest** or that seriously limits activity can be said to affect mobility. Immobility is where a person's movement is constrained or restricted.

Joint problems

Joint problems can affect the individual's ability to move. Health conditions that affect joints are described in Figure 12.2 below.

Key terms

Bed rest: continuous confinement to bed

Joint: connection, such as the knee, elbow and wrist, which allows for the movement of parts of the body

Figure 12.2 Health conditions and their effects on mobility

Causes of immobility	How mobility is affected
Arthritis	Arthritis is the name given to a group of conditions, including rheumatoid arthritis and osteoarthritis, that involve damage to the joints. Arthritis makes it difficult for the person to be active, and causes pain, swelling of the joint and stiffness. It can result in inability to use the hands or even to walk.
Torn ligament	A sprained ankle is an example of damaged ligaments. Sprains occur when the ankle is twisted or rolled more than usual – such as when it is placed on an uneven surface. The ligaments, which hold the bone and joint in place, are stretched into an abnormal position. The person may not be able to walk unaided and may have a limp for a while.
Joint swelling	Knee effusion – or 'water on the knee' – is an example of a swollen joint. It occurs when excess fluid gathers around the knee. The individual may need help from a walking aid, and should not take part in vigorous activity.
Bone fractures	These are caused by a break in the bone. There are different kinds of fracture, including: complete fracture, where the bone is snapped; incomplete fracture, where the bone is still joined together but cracked in some way. In the case of legs or arms, the bones are usually protected in a plaster cast until they are mended. With a fractured leg bone the person may not be able to walk at all for a few weeks and then will need an aid, such as a crutch, to walk.
Infections	A bacterial infection of a joint can cause a severe form of arthritis known as septic arthritis. Other forms of joint infection are caused by knee or other joint replacement – the person has an artificial joint infection. Symptoms may include pain and fever. It is painful to bear weight on the joint, affecting the individual's ability to walk.

Case study

Ingrid, aged 88, has complained to her daughter that she is finding it more and more difficult to get to the shops, even though they are only 100 metres down the road from her flat. Her knees and hips hurt when she moves. For a number of years Ingrid's joints have been becoming swollen and stiffening. At first Ingrid just accepted the pain as something that came with age, but now it is severely restricting her mobility. She does not want to see a doctor about it because she fears having to have an operation. Instead she has tried taking pain killers and anti-inflammatory medicines she buys over the counter. These worked for a short time, but did not stop the deterioration. Her daughter suspects what might be the cause of Ingrid's pain and restricted mobility, but as she knows her mother is afraid of involving the medical profession she doesn't want to say what she thinks the problem is.

1. What joint problem do you think Ingrid might be suffering from?
2. How does this joint problem affect individuals?
3. What other types of joint problems are there?

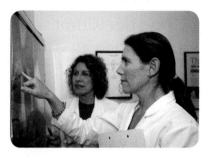

Key terms

Complete injury: the term for a spinal cord injury resulting in paralysis below the point of injury

Figure 12.3 Other causes of immobility and their effects

Cause of immobility	How mobility is affected
Stroke	Strokes are a disturbance of the blood supply to the brain due to lack of blood flow or a leaking of blood in the brain. The person usually loses the use of one side of their body. This can mean they lose the ability to walk.
Depression	Depression is a form of mental disorder in which the person feels very sad over a long period, thinks negatively and lacks the will power to be active. It may mean that they stay in bed, or don't move, because nothing seems worthwhile.
Dementia	Dementia is a term given to a cognitive disorder in which there is a gradual loss of ability to think and remember, so that the person forgets to move about – for example, to make a meal or use the toilet. Dementia usually affects older people.
Ulceration	This is an area of skin erosion, often found on the leg, in which a sore becomes infected. Ulcers can be caused by bed sores, such as when an older person is left lying in the same position for a long time. Ulcers can result in pain and difficulty in moving unaided.
Muscular sclerosis (MS)	Muscular sclerosis affects the ability of the brain cells and cells in the spinal cord to communicate with each other. It can lead to numbness and muscular weakness, with the individual having to use a wheel chair.
Spinal cord injury	Spinal cord injury is often a result of an accident or injury. There are two main classifications: • **complete injury**, in which the nerve connection below the point of damage is lost, causing paralysis with little chance of total recovery • incomplete injury, where there is still some sensation below the point of damage, so the person can move a bit, and will probably improve.

The effects that reduced mobility may have on an individual's wellbeing

Reduced mobility may have many effects on an individual's wellbeing.

Psychological and emotional effects

Reduced mobility may have a significant psychological and emotional impact on a person. The psychological and emotional effects cannot always be seen, but may be discovered by talking to a person with reduced mobility.

Figure 12.4 Psychological and emotional effects of immobility

Psychological and emotional aspects	Effects
Confidence	An older person who has fallen when walking about the house may fear falling again, and then become less confident walking alone or unaided.
Depression and anxiety	Depression can affect anyone of whatever age when their mobility is reduced. People can become unhappy and frustrated when they cannot do what they are used to doing. Inactive people may have higher anxiety levels than people who exercise regularly.
Loneliness and isolation	Reduced mobility can lead to loneliness and isolation, especially if the individual cannot leave the house. There is the danger that the individual becomes housebound and isolated, spending more time than they want alone.

Practical and financial effects

As a result of reduced mobility, individuals may experience a range of financial and practical difficulties.

Figure 12.5 Practical and financial effects of immobility

Practical and financial aspects	Effects
Unemployment	Reduced mobility leads to fewer job opportunties. Children and young people with reduced mobility are less likely to be in education, training or employment, thus having fewer chances of getting a good job.
Inactivity	Reduced mobility can affect an individual's ability to do things they enjoy, such as gardening, and everyday activities that people generally do without thinking, such as carrying the rubbish to the bin.
Inability to access services	Being unable to stand for long periods, such as when waiting for a bus, can mean it is harder for people with reduced mobility to access services that other people take for granted.
Expense	Reduced mobility can mean the individual has to buy aids and appliances to help them walk. This can be expensive.

Physical effects

There are numerous ways that reduced mobility affects the physical wellbeing of individuals.

Figure 12.6 Effects of immobility on physical wellbeing

Physical aspects	Effects
Cardiovascular	Cardiovascular problems that are caused or made worse by lack of exercise may lead to more serious heart conditions and strokes.
Muscular and joint stiffness	Muscular and joint stiffness can be made worse by lack of exercise, leading to further weakness.
Pain	Pain is a big problem that can make the individual less likely to try to be mobile.
Balance	Balance can be affected so that the individual is more likely to fall or bump into things like furniture.
Obesity	Obesity can be made worse as the person's lack of movement and exercise leads to the build-up of fat.
Medication	Some medications that people take for health problems can cause the individual to feel dizzy, lethargic and unmotivated.

Key terms

Cardiovascular: the term for anything that relates to the lungs and heart

Obesity: a recognised medical condition in which excess fat has accumulated to the point of negatively affecting an individual's health

Case study

Evelyn has muscular sclerosis (MS), which she contracted when she was 25. The illness has left her with muscle weakness in her legs so that she cannot stand for long periods or walk more than a few paces. The illness is slowly getting worse, making her more reliant on other people to do the things she once did independently. She lives by herself in a small ground floor flat, and uses a wheelchair to get about the local area. She can only work occasionally due to her health problem. A friend takes her shopping once a week, and another friend drives her to church on Sunday mornings. At other times Evelyn uses a local taxi service as the nearest bus stop is too far to reach unaided. While Evelyn appreciates the help, it makes her feel over-dependent on her friends. She also feels vulnerable in crowded places such as busy shops.

1. Describe one possible psychological and emotional effect of her reduced mobility.
2. Describe one possible practical and financial effect of her reduced mobility.
3. Describe one possible physical effect of her reduced mobility.

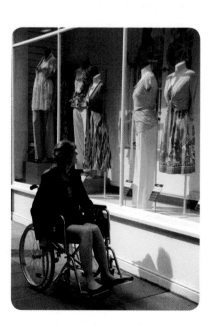

The benefits of maintaining and improving mobility

Your assessment criteria:

1.4 Describe the benefits of maintaining and improving mobility

There are many benefits to maintaining and improving mobility. These can be divided into psychological and emotional benefits, financial and practical benefits, and physical benefits.

Psychological and emotional benefits

By trying to maintain and improve mobility an individual can become more confident, overcome depression and feel less anxious. They are also less likely to be isolated in their own home. A person who is able to maintain or improve mobility following, or despite, a period of ill health, is likely to experience a boost in their self-esteem.

Practical and financial benefits

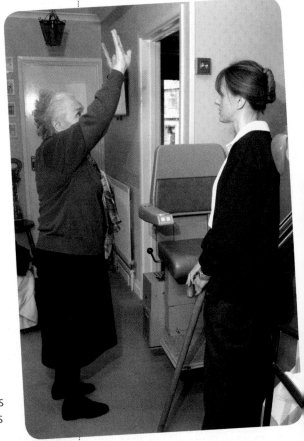

The practical and financial benefits of being more mobile can lead to opportunities to attend college, undertake work training or to take a job. This in turn will make it more likely that the individual will earn money that enables them to buy things they want and travel both in their local areas and further afield. A person who is able to improve their mobility will also not have to spend their income on aids and appliances to help them walk or travel around.

Physical benefits

The physical benefits are that the individual can keep fitter and healthier so that other health conditions that can make mobility even harder to achieve, such as obesity and heart disease, are avoided. Moving also helps loosen and tone muscles, which can help reduce stiffness and pain, and also improve balance.

Reflect

Reflect on what it might be like if, following mobility activities, there is no improvement in mobility. Is the individual likely to have more severe psychological and emotional effects?

Case study

Audrey was 60 years old last birthday. She has recently been diagnosed with diabetes and has developed an ulcer on her leg, which means she sits in her chair most of the day. The nurse told her she was overweight and needed to lose several stone to improve her chances of leading a full life. At first Audrey ignored the nurse's advice, but then thought about the benefits of losing some weight. She could do more than sit around watching day-time TV. She could visit her grandchildren, who always made her feel better. She would be able to walk to the bus stop again. After all, the buses are a lot cheaper than taking a taxi. She might even meet a new man at a weight loss class – with all the possibilities that that could bring. There seemed to be more benefits than the nurse talked about!

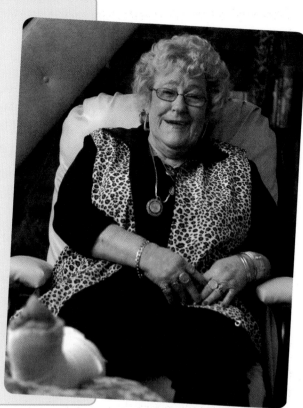

1. What psychological and emotional benefits of improving her mobility are there for Audrey?

2. What financial and practical benefits are there for Audrey of improving her mobility?

3. What physical benefits are there for Audrey of improving her mobility?

Knowledge Assessment Task — 1.1 1.2 1.3 1.4

Health and social care practitioners who work with older people, those who are physically frail, disabled or experiencing a period of ill health, need to understand the importance of mobility for the person they are working with. In this activity you are required to design and write a short booklet about supporting mobility.

1. Describe what 'mobility' means.

2. Use three examples to explain how different health conditions may affect and be affected by mobility.

3. Outline three effects that reduced mobility may have on an individual's wellbeing. Give examples for each of the effects.

4. Describe the benefits of maintaining and improving mobility, giving one example for each of the following aspects: psychological and emotional, financial and practical, physical.

Keep a copy of the written work that you produce as evidence for your assessment.

Discuss

Discuss with an individual in your care the physical benefits of maintaining or improving mobility. Are there any benefits you do not know about?

Preparing for mobility activities

Being prepared

It is important, when you are in your work setting, that you are prepared to support mobility activities with individuals. Before you begin, though, there are four principles that you must understand:

1. You must always put the safety of the individual in your care first.

2. You must only help someone if you have their consent to do so.

3. Any mobility activities must be for the benefit of the individual in your care.

4. You must not harm any individual in your care when providing support for their mobility.

These four principles must be thought about every time you take part in a mobility activity.

Agreeing mobility activities with individuals and others

Before you provide support to an individual for their mobility, you must agree with them what you are going to do.

Your assessment criteria:

2.1 Agree mobility activities with the individual and others

Key terms

Consent: this involves an individual giving informed permission

Vicarious consent: consent given on behalf of an individual legally unable, or lacking the capacity, to give consent – a child or a person in a coma, for example

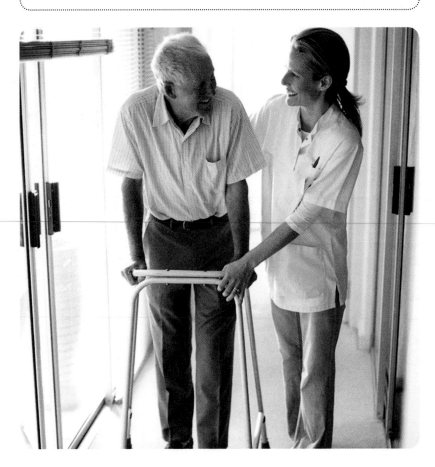

There are a number of different types of consent.

Figure 12.7 Forms of consent

Written consent	Written consent can be in the form of a letter or signed form saying consent or permission is given. This is the case when people go into hospital for an operation: they give consent for the operation.
Verbal consent	The person says to you that they want you to help them. This is the case in many social care situations when the person may say something like, 'Yes please. I would like you to help me walk to the bathroom.'
Implied consent	Consent can be implied. This is the case where someone does not say they want you to help them, but may hold your hand or arm when walking. By their action they imply they want you to help them.
Vicarious consent	This is where another person such as a parent of a child gives consent on their behalf.

What next?

After you have gained consent, and before you help the individual with their mobility, you should explain to them what you are going to do, and why. You should ask the person if they are happy for you to help them in this way, or if they would prefer to be supported in another way.

Case study

Maxine had a stroke, leaving her partially paralysed down her left side and unable to walk unaided. She is being treated in a rehabilitation centre where you work. It is part of her care plan that she be encouraged to walk three times a day. You are asked to support her. At the time for her exercise you go over to Maxine as she rests in the day room. You greet Maxine warmly and say you have been asked to support her with her mobility. She looks at you, seeming not to understand what you mean. You then remind her that her care plan says she should be assisted to walk a short distance three times a day, each day the walk being a little further to build up her strength. You then remember that she must agree to you helping her so you ask if it is all right to support her now. Maxine nods her head and lifts her good hand to take your arm.

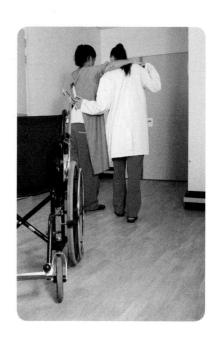

1. What difficulties might a person with a stroke have with mobility?
2. How do you make sure Maxine gives consent to supporting her?
3. What other ways of gaining consent are there?

Removing or minimising hazards in the environment before a mobility activity

Potential hazards

Before a mobility activity any hazards in the environment should be removed or minimised, thus ensuring that you abide with the first principle of supporting mobility: that is, safety must come first. There are plenty of **potential hazards** in health and social care environments, including:

- loose carpets and rugs in an older person's flat
- trailing electricity cables around computer and audiovisual equipment in a house
- other clients walking in a residential home for older people
- cluttered living space
- walking aids not being used properly
- untrained helpers
- stairs and unsupervised lifts
- unsafe or inappropriate clothing and footwear.

Suitability of clothing and footwear

Clothing and footwear can be a hazard when supporting an individual with mobility needs. Hazards can include:

- trailing dressing gown cords
- unsuitable slippers or shoes that are too tight or too large
- dresses and other clothing that drag along the floor
- scarves and ties that interfere with mobility aids and appliances.

Safety and cleanliness of mobility equipment and appliances

It is very important to ensure that all equipment and appliances that are used to support mobility are safe and clean. Dirt, grease or other unclean matter can hide imperfections, such as cracks in a walking stick, or lead to accidents, such as a hand slipping off a walking frame.

Key terms

Potential hazard: the possibility that a person, object or environment will cause an individual to be harmed

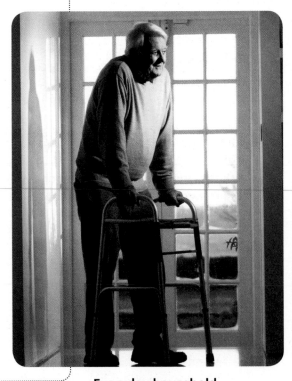

Everyday household environments can contain potential hazards

Case study

Mahmoud, 83, uses a walking frame to get about his house. He is very fond of gardening and likes to grow his own vegetables. Every day since his retirement he has walked around his garden, being supported by the walking frame, and will still get down on his knees to do digging and weeding. One day Greta, his daughter-in-law, visits to find him barely alive in the garden. Mahmoud says he has been lying on the ground in the garden for two days and nights. Nobody heard his cries for help. On investigating how he fell it seemed that the handle of the walking frame was covered in wet mud and that Mahmoud had lost his grip.

1. What are the potential hazards that pose a risk to Mahmoud?
2. How can potential hazards be removed or reduced?
3. What further steps can be taken to make Mahmoud safer in his garden?

Practical Assessment Task   2.1   2.2   2.3   2.4

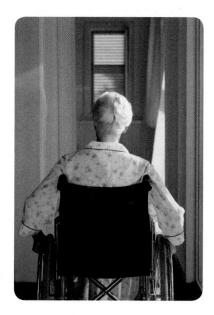

In this task you must demonstrate that you are able to prepare for mobility activities in your work environment.

With the permission of your supervisor and the consent of an individual in your care, prepare to provide support for mobility with a client or service user.

As preparation for carrying out the mobility activity you must discuss what you plan to do with the assessor, and then:

▶ ensure it is part of the care plan
▶ gain the consent of the service user
▶ explain what you are going to do with the service user.

Now prepare to provide support for the service user's mobility.

1. Demonstrate to your assessor how you will identify, remove or minimise any hazards in the environment in preparation for the mobility activity.
2. Check that the individual you are going to support in their mobility is wearing suitable and safe clothing and footwear. Discuss this with your assessor.
3. Check that any equipment and appliance you are going to use for the mobility activity is safe and clean, and appropriate for the mobility activity. Explain what you do and why you are doing this.
4. Provide a list of:
    ▶ three potential hazards in the individual's environment, and how you can remove or minimise these hazards
    ▶ three potential risks from unsuitable clothing and footwear
    ▶ three ways that mobility aids can be dangerous if broken or unclean.

Access, support and promotion

Individuals have the right to participate in activities and relationships of everyday life as independently as possible. The individual is regarded as an active partner in their own care or support, rather than as a passive recipient of care by others.

One of the key aims in supporting people with mobility is to help them stay mobile. To do this you need to prepare people to take an active part in their mobility, assist them to use mobility equipment and appliances if appropriate, and give them feedback and encouragement during and after mobility activities.

The promotion of active participation in a mobility activity

Active participation is about including the individual in their care. It is a way to make sure that the individual with whom you are going to do a mobility activity is involved in the activity. By being involved they are more likely to learn and the mobility activity will go better and be more effective.

Figure 12.8 Benefits of active participation

Key aspects	Benefits
Effective activity	It is the individual who should gain from support with mobility. It will be more effective if they take an active part instead of it being 'done to them'.
Inclusion	The individual is included by being made aware of the purpose of the mobility activity.
Explaining the activity	Explanation of the purpose of the mobility activity and the assistance offered helps reassure and support the individual.
Showing the activity	Demonstrating what is going to happen during a mobility activity is a good way to teach the individual about what they are going to do.
Doing the activity	When an activity is learned it is easier to repeat. The individual will learn quicker if they participate than if they do not.
Learning from and correcting mistakes	When the individual makes mistakes, it is an opportunity to you to correct an activity and adjust the care plan if necessary.

Your assessment criteria:

3.1 Promote active participation during a mobility activity

Key terms

Active participation: a way of including people in their own care

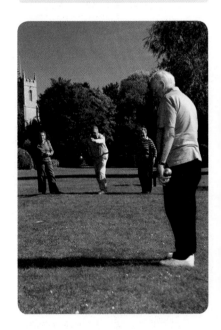

Case study

Amy lives in a residential home for older people. Following a stroke she is getting used to walking again. One of the mobility activities the occupational therapist, Lucy, wants her to do is to use a walking frame. Lucy helps Amy stand and shows her how to hold the walking frame. As she helps Amy, Lucy explains what she is doing. When Amy tries to hold the frame with only one hand, Lucy explains this is not a safe way to walk and shows her where to put both hands. This gives Amy more confidence and the activity is successful and effective in getting Amy to walk again.

1. How did Lucy include Amy in the activity?
2. How did Lucy correct Amy's mistake?

Key terms

Occupational therapist: a therapist trained in enabling individuals with physical or mental disabilities to participate in daily activities

Reflect

Can you think of ways to encourage the active participation of individuals? Have you observed these methods in use?

Discuss

Discuss with your line manager or supervisor how they promote active participation by individuals in their care.

Explaining the purpose of a mobility activity helps reassure and support the individual

Assisting to use mobility appliances correctly and safely

For some individuals keeping mobile means using **mobility appliances**. Without them they will not be able to do what they want to do. It is important that they are able to use mobility appliances correctly and safely to minimise the risk of hurting themselves or other people.

What are mobility appliances?

Mobility appliances are aids that help people walk or to improve their mobility.

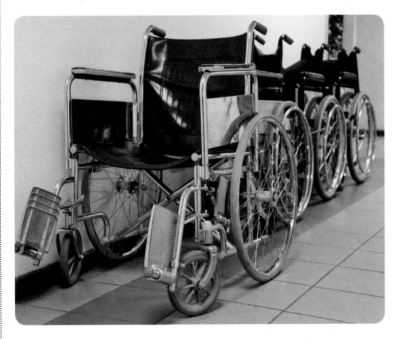

Many mobility appliances are used to aid walking.

Figure 12.9 Mobility aids and their uses

Your assessment criteria:

3.2 Assist an individual to use mobility appliances correctly and safely

Key terms

Mobility appliance: a piece of assistive equipment designed to enable greater movement for the user

Investigate

In your workplace look for manufacturer instructions for using mobility appliances. What kind of information do they give about the correct and safe use of the appliance? Is the information clear, straightforward and easily understood?

Discuss

Discuss with your line manager or supervisor any instances when an individual did not use an mobility aid correctly or safely. What action was taken?

Mobility aid	Uses
Walking sticks	Walking sticks or canes are a simple form of walking aid. They are held in the hand and used for balance or to support the individual as they walk.
Crutches	Crutches are a walking aid that is held under the armpit or elbow and by the hand.
Quad stick	Quad sticks are like walking sticks except they have four points of contact like feet on the ground.
Walking frames	Walking frames are more stable and are made of a metal framework with three or more points of contact, which the individual moves in front of them and then grips as they move forward.

Other mobility appliances

Other types of appliances are used if the person has to go a longer distance than they can walk. These include:

▶ wheelchairs   ▶ mobility scooters

Individuals may need assistance to use mobility appliances correctly and safely because for some people whom you look after it will be their first time using them. They will not know how to use them correctly and they must be able to use them safely.

How do you assist in the use of mobility appliances?

There are things you must do to make sure that any mobility appliance is used correctly and safely. Not doing so can cause hazards and put the individual at risk.

Figure 12.10 Responding to hazards

Hazard	Example of hazard	Response to hazard
Broken mobility aid	Walking stick with a broken handle	Do not use it; replace the walking stick
Dirty appliance	Walking frame with grease on the arm	Clean the walking frame before use
New aid	The individual has not used a mobility aid before	Ensure the person knows how to use it correctly and safely
Incorrect mobility aid	An older person using a mobility scooter when they have poor vision	Ensure the correct aid is used and that the individual is able to use it safely
Discomfort	A crutch designed for a small adult, but used by a tall man with a broken leg	Ensure the correct size of mobility aid is used
Bags	An older woman ties her shopping bag to her walking frame causing it to lean to one side	Use another mobility aid, such as a trolley with space for shopping

Case study

Cora uses a walking frame to get about her warden-controlled flat, and to do some shopping. A trainee, Rita, from a local college, on placement at the warden-controlled flats, offers to help Cora with her shopping. Aware that she must make sure Cora can use the walking frame correctly and safely, Rita asks Cora if she can manage the walking frame, checks it for any damaged parts, sees that Cora can use it properly and is comfortable. Rita then goes out of the flat and a second later hears Cora cry out and fall. She rushes back into the flat to see Cora on the floor, clutching her shopping bag.

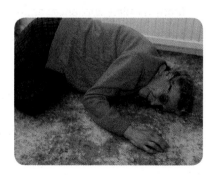

1. What steps did Rita take to make sure Cora is using the walking frame correctly and safely?
2. What did she forget to do?
3. Reflect on occasions when you have used an everyday appliance for the first time.

Giving feedback and encouragement to the individual during mobility activities

It is important that you give feedback and encouragement to individuals during mobility activities. By giving feedback the individual knows:

▶ what they are doing correctly and safely

▶ what they are not doing correctly and safely

▶ what they need to do to carry out the mobility activity correctly and safely.

Giving encouragement is also important because:

▶ when individuals lose their mobility, even for a short time, it can make them lose confidence in their ability to walk

▶ it can help people regain their confidence.

Your assessment criteria:

3.3 Give feedback and encouragement to the individual during mobility activities.

Case study

Ben is six years old. He broke his leg climbing in the park and it is in a plaster cast. Today the physiotherapist wants him to put some weight on the leg. As he first tries to stand up and then walk a few steps she tells him how well he is doing and that he will soon be running about with his friends. When he looks like he might fall over, she suggests he hold his mother's hand to give him a bit more confidence. He holds his mother's hand and is able to walk across the room. When he finishes the mobility exercises his mother hugs him and tells him that she is very proud of what he has done. The physiotherapist is also pleased and she sticks a star onto his plaster. This is so that he can show everyone how well he did.

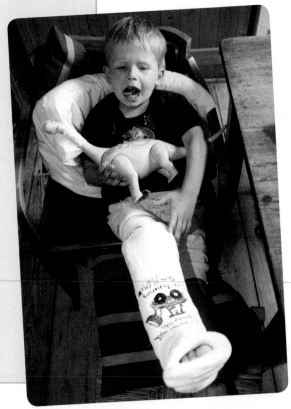

1. What feedback and encouragement did the physiotherapist give Ben?

2. What other ways are there to give feedback and encouragement to Ben?

3. Why would this feedback and encouragement not be suitable for everybody ?

Practical Assessment Task   3.1   3.2   3.3

In this practical assessment task you must demonstrate that you are able to support individuals to keep mobile. With the consent of an individual and the permission of your supervisor you must:

▶ demonstrate how you promote active participation during a mobility activity

▶ assist two individuals to use two different mobility appliances correctly and safely

▶ show how you give feedback and encouragement to the individuals during mobility activities.

Your assessor may also ask for written testimony from your manager or supervisor that you are able to:

▶ promote active participation during mobility activities

▶ assist people to use mobility appliances correctly and safely

▶ give adequate feedback and encouragement to people during mobility activities.

Investigate

Research on the internet how people gain confidence. How can you use these techniques when giving feedback and encouragement during mobility activities?

Discuss

Discuss with your line manager or supervisor the type of feedback and encouragement that they give. Do they adapt their feedback according to the individual's age, gender, occupation, social status or other factors?

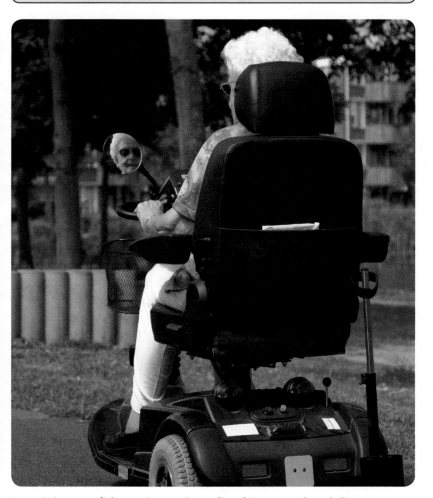

Regaining confidence is one benefit of increased mobility

Observing changes and responses

When you provide support for an individual who is carrying out a mobility activity it is important that you observe, record and report to others on how the activity was carried out. It is important to observe to make sure the individual is carrying out the mobility activity correctly and safely, and, if not, to show the individual how to do so. You observe by watching and listening as the mobility activity is carried out.

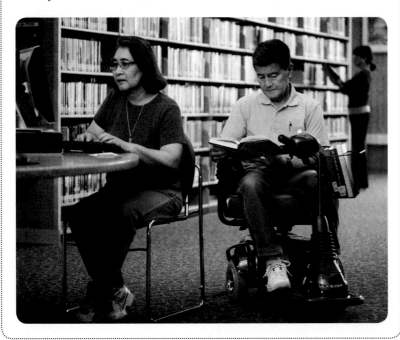

Your assessment criteria:

4.1 Observe an individual to monitor changes and responses during a mobility activity

4.2 Record observations of mobility activity

Case study

Amir has a painful ulcer on his leg and up until now has been using a quad stick to support himself as he walks. Recently he has found this more difficult and has bought a mobility scooter, which he uses to help him move around the gardens at the block of flats where he lives with other older people. Coraline, a worker who has not worked in care before, is asked to report to the care team as to how Amir is managing with the scooter. With Amir's agreement, Coraline follows him around the gardens. She notes that he maintains a modest speed and is aware of obstacles, and she talks to him about the bends and patches of uneven surfaces on the path.

1. How does Coraline observe Amir using the scooter?
2. How does Amir respond to the change from using a quad stick to using a scooter?
3. After observing Amir what should Coraline do to complete what was asked of her?

Recording observations on mobility activities

When reporting on mobility activities, there are three stages:

1. **Observe**
2. **Record**
3. **Report**

It is important to record your observations of an individual's mobility activity so that there is a record of what the individual did and how well the activity went. This is so that any care plan the person has can be kept up-to-date and action can be taken if necessary to make sure the individual remains safe. When making a record of a mobility activity you must:

▶ record what happened, including where it happened, who was involved, and what appliances were used

▶ write clearly so the record can be read by other people

▶ sign the record and print your name so it is clear who wrote the record

▶ include the time and date so that it is clear when the record was written.

Case study

Amir has recently started using his new mobility scooter. His care worker, Coraline, observes him using it in the gardens of the block of flats where he lives. When this mobility activity is over, Coraline looks for her supervisor to make sure she is recording the correct information. She is not sure exactly what to write. However, not being able to find her supervisor she decides to write some notes in Amir's file about what she saw Amir do. In the notes she uses a pen to write about how Amir used the scooter correctly and how he was safe, saying that he was aware of potential hazards on the path. She signed and dated the record.

1. Should Coraline report on what she observed or should she write about what she thought about Amir in the garden?

2. Exactly what did Coraline observe?

3. Does it matter if Coraline signs the record? Why does it matter?

Reflect

Reflect on an occasion, in your own work or training, when a service user began to use a different mobility aid. What were the challenges and benefits of this change?

Investigate

Investigate care records where you work for evidence of signatures and dates.

Discuss

Discuss with a friend or colleague about how they record and report care activities.

Reporting on progress

You must always report on any mobility activity that you provide support for so that other people involved in an individual's care know how that individual is managing. This is particularly important if:

▶ there is a change in the person's mobility

▶ there is a change of mobility appliance

▶ the individual is changing the way they use a mobility appliance

▶ the individual is not using appliances correctly and safely

▶ the person is being shown how to use a mobility appliance correctly and safely.

When reporting, it is necessary to bear in mind that either progress or problems can arise from a mobility activity, concerning:

▶ the choice of activity

▶ any equipment or appliance that is used to aid mobility

▶ the kind of support that is needed.

Your assessment criteria:

4.3 Report on progress and/or problems relating to the mobility activity including: choice of activities, equipment, appliances, and the support provided

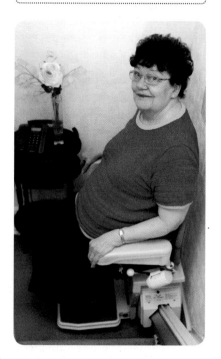

Practical Assessment Task | 4.1 | 4.2 | 4.3

In this task you are required to demonstrate that you can observe, record and report the outcome of a mobility activity with an individual.

1. With the permission of your supervisor, prepare an individual for a mobility activity and then observe them carrying out the activity, making sure they remain safe.

2. Make a complete and accurate record of the mobility activity, ensuring you write clearly, sign the record and date it as required in the person's records.

3. Identify who else needs to know about the mobility activity, and inform them.

Are you ready for assessment?

AC	What do you know now?	Assessment task	✓
1.1	The definition of mobility	Page 317	
1.2	How different health conditions may affect and be affected by mobility	Page 317	
1.3	The effects that reduced mobility may have on an individual's wellbeing	Page 317	
1.4	The benefits of maintaining and improving mobility	Page 317	

AC	What can you do now?	Assessment task	✓
2.1	Agree mobility activities with the individual and others	Page 321	
2.2	Remove or minimise hazards in the environment before a mobility activity	Page 321	
2.3	Check the suitability of an individual's clothing and footwear for safety and mobility	Page 321	
2.4	Check the safety and cleanliness of mobility equipment and appliances	Page 321	
3.1	Promote active participation during a mobility activity	Page 327	
3.2	Assist an individual to use mobility appliances correctly and safely	Page 327	
3.3	Give feedback and encouragement to the individual during mobility activities	Page 327	
4.1	Observe an individual to monitor changes and responses during a mobility activity	Page 330	
4.2	Record observations of mobility activity	Page 330	
4.3	Report on progress and/or problems relating to the mobility activity including: choice of activities, equipment, appliances and the support provided	Page 330	

13 | Support individuals to eat and drink (HSC 2014)

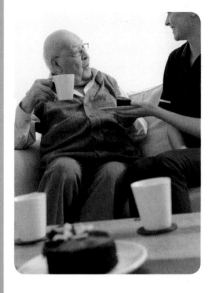

Assessment of this unit

Every human being needs to eat and drink in order to survive. Inadequate fluid and food intake can harm the body. Most people do consume the right amount of food and fluids to maintain a healthy body and are able to eat a healthy and nutritious diet without requiring assistance with feeding and drinking. However, some individuals receiving care and support within health and social care settings do need support and assistance to eat and drink. This unit introduces you to a range of issues relating to the provision of support for eating and drinking. You will need to be able to:

▶ support individuals to make choices about food and drink

▶ prepare to provide support for eating and drinking

▶ provide support for eating and drinking

▶ clear away after food and drink

▶ monitor eating and drinking and the support provided.

The assessment of this unit is entirely competence-based (based on activities in the real work environment). To successfully complete this unit, you will need to produce evidence of your practical competence in providing support for individuals to eat and drink. The table below outlines what you need to do to meet each of the assessment criteria for the unit.

Your tutor or assessor will help you to prepare for your assessment, and the tasks suggested in the unit will help you to create the evidence that you need.

AC	What you need to do
1.1	Establish with an individual the food and drink they wish to consume
1.2	Encourage the individual to select suitable options for food and drink
1.3	Describe ways to resolve any difficulties or dilemmas about the choice of food and drink
1.4	Describe how and when to seek additional guidance about an individual's choice of food and drink
2.1	Identify the level and type of support an individual requires when eating and drinking

2.2	Demonstrate effective hand washing and use of protective clothing when handling food and drink
2.3	Support the individual to prepare to eat and drink, in a way that meets their personal needs and preferences
2.4	Provide suitable utensils to assist the individual to eat and drink
3.1	Describe factors that help promote an individual's dignity, comfort and enjoyment while eating and drinking
3.2	Support the individual to consume manageable amounts of food and drink at their own pace
3.3	Provide encouragement to the individual to eat and drink
3.4	Support the individual to clean themselves if food or drink is spilt
3.5	Adapt support in response to an individual's feedback or observed reactions while eating and drinking
4.1	Explain why it is important to be sure that an individual has chosen to finish eating and drinking before clearing away
4.2	Confirm that the individual has finished eating and drinking
4.3	Clear away used crockery and utensils in a way that promotes active participation
4.4	Support the individual to make themselves clean and tidy after eating or drinking
5.1	Explain the importance of monitoring the food and drink an individual consumes and any difficulties they encounter
5.2	Carry out and record agreed monitoring processes
5.3	Report on the support provided for eating and drinking in accordance with agreed ways of working

This unit also links to some of the other units:

HSC 027	Contribute to health and safety in health and social care
HSC 2013	Support care plan activities
HSC 2028	Move and position individuals

Some of your learning will be repeated in these units and will give you the chance to review your knowledge and understanding.

Consuming a balanced diet

Care practitioners have a responsibility to encourage individuals to make choices regarding their food and drink, whilst also seeking to provide a fully **balanced** nutritional diet. You should find out about what the person likes to eat and drink, and then give them menu cards or explain what choices are available at mealtimes to let each person choose their preferred foods and drinks. Make a note of their preferences regarding:

▶ fish, poultry, red meat, seafood

▶ fruit and vegetables – for example, apples, pears, oranges, carrots, potatoes

▶ drinks – tea, coffee, milk, alcohol or other beverages – the person may like a glass of wine or beer with a meal but you will need to check this with the person in charge

▶ cakes and biscuits – does the person has a 'sweet tooth' and like particular treats?

▶ dairy products.

You will also need to find out if the individual is a vegetarian or on a special diet for medical or religious reasons.

The above list is evidence of the huge range of foods that are available. Try to influence the menus when these are prepared so that the individual has a real choice and does not have simply to accept what is being served. If the individual cannot communicate this information then a close friend, partner or relative may be able to inform you of their likes or dislikes.

Your assessment criteria:

1.1 Establish with an individual the food and drink they wish to consume

1.2 Encourage the individual to select suitable options for food and drink

Key terms

Balanced: refers to a diet containing a suitable amount and range of protein, carbohydrate, vitamins, minerals and water

Reflect

How do you encourage individuals within your care setting to make choices regarding the food and drink that they wish to consume? Do you think about balanced diet when doing this?

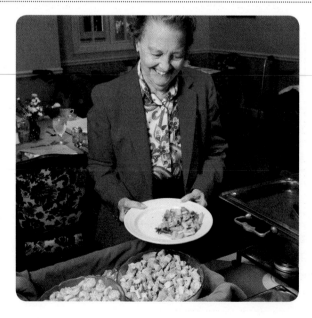

Choosing healthy options at mealtimes is a good way of encouraging others to eat a balanced diet

Encouraging individuals to select suitable options

Individuals need to be encouraged to eat a balanced diet to maintain good health. It is recommended that everyone should eat five portions of fruit and vegetables daily plus a selection of protein and a moderate amount of dairy products and grains. The Food Standards Agency suggests that people should drink six to eight glasses of fluid daily. Older adults, in particular, need to eat large amounts of fibre to prevent constipation. Fibre is contained in breads (particularly, whole grain breads), cereals, fruit and vegetables, and you should encourage individuals to eat these.

Offer tea and coffee without sugar first, then ask whether the person takes sugar or uses a sweetener. Clients may be allowed to drink alcohol in moderation but you will first need to request permission from the person in charge.

Some individuals may be vegetarian or vegan, meaning that they don't eat meat. Vegetarians eat dairy products, milk and eggs, whereas vegans only eat plant foods (including soya-based alternatives to dairy products). Their diets will need to contain protein, vitamin and minerals, and you should find out whether food supplements are necessary to ensure a healthy diet.

A balanced diet should contain a selection from the five food groups below:

► **milk and dairy foods** – e.g. cheese, milk – these should be eaten in moderation due to high saturated fat content but they are an important source of calcium for bones

► **meat and alternatives** – meat, fish, pulses, soya products are good sources of protein that are essential for the growth and repair of body tissues and are a source of energy

► **fruit and vegetables** – e.g. apples, pears, lettuce, tomatoes – good source of nutrients (minerals and vitamins) and fibre

► **carbohydrates/starch** – grains (made into bread and cereal, rice, pasta) and starches (e.g. potatoes) are the body's main source of food energy

► **fats and sugar/alcohol** – foods and drinks high in fats and sugar are energy-rich, but should be eaten sparingly. They contain few nutrients, and too much fat can lead to heart disease or stroke.

Investigate

Find out who plans the menus of the people who use your care setting. If possible ask them how they ensure that everyone has a balanced diet regardless of their personal preferences and special dietary needs.

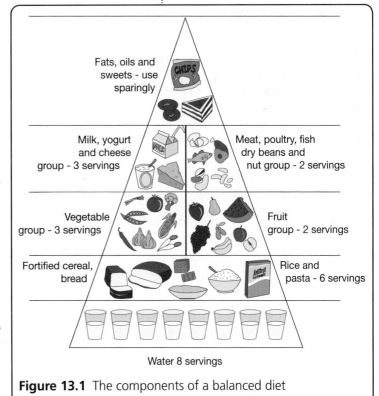

Fats, oils and sweets - use sparingly

Milk, yogurt and cheese group - 3 servings

Meat, poultry, fish dry beans and nut group - 2 servings

Vegetable group - 3 servings

Fruit group - 2 servings

Fortified cereal, bread

Rice and pasta - 6 servings

Water 8 servings

Figure 13.1 The components of a balanced diet

Resolving dilemmas about the choice of food and drink

Some individuals may make poor food choices that could cause harm to the body. It is easy for people to get into the habit of eating unhealthy foods, particularly if they are unaware of the possible effects of a particular diet or because they develop a preference for sugary, salty or fatty food. The government has created clear guidelines on healthy eating, but we are also bombarded with advertisements for unhealthy foods and drink – for example, television adverts for fast foods and fizzy drinks.

Diet and health problems

The individual's preferences may, on occasion, contradict the advice that is being given by the care practitioner. If the individual has a long-term condition, such as type 2 diabetes, they may have to restrict their diet in various ways. The individual will need the support of their care practitioner to encourage and guide them in choosing food and drink that meets the restrictions of their diet.

Your assessment criteria:

1.3 Describe ways to resolve any difficulties or dilemmas about the choice of food and drink

Key terms

Diabetes: a metabolic disorder that causes high glucose levels in the blood

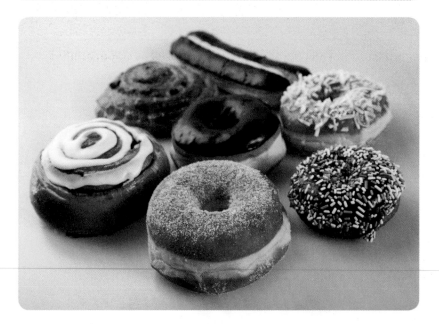

Foods that are high in fat and sugar should only be consumed occasionally to avoid over-consumption of calories. They should be avoided by individuals with diabetes or weight problems

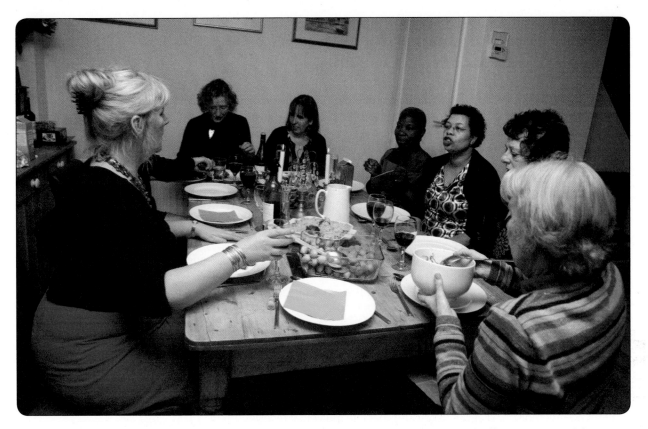

Meals are social occasions and opportunities to celebrate special events as well as opportunities to 'refuel' the body

Encouraging dietary change

People do not find it easy to change their established diets. The care practitioner can help by highlighting the wide selection of foods that are available – and perhaps even offer tasting sessions. The key is to make alternative options attractive and appetising, and encourage people to eat less healthy foods in moderation. In the case of alcohol, it may be perfectly acceptable for an individual to have a glass of wine or a beer with a meal, unless the person is on medication. However, if the person is used to drinking excessively then this will require sensitive handling.

Meeting cultural needs

People from black and minority ethnic groups may have particular habits and preferences regarding their diet. Many care homes will not provide meals that meet the needs of these diverse groups, unless special provision has been made, and the individual may therefore refuse to eat the meal that has been provided. To avoid this problem, the care practitioner should make sure to find out about dietary preferences, and try to ensure that these are reflected in the meals that are on offer. Family members can normally offer advice, or even bring in an occasional meal for the individual, though this should not be relied on.

Reflect

Write an account of how you would meet the needs of individuals from black and minority ethnic groups regarding their choice of food and drink.

Seeking guidance about an individual's choice of food and drink

It is important to seek additional guidance regarding an individual's choice of food and drink if the person has specific physical problems or cultural requirements.

Physical conditions affecting diet

Individuals who have difficulty in swallowing may have developed a condition known as dysphagia. You may need, in these cases, to seek guidance regarding the type of food that the person can tolerate. Eating can become a challenge for the individual as they have problems swallowing liquids and eating food, which can become lodged in the throat. A speech and language therapist and a dietician can offer guidance regarding the types of foods and drink that can be consumed safely.

Inadequate food and fluid intake may be the result of chronic illness or may occur for other unexplained reasons. For example, a person may be losing weight as a result of a condition like cancer or liver disease. This can also alter the individual's choice of what to eat so the care practitioner may need to seek guidance from a speech and language therapist or dietician to ensure that the individual receives a nutritionally balanced diet.

Symptoms of gastrointestinal problems, such as nausea, vomiting, diarrhoea and constipation, are other factors that limit the choice of food and drink. If these problems are persistent then the doctor will need to be notified so that appropriate action can be advised. Normally, clear fluids are given if the person continues to vomit, until the vomiting has subsided. For constipation, the individual should drink plenty of fluids and eat foods that contain fibre. In cases of diarrhoea, the individuals should drink plenty of liquids and avoid eating any solid foods until the diarrhoea ceases.

Cultural and religious practices

Many people have religious beliefs which influence the food they will or won't eat. Jews, Moslems, Hindus and other faith groups have dietary rules regarding certain foods (such as the Jewish and Moslem prohibition on the eating of pork), which you will need to be aware of if any individuals in your care are members of

Key terms

cultural: refers to practices and beliefs shared by groups of people

Dysphagia: difficulty in swallowing

Speech and language therapist: specialist who assesses people who have problems with swallowing

Dietician: specialist who assesses individuals for special dietary needs

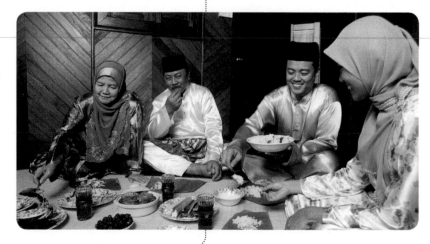

these faiths. Seek guidance on this from the individual or family members.

Food preferences are also strongly influenced by cultural background. People who grew up in the Caribbean, for example, will probably enjoy different foods, and flavours, to individuals from southeast Asia. The individual's food and drink should reflect, as near as possible, the food they eat at home. Again, seek guidance on this from the individual or their family members.

Case study

Naina is a resident in a care home. She is a strict Moslem and dislikes the food and drink that is being provided for her. She misses her usual diet of curries, rice and dhal and does not drink tea or coffee. The staff on your placement have expressed concern regarding Naina's loss of appetite.

1. What suggestions would you make regarding Naina's diet?

2. How would you assist Naina in getting the meals and drinks she wants?

3. How would you involve her family in meeting her nutritional needs?

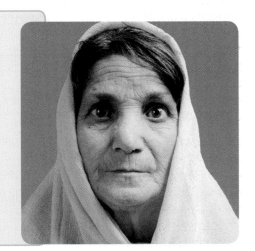

Practical Assessment Task   1.1   1.2   1.3   1.4

With the permission of your supervisor and the person concerned, select an individual from your work or placement setting who requires support to make choices about food and drink. Spend some time talking with the individual about their food preferences and diet. You could do this by discussing the forthcoming week's menu with the person. You need to show that you are able to:

▶ establish with the individual the food and drink they wish to consume

▶ encourage the individual to select suitable options for food and drink

▶ describe ways of resolving any difficulties or dilemmas about the person's choice of food or drink

▶ describe how and when to seek additional guidance about the individual's choice of food and drink.

Your evidence for this task must be based on your practice and experience in a real work environment. Keep any written work that you produce for this activity as evidence towards your assessment. Your assessor may also want to observe or ask you questions about the way you support individuals to make choices about food and drink in the care setting.

Providing support for eating and drinking

The support an individual requires will vary: a careful assessment of the individual's needs should be made at the beginning of the care period, and reviewed on a regular basis. Some individuals may just need encouragement and support when eating and drinking but are independent to feed and to drink on their own. Others may need reminders or cues from the care practitioner – for example, 'would you like to try some of the vegetables on the plate?'

Assessing individual's support needs

Some individuals may need a lot of help and support with eating and drinking. Bear the following points in mind:

► Ensure individuals have the right cutlery, crockery and any necessary aids.

► Support individuals who are confused or feeling too weak to feed themselves. Offer to feed them if they have lost the ability to bring the food from the plate to their mouth.

► Offer to cut up food and assist with drinking when necessary.

► Give the attention the person requires so that they feel valued.

► Allow them enough time to feed themselves.

Your assessment criteria:

2.1 Identify the level and type of support an individual requires when eating and drinking

2.2 Demonstrate effective hand washing and use of protective clothing when handling food and drink

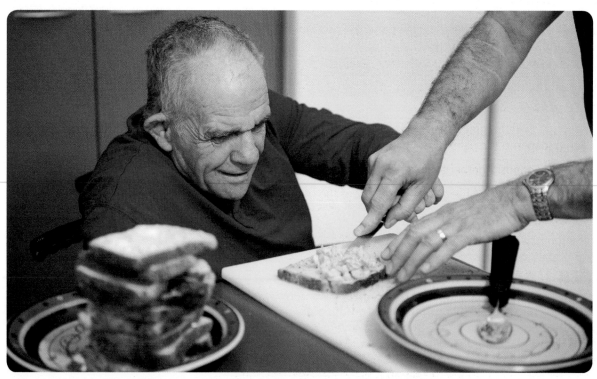

It is important to check how much support with eating and drinking an individual needs and wishes to have

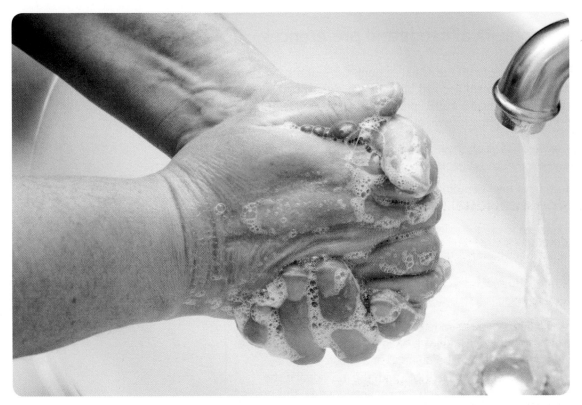

Clean hands are a vital part of food hygiene and safety practices in care settings

Safe handling of food and drink

Anyone handling food needs first to wash their hands thoroughly to reduce the spread of infections from one person to another. As a care practitioner you will be handling food when preparing and serving meals. The Food Standards Agency suggests a series of steps that a person should follow when handling food:

1. Wet hands thoroughly under warm running water and squirt liquid soap into the palm of the hand.

2. Rub your hands together to make a lather.

3. Rub the palm of one hand along the back of the other and along the fingers. Then repeat with the other hand.

4. Rub in between each of the fingers on both hands and around the thumbs.

5. Rinse off the soap with clean water.

6. Dry hands thoroughly on a disposable towel.

It is also important to wear protective clothing such as an apron when handling food, which should be removed when no longer required. Hair should be tied back and care taken to ensure that strands of hair do not fall into food that is being prepared or served.

Discuss

Discuss with your colleagues how you can promote good hand washing techniques related to food handling among staff and residents in your workplace.

Meeting individual needs and preferences

Individuals who cannot manage to eat or drink without assistance may suffer embarrassment and loss of dignity. It is important, therefore, to take particular care in preparing for mealtimes. You may need to consider the following:

- ▶ Do they need to wash their face and hands? You may have to assist if the person is unable to do so.
- ▶ Do they have their dentures in? Ensure these have been cleaned or provide oral hygiene.
- ▶ Do they need to use the toilet, commode or urinal before the meal?
- ▶ Make sure they have put on protective clothing if that is required.
- ▶ Do they need to be helped to the table, and to a particular seat?
- ▶ Who would they like to sit with?

As a care practitioner you need to check if the individual is on a special diet or has any difficulty with eating and drinking. Discuss the menu with the individual beforehand and ensure that they receive what has been ordered. Check with the individual if she would like to be fed or can eat and drink independently. This needs to be managed sensitively.

Your assessment criteria:

2.3 Support the individual to prepare to eat and drink in a way that meets their personal needs and preferences

2.4 Provide suitable utensils to assist the individual to eat and drink

Reflect

How can you help individuals to satisfy their eating and drinking preferences whilst also protecting their dignity and self-esteem?

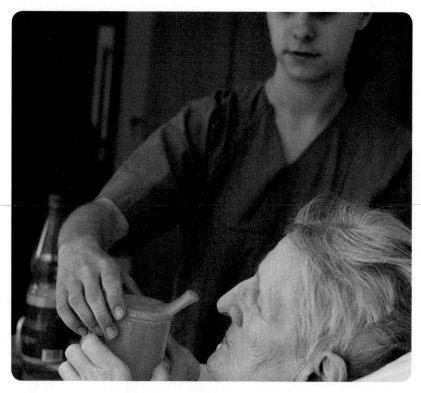

Adapted utensils and cups are sometimes needed to enable people to eat and drink effectively

Utensils to aid eating and drinking

Normal cutlery and crockery should be used whenever possible for individuals who require assistance with eating and drinking. For those who require additional assistance with drinking, cups with straws can be used to enable the person to drink easily and without spilling. Aids that can be helpful for eating include:

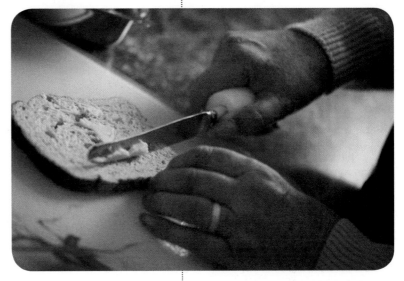

Adapted cutlery may be all that some individuals need to eat and drink independently

▶ plate guards – useful for keeping the food on the plate and for those who can only use one hand, or whose hands shake or are weak

▶ place mats – help with keeping plates and cups from moving around on the table

▶ cups with special handles which the individual can use independently or can be assisted with

▶ knives, forks and spoons with wide handles

▶ plates with rims and plastic non-slip mats.

Practical Assessment Task   2.1   2.2   2.3   2.4

Some of the people who use or are resident in your care setting may require support for eating and drinking. Choose a suitable person or small group to work with and demonstrate that you are able to:

▶ identify the level and type of support that an individual requires when eating and drinking

▶ demonstrate effective hand washing and use of protective clothing when handling food and drink

▶ support the individual to prepare to eat and drink, in a way that meets their personal needs and preferences

▶ provide suitable utensils to assist the individual to eat and drink.

Your evidence for this task must be based on your practice and experience in a real work environment. Keep any written work that you produce for this activity as evidence towards your assessment. Your assessor may also want to observe or ask you questions about the way you prepare to provide support for eating and drinking in the care setting.

Investigate

Using the internet and other resources, conduct a search on the type of utensils that can be used to assist individuals with eating and drinking.

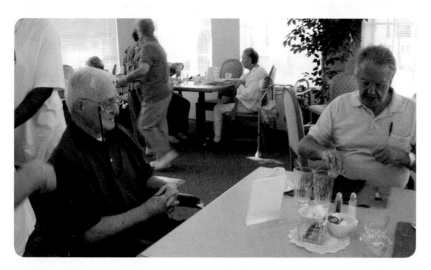

Mealtimes are occasions many people look forward to in care settings

Factors affecting dignity, comfort and enjoyment

There are a number of factors that need to be considered in promoting the individual's comfort and enjoyment while eating and drinking. The food should be presented in an attractive and appetising manner and the environment where the meals are being eaten should be relaxed, attractive and clean, with comfortable seating arrangements and no bad odours. Nutritional screening needs to take place to record and check dietary needs and preferences.

You should also consider the following suggestions and issues:

▶ Set up the dining room so that it looks homely and inviting.

▶ Ensure the food is at the right temperature – hot food should be hot and cold food should be kept cold.

▶ If the texture of the food is difficult for the person to swallow, the speech and language therapist or dietician may be able to suggest how to present the meal in a more attractive way. Not all foods should be pureed as these meals can look very unattractive. There are also appetising milkshakes or soups that are equally nutritious if a full meal cannot be tolerated.

▶ Are second helpings on offer?

▶ Make sure that drinks and healthy snacks are made available throughout the day, not just at mealtimes.

▶ Offer privacy to those who have difficulties with eating so that they do not feel embarrassed or lose dignity if they make a mess.

Reflect

What factors do you think affect an individual's dignity, comfort and enjoyment while they are eating and drinking?

- ▶ Encourage family members, carers and partners to visit during mealtimes. They can be a great source of help in feeding a family member.

- ▶ Ensure that the environment is well staffed so that the individual can obtain the full attention of a carer during mealtimes.

- ▶ Do not make assumptions regarding what people should eat. Ask the individual what their preferences are.

- ▶ Raise awareness of the importance of maintaining good nutritional care.

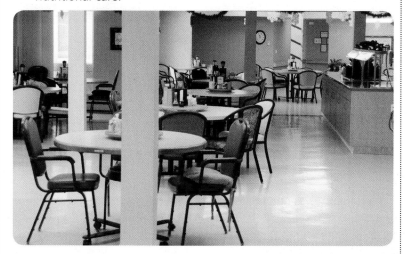

The dining area of a care setting should be clean, welcoming and accessible

Supporting the individual to eat and drink.

You should always aim to provide food in a way that will enable the individual to eat. Consider beforehand if the individual has any problems with eating and drinking then serve small manageable amounts of food on a plate. This can look more appetising than a crowded plate, which can appear daunting. If you are feeding an individual:

- ▶ select a small portion to put in the person's mouth and allow them to chew as long as is required

- ▶ do not hurry the person to finish; allow ample time for the individual to eat and then offer a drink

- ▶ vary the selection of food so that the individual has, for example, some meat, a vegetable and then potato or rice

- ▶ explain to the individual what foods you are feeding them with

- ▶ rest in between and talk to the person while you are feeding them: make it a pleasant interactive process.

You should also enquire what the person would prefer to drink – for example, tea, coffee, juice or water.

Investigate

When you are next in the workplace or placement setting, review the layout of the dining area and consider whether it is welcoming and accessible. Comment on the positive aspects of the dining area and highlight any possible improvements that could be made.

Reflect

Practise feeding another student and vice versa. How did it feel to be fed? Reflect on the experience and make notes.

Encouraging unwilling eaters and drinkers

The care practitioner should first try to establish the reasons for the individual not eating or drinking. The individual may be experiencing pain or feel rather unwell due to other circumstances. If, for example, the loss of appetite is due to pain then the individual may require an analgesic. The following suggestions may also be useful:

▶ Offer attractive and tasty foods.

▶ Offer a good selection of hot and cold drinks throughout the day.

▶ Encourage the individual to drink whenever you come into the room.

▶ Try playing some soft music, especially something the person likes.

▶ Make sure you are sitting at the right level so you can assist the person with eating.

▶ Make sure the person is comfortable, and in a good sitting position.

▶ Use finger foods so the person can feed themselves and feel more independent – they may dislike being fed.

▶ Offer food supplements, but only on advice from the dietician and as a last resort.

▶ Ask a relative, friend or partner to bring in a home-cooked meal and favourite drink that could encourage individual to eat and drink. You should avoid, however, making this a regular practice.

Dealing with spillages

If food or drink is spilt on the individual's clothes, help the individual to clean themselves while offering any assistance that may be necessary. If the person can successfully clean themselves without your help this will help them to preserve their dignity and sense of independence. Crucially, the person must not be treated as a child, particularly in front of other individuals who may be eating their meals. This could be a humiliating and upsetting experience for the individual.

Key terms

Analgesic: medicine used to relieve pain

Reflect

Write an account of about 100 words on how you would support an individual who has spilt food and drink on their clothes while in the dining room. Consider how you would retain the person's dignity.

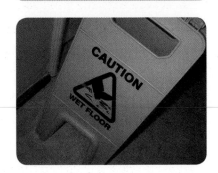

Practical Assessment Task | 3.1 | 3.2 | 3.3 | 3.4 | 3.5

Health and social care practitioners are sometimes required to provide practical assistance to enable individuals receiving care to eat and drink. In this assessment activity you need to demonstrate that you are able to provide appropriate support for eating and drinking. You will need to:

▶ describe factors that help promote an individual's dignity, comfort and enjoyment while eating and drinking

▶ support the individual to consume manageable amounts of food and drink at their own pace

▶ provide encouragement to the individual to eat and drink

▶ support the individual to clean themselves if food or drink is spilt

▶ adapt your support in response to an individual's feedback or observed reactions while eating and drinking.

Your evidence for this task must be based on your practice and experience in a real work environment. Keep any written work that you produce for this activity as evidence towards your assessment. Your assessor may want to observe or ask you questions about the way you provide support for eating and drinking in the care setting.

Your assessment criteria:

3.5 Adapt support in response to an individual's feedback or observed reactions while eating and drinking

Obtaining feedback on eating behaviour

You should regularly ask individuals in your care about their eating and drinking, whilst also paying close attention to their behaviour at mealtimes and between meals. Your questions could be in a form of a short consultation or evaluation exercise. You might ask, for example:

▶ Do you enjoy the meals you are given?

▶ What do you think of the quality of the food?

▶ Are there any other types of food and drink that you might like to see on the menu?

▶ Is there enough variety to choose from?

▶ Would you like to help in the preparation of the food?

▶ Do you have any other ideas or comments?

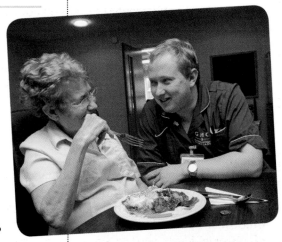

If the individual is unable to communicate their needs the care practitioner may obtain feedback through observing their behaviour. An example of this could be the individual's refusal to eat or negative responses received from family members. Try to ensure variety in the food that is on offer and if possibly encourage the individual to participate in preparing food for mealtimes. You should always adapt the eating and drinking support you provide for an individual in response to their feedback (What, do they say, helps? What doesn't help?) and how they respond to what you do.

Reflect

Consider how feedback regarding food and drink is managed in your workplace.

▶ How do staff consult with service users?

▶ What do they do with the feedback?

▶ Have you observed any changes being made as a result of feedback?

Managing mealtimes appropriately

Mealtimes are an important social event and are often the focus of the day for people in care. It's important, for this reason, to make the individual feel comfortable and at ease, and not to rush them. You will also need time to ensure that the person has had a balanced meal.

Some individuals may need a longer time to swallow food or drink due to physical problems so the whole event may take much longer than anticipated. Taking solid food can be tiring for frail individuals; mealtimes can require sensitivity and patience on the part of the care practitioner.

Confirming that the individual has finished eating and drinking

This can sometimes be difficult to gauge. The person may refuse to eat anymore if they are eating independently and actually state this, or if being fed may indicate by shaking their head. You may be able to encourage the person to eat a little more from the plate or accept another spoonful if being fed; however, eventually the individual will refuse to eat any more. This is the moment to stop persuading the individual to eat or drink and accept that the individual has finished eating.

Clearing away used crockery and utensils

When meals are finished, you can use this time effectively to involve individuals in clearing away the crockery and utensils. This type of activity encourages everyone to participate regardless of any disability, helping to empower individuals and promote their self-esteem. You will need to assess who is able to carry out certain tasks – for example, people who are independent and mobile may be able to collect plates, dishes, knives and forks and remove all the excess food, though all will require supervision while undertaking these tasks. People with less mobility can still help to wipe the tables and mats. You could develop a rota system so that all individuals have the opportunity to carry out different tasks at different meals.

Your assessment criteria:

4.1 Explain why it is important to be sure that the individual has chosen to finish eating and drinking before clearing away

4.2 Confirm that the individual has finished eating and drinking

4.3 Clear away used crockery and utensils in a way that promotes active participation

Discuss

Discuss with colleagues in your workplace how you would confirm that an individual has finished eating and drinking.

Discuss

Discuss with colleagues how you (and they) can promote active participation in clearing up after meals.

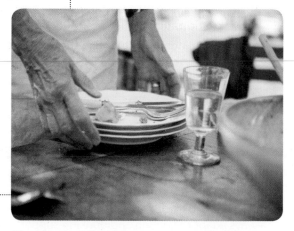

Clearing up should occur promptly but shouldn't cause people to feel rushed to finish their meal

Supporting individuals to make themselves clean and tidy

Following a meal every effort should be made to make the individual feel clean and comfortable. You may need to remind the person to tidy themselves; others may require more assistance. If that is the case, the person should be escorted to their room for privacy so they can either clean up their existing clothes or put on fresh clothing. Below are examples of good practice:

▶ Check the person's mouth after the individual has finished eating and remove any excess food.

▶ Help the individual to remove any food that may be on their clothes.

▶ Encourage the individual to rinse their mouth after the meal.

▶ If wearing dentures, take these out and rinse or brush teeth following the meal.

▶ Assist the individual in washing and drying their hands.

▶ Remove their apron and clean it ready for the next meal.

▶ Offer to assist with a change of clothes if that is required. Maintain privacy throughout.

Reflect

Why it is important to be certain that an individual has finished eating before clearing away? What are the implications if a person's food is taken away too quickly?

Practical Assessment Task | 4.1 | 4.2 | 4.3 | 4.4 |

Ending a meal appropriately and cleaning away after food and drink are important aspects of the routine of mealtimes in care settings. In this assessment task you need to:

▶ explain why it is important to be sure that an individual has chosen to finish eating and drinking before clearing away

▶ confirm that the individual has finished eating and drinking

▶ clear away used crockery and utensils in a way that promotes active participation

▶ support the individual to make themselves clean and tidy after eating or drinking.

Your evidence for this task must be based on your practice and experience in a real work environment. Keep any written work that you produce for this activity as evidence towards your assessment. Your assessor may also want to observe or ask you questions about the way you clear away after food and drink has been consumed in the care setting.

The importance of monitoring food and fluids

Monitoring a person's food and drink is vitally important as the individual could develop **malnutrition** if they do not consume the right amount of food to satisfy the needs of the body or **obesity** if they consume too much food and drink. You will need to establish the reasons why the person may be under- or overeating, and make a note of the fluid intake and food eaten. The aim is to recognise who is vulnerable and to treat any malnutrition or obesity problems before they become too advanced causing the individual severe distress and leading to illness.

The person can also become **dehydrated** as a result of not taking in sufficient fluids. If the individual refuses to drink they may have to be referred to the GP in case they require hospitalisation to be given **intravenous fluids**. An individual about whom there are dietary concerns can be referred to a dietician who will conduct a nutritional assessment. The assessment will identify the most appropriate diet for the individual and calculate the protein and fluid content required.

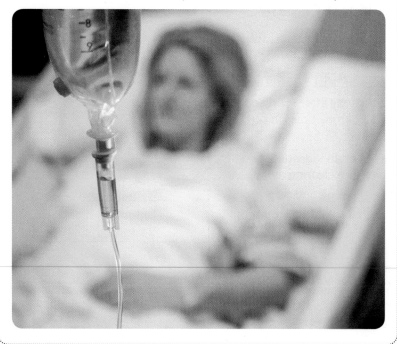

Your assessment criteria:

5.1 Explain the importance of monitoring the food and drink an individual consumes and any difficulties they encounter

5.2 Carry out and record agreed monitoring processes

Key terms

Malnutrition: inadequate nutrition caused by over- or under-eating or a diet that lacks nutrients

Obesity: excess body fat leading to a body mass index equal to or above 30

Dehydrated: experiencing a lack of body fluids

Intravenous fluids: fluids administered to the individual through the circulatory system

Carrying out and recording an agreed monitoring process

The care setting where you work should have an agreed way of monitoring the range and quantity of food and drink that each individual consumes. To assess for malnutrition, weight and height are checked to get a body mass index (BMI) score. The Malnutrition Universal Screening Tool (MUST) is a complex analytical tool that can be used to identify adults who are malnourished, at risk of malnutrition, or obese. It is used in a range of settings.

There are, however, signs that are easily recognisable for malnutrition and dehydration that the care practitioner can identify. These include:

▶ noticeable weight loss

▶ lack of energy

▶ restlessness

▶ aggressive behaviour

▶ problems with absorbing food.

In cases of dehydration due to lack of fluids the individual may:

▶ show persistent tiredness

▶ have a dry mouth

▶ feel nauseous

▶ be confused

▶ feel dizzy

▶ have dry eyes

▶ have headaches

▶ have constipation

▶ pass urine that is dark in colour.

To monitor for weight loss or gain:

▶ consider if there has been a noticeable change in the individual's weight

▶ create food and fluid charts to record intake over a week

▶ weigh the individual weekly

▶ if there is an underlying condition this should be treated and the individual provided with appropriate food and drink

▶ special dietary needs should be documented and maintained until weight improves.

Key terms

Body mass index (BMI): a formula used to calculate weight loss or weight gain

Malnutrition Universal Screening Tool (MUST): analytical tool used to identify adults who are malnourished

Reflect

Why do you think it is important to monitor the food and drink an individual consumes? What difficulties might you encounter as you monitor the individual?

Agreed ways of working

The Alzheimer's society has put forward guidelines regarding support with eating and drinking for those with Alzheimer's disease. A report by Age UK on malnutrition in hospital (2006) found that an unacceptable number of individuals were malnourished when in hospital because they were either not being given the food to eat or help to eat it.

Department of Health guidance

The Department of Health (DOH) issued national standards (2003) that care homes and other caring institutions should adhere to when supporting individuals with eating and drinking. The standards state:

'Older people national minimum standards require each individual to have a needs assessment which includes details of weight, diet and diet preferences, and oral health. Any unexplained swallowing disorder or other eating problems should be assessed by a speech and language therapist, doctor or dentist. There should be regular checks to look at residents' food and beverage likes and dislikes, food and drink wastage and access to second helpings.'

The DOH also stated that extra time should be allowed for slow eaters. Residential and nursing care staff should watch for the following warning signs:

▶ changes in eating habits

▶ food or drinks left over at mealtimes and at snacks between meals

▶ loss of independence in eating

▶ difficulties with swallowing

▶ visible signs of tight-fitting or loose clothes, which could indicate weight gain or loss.

Investigate

Using the internet, your local library and other resources, find the guidance written by DOH (2003) regarding the extra time that should be given to individuals when they are slow eaters. Check if your workplace or placement setting is aware of this guidance and share your findings with your colleagues.

Reflect

Why is it important to have agreed ways of working regarding eating and drinking support for those that have dementia-related conditions? Think about the challenges and significance of this area of practice as well as the possible consequences of poor practice.

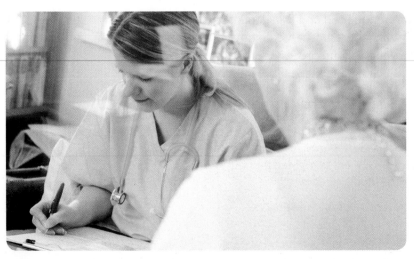

Documenting information about individuals' dietary needs and eating patterns can be an important part of care practice

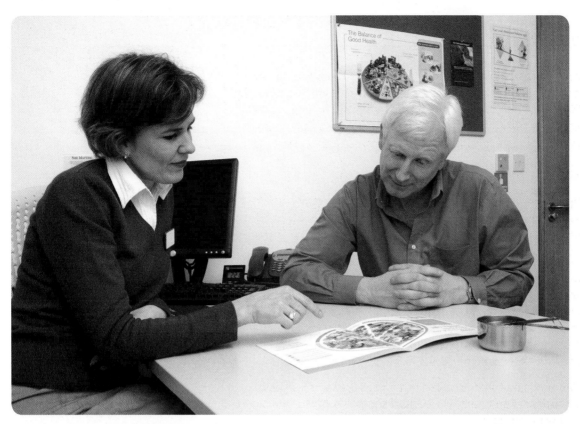

Health and social care practitioners may provide advice on diet and nutrition to people with particular needs or conditions

Practical Assessment Task   5.1 5.2 5.3

Health and social care practitioners often need to monitor and manage the diet that service users consume to ensure that it is nutritionally balanced and sufficient or appropriate for their dietary and medical needs. In this assessment activity you need to show that you can:

▶ explain the importance of monitoring the food and drink an individual consumes and any difficulties they encounter

▶ carry out and record agreed dietary monitoring processes

▶ report on the support provided for eating and drinking in accordance with agreed ways of working.

Your evidence for this task must be based on your practice and experience in a real work environment. Keep any written work that you produce for this activity as evidence towards your assessment. Your assessor may also want to observe or ask you questions about the way you monitor eating and drinking and the support provided in the care setting.

Are you ready for assessment?

AC	What can you do now?	Assessment task	✓
1.1	Establish with an individual the food and drink they wish to consume	Page 339	
1.2	Encourage the individual to select suitable options for food and drink	Page 339	
1.3	Describe ways to resolve any difficulties or dilemmas about the choice of food and drink	Page 339	
1.4	Describe how and when to seek additional guidance about an individual's choice of food and drink	Page 339	
2.1	Identify the level and type of support an individual requires when eating and drinking	Page 343	
2.2	Demonstrate effective hand washing and use of protective clothing when handling food and drink	Page 343	
2.3	Support the individual to prepare to eat and drink, in a way that meets their personal needs and preferences	Page 343	
2.4	Provide suitable utensils to assist the individual to eat and drink	Page 343	
3.1	Describe factors that help promote an individual's dignity, comfort and enjoyment while eating and drinking	Page 347	
3.2	Support the individual to consume manageable amounts of food and drink at their own pace	Page 347	
3.3	Provide encouragement to the individual to eat and drink	Page 347	
3.4	Support the individual to clean themselves if food or drink is spilt	Page 347	
3.5	Adapt support in response to an individual's feedback or observed reactions while eating and drinking	Page 347	
4.1	Explain why it is important to be sure that an individual has chosen to finish eating and drinking before clearing away	Page 349	

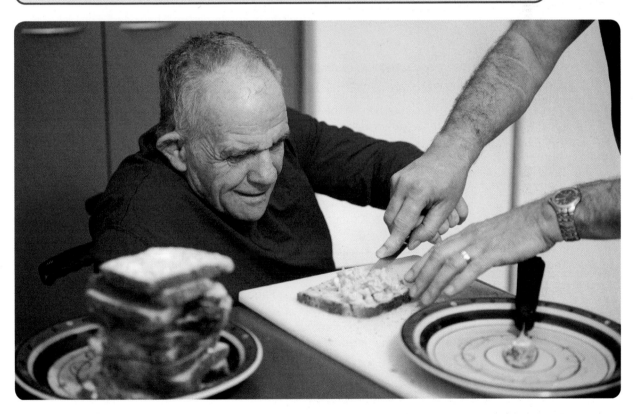

14 | Support individuals to meet personal care needs (HSC 2015)

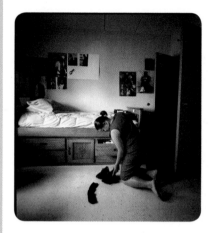

Assessment of this unit

This unit introduces you to the topic of supporting individuals with their personal care needs. It provides the knowledge and skills needed to support individuals to use toilet facilities, maintain personal hygiene and manage their personal appearance. You will need to be able to:

▶ work with individuals to identify their needs and preferences in relation to personal care

▶ provide support for personal care safely

▶ support individuals to use the toilet

▶ support individuals to maintain personal hygiene

▶ support individuals to manage their personal appearance

▶ monitor and report on support for personal care.

The assessment of this unit is entirely competence-based. You are assessed on the things you need to do in the work environment. To successfully complete this unit, you will need to produce evidence of your competence in supporting individuals to meet their personal care needs. The table below outlines what you need to do to meet each of the assessment criteria for the unit.

Your tutor or assessor will help you to prepare for your assessment, and the tasks suggested in the unit will help you to create the evidence that you need.

AC	What you need to do:
1.1	Encourage an individual to communicate their needs, preferences and personal beliefs affecting their personal care
1.2	Establish the level and type of support and individual needs for personal care
1.3	Agree with the individual how privacy will be maintained during personal care
2.1	Support the individual to understand the reasons for hygiene and safety precautions
2.2	Use protective equipment, protective clothing and hygiene techniques to minimise the risk of infection
2.3	Explain how to report concerns about the safety and hygiene of equipment or facilities used for personal care

2.4	Describe ways to ensure the individual can summon help when alone during personal care.
2.5	Ensure safe disposal of waste material
3.1	Provide support for the individual to use toilet facilities in ways that respect dignity
3.2	Support individuals to make themselves clean and tidy after using toilet facilities
4.1	Ensure room and water temperatures meet individual needs and preferences for washing, bathing and mouth care
4.2	Ensure toiletries, materials and equipment are within reach of the individual
4.3	Provide support to carry out personal hygiene activities in ways that maintain comfort, respect dignity and promote active participation
5.1	Provide support to enable individuals to manage their personal appearance in ways that respect dignity and promote active participation
5.2	Encourage the individuals to keep their clothing and personal care items clean, safe and secure
6.1	Seek feedback from the individual and others on how well support for personal care meets the individual's needs and preferences
6.2	Monitor personal care functions and activities in agreed ways
6.3	Record and report on an individual's personal care in agreed ways

All of the assessment criteria relating to this unit must be assessed in a real work environment.

This unit also links to some of the other units:

HSC 027	Contribute to health and safety in health and social care
IC 01	The principles of infection prevention and control
HSC 026	Implement person-centred approaches in health and social care

Some of your learning will be repeated in these units and will give you the chance to review your knowledge and understanding.

Identifying needs and preferences

You are expected to be able to work with individuals to identify their needs and preferences in relation to personal care. Personal care includes:

▶ using toilet facilities

▶ bathing, washing and mouth care

▶ individuals managing their own appearance.

What is meant by 'communicating needs'?

Communicating care needs is about how individuals let others know they have a need or preference in care; or about others communicating that they are aware the individual has a care need or preference.

Communication is an important aspect of care. Sometimes people are embarrassed about saying what their needs are, especially if they refer to wanting to use the toilet. It is therefore important that care workers are sensitive to issues involving personal care.

Care workers should also be aware that individuals might need encouragement to communicate their personal care needs and preferences. This may be because they:

▶ are not aware they have a care need

▶ are not aware they can be supported with a care need

▶ do not like to ask for support

▶ are embarrassed at their care need

▶ feel their care need is undignified.

How can individuals communicate personal care needs?

Personal care needs can be established either through communication started by the individual or begun by another person, such as a care worker or a family member. For example:

▶ *started by the individual* – Marcus (17) has learning difficulties. For his birthday he was given a new electric razor which he now wants to use. He asks you to help him.

▶ *started by another person* – Hazel, a home care worker, notices that Fred (85) has not shaved for a week. She asks him if he would like help shaving.

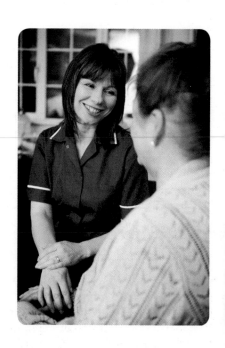

How is the level and type of support established?

The level and type of support is established by finding out what individuals prefer and by working in agreed ways, in accordance with policies and procedures.

Key terms

Prosthetic: artificial (used for artificial limbs or parts of limbs)

Figure 14.1 Levels of need

Example of need	High level	Low level
Unable to wash and dress unsupported	Needs support to use soap and shampoo, pour water and get in and out of a bath safely	Needs help pouring bathwater and ensuring it is at a safe and comfortable temperature
Unable to use the toilet unsupported	Needs help to sit on the toilet, clean afterwards, adjust clothing and wash hands	Help provided to make sure the person can find the toilet
Unable to attach prosthetic leg unsupported	Needs to have the prosthetic limb attached and made comfortable	Individual is shown how the limb is attached

The level and type of support is established in three ways:

▶ preference

▶ policy and procedure

▶ level and type of need.

Reflect

Reflect on what you think about helping others with their personal care.

Figure 14.2 Establishing the level and type of support

Need	Preference	Policy and procedure	Level and type of need
Fran, who lives in a residential home for older people, is incontinent of urine every night.	She prefers to wear a clean night dress every night.	The policy is that all residents wear their own clothes.	Fran is woken in the night to be supported with toileting and changing into a clean night dress if necessary.
Holly, who has Down's syndrome, is encouraged to take part in normal community activities like shopping, but has problems dressing appropriately.	When out she likes talking to men she doesn't know about what she wears.	The policy is that individuals are supported in choosing clothes to wear and accompanied when they leave the home.	Holly is encouraged to be as independent as possible, but with the awareness that she is at risk.
Jason (8) is over hyperactive and needs one-to-one attention at school. He likes to jump in puddles.	He prefers to run around the playground getting wet than sit in lessons.	The policy is that children have three hours of teaching in a classroom every day and that three playtimes are worked into this time.	Jason has a coat and Wellington boots to go outside in, and is observed from a distance by a member of staff.

Privacy

Care situations may occur in public where individuals are not alone.
They might often be in a hospital day room or ward with others,
or be at a day centre or training college. Maintaining **privacy** is
therefore an issue, and is important because:

▶ it affects the individual's **dignity** and self-respect

▶ the individual might be vulnerable

▶ the individual might feel they are a burden.

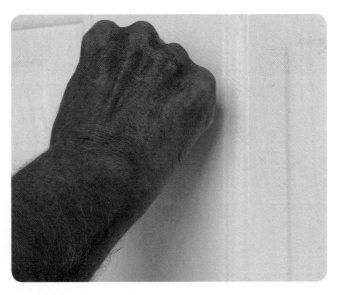

It is therefore important that care workers:

▶ understand how individuals might feel

▶ show respect

▶ protect the individual's dignity.

How can privacy be maintained?

Individuals should always have privacy when personal care is being
provided. When washing, dressing, bathing, or attending to other
personal care needs, they should always be out of sight and – if
possible – out of earshot of other people.

How you achieve this should be agreed with the individual. The
points that need to be agreed are as follows:

▶ the bathroom or toilet door should be closed and/or locked

▶ curtains or a screen should be pulled around a bed

▶ the individual should not be left partially dressed in view of others

▶ staff and visitors should knock before they enter a private area

▶ you should talk quietly so others can't overhear you.

Your assessment criteria:

1.3 Agree with the individual how privacy will be maintained during personal care

Key terms

Privacy: an individual's right to have personal information, activities and property kept from others

Dignity: an individual's right to personal privacy and to be treated with respect by others; presenting a clean, decent personal appearance is important to maintaining the individual's dignity and self-esteem

Reflect

Reflect on a time when you were involved in a sensitive personal care situation. How did you feel about either providing or receiving support?

Case study

Sotina is receiving end of life care in a hospice. She is unable to speak due to a brain tumour and spends much of the day in a chair. When she wants something she uses flashcards. The set of flashcards helps her communicate when she is hungry, wants to brush her hair, or for any other issues that are important to her wellbeing and comfort. Daniel, a care worker, is aware that the flashcards are used by Sotina when she wants to use the toilet. During the morning Daniel notices that Sotina is looking at him. He goes over to Sotina and suggests she uses the flashcards to indicate if she wants something. At first Sotina looks embarrassed, but then shows Daniel the card with a picture of a toilet on it. Daniel is about to help take Sotina to the toilet, when he remembers something else. He shows Sotina the card with a picture of a woman on it. Sotina smiles and nods her head. Daniel then goes to ask his colleague Marianne to help Sotina. When using the toilet Marianne leaves Sotina alone and knocks on the door after a few minutes to see if Sotina is finished before helping her back to her chair.

1. Why might Sotina be reluctant to tell Daniel about her personal care needs?

2. How does Daniel encourage Sotina to communicate her care needs?

3. How does Marianne help maintain Sotina's privacy?

Key terms

Flashcard: a card with key information printed on it; it can contain words, pictures or symbols

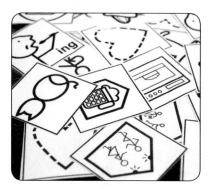

Practical Assessment Task   1.1   1.2   1.3

Health and social care practitioners should provide personalised care and support for people that meets their individual needs. In this practical assessment task you must demonstrate the ability to identify the needs and preferences of individuals in relation to personal care. When you are in your work setting, select a client or service user, and – with their consent and with the agreement of your supervisor or line manager – carry out the following task:

1. Find out the personal care needs and preferences of an individual by encouraging them to communicate them to you.

2. Establish what type of support they require for their personal care needs, and the level they need it at.

3. Agree with the individual how their privacy should be maintained during support with personal care.

4. Write an account of what you did at each stage.

5. Discuss your task with your assessor.

Your evidence must be based on your practice in a real work environment and must be witnessed by, or be in a format acceptable to, your assessor.

Investigate

Investigate how individuals in your work setting are supported with their personal care.

Why support precautions?

Providing support for personal care involves helping the individual to understand the reasons for hygiene and safety precautions. This is important because:

▶ maintaining safety is a key aspect of health and social care work

▶ some individuals do not always understand they are at risk

▶ some individuals are not always aware of their personal cleanliness

▶ care workers also need to stay safe and well.

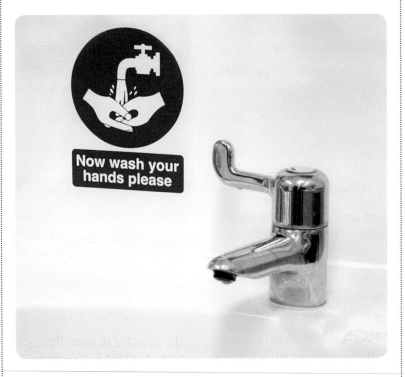

Who is at risk?

Everyone in the care environment is at risk and should take precautions. Some individuals and groups are at particular risk because of their care needs. At-risk groups may include:

▶ children

▶ older people

▶ people with physical disabilities

▶ people with mental health problems

▶ people with learning disabilities.

Your assessment criteria:

2.1 Support the individual to understand the reasons for hygiene and safety precautions

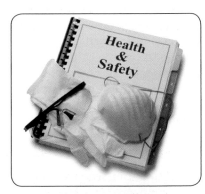

Reflect

Reflect on potential risks when you perform personal care activities with individuals.

Discuss

Discuss with a friend or colleague ways to help individuals understand reasons for hygiene and safety precautions.

Investigate

Investigate in your work area ways individuals are helped to understand reasons for hygiene and safety precautions.

How is understanding supported?

Health and safety involves balancing the needs and preferences of the individual with the health and safety of others. A risk assessment of the care environment, and of the individual's ability to carry out personal care activities, will need to be undertaken. This includes managing your own safety and personal hygiene.

The individual's needs may create a risk which requires specific precautions (see figure 14.3 for examples). It may also be necessary to help the individual understand the risks and ways to minimise or prevent them.

Figure 14.3 Risks and precautions

Personal care need and risk	Precaution taken	Support understanding
Need: Jason, who has no arms, needs help using the toilet Risk: care workers risk cross-infection from assisting with toileting and cleaning Jason	Care workers wear protective gloves and wash their hands afterwards	Show Jason what you are doing and explain about the risks as you do it
Need: Gilbert has lice in his hair Risk: infestation of other individuals and care workers	Gilbert is helped to treat the infestation and check his hair for lice daily	Group teaching session to explain about infestation
Need: Carter uses a mobility scooter but isn't aware of all hazards Risk: to others and to Carter himself, as in his garden at home there are steps down to the lawn	The steps down to the lawn are fenced off, and he is observed in the garden	Explain the risks with the aid of a safe use of mobility scooter video
Need: Carla doesn't understand how to talk to people she doesn't know. Risk: sexual and other kinds of abuse	She is accompanied when doing activities away from her home	Use role play to show the risks of talking to strangers

Practical Assessment Task — 2.1

For this practical assessment task you must demonstrate that you are able to provide individuals with support for personal care. With the permission of your manager or supervisor, and the consent of an individual, explain the reasons for hygiene and safety precautions at a time when you are providing this kind of support.

Your evidence must be based on your practice in a real work environment and must be witnessed by, or be in a format acceptable to, your assessor.

Protection and techniques to minimise risk

Why is protection necessary?

It is necessary to protect yourself and others to: safeguard clients and service users from infection; maintain a safe working area; ensure safe working practices; comply with health and safety laws.

What risks are there?

All work environments have risks that must be protected against. In health and social care there are particular risks. These include:

▶ MRSA and other infections

▶ skin diseases

▶ infections from exposure to bodily fluids

▶ infections spread through contact with mobility and handling equipment.

How is protection carried out?

Protection is carried out by the use of protective equipment, protective clothing and hygiene techniques.

What protective equipment is used?

Protective clothing includes:

▶ disposable gloves to protect hands

▶ face masks to protect mouth and nose

▶ goggles to protect eyes

▶ disposable plastic aprons.

The type of protective equipment used depends on the risk. Figure 14.4 shows what to wear to protect against risks from bodily fluids.

What hygiene techniques are used?

The appropriate hygiene techniques are: hand washing, safe handling and disposal of bodily fluids, and safe handling and disposal of protective equipment.

Bodily fluids include: urine; faeces; vomit; blood; saliva; seepages from wounds.

Figure 14.4 Protecting against risks from bodily fluids

Example of situation	Bodily fluid risk	What to wear
Escorting a client to the toilet	No exposure to bodily fluids	No protection necessary
Escorting client to the toilet and supporting them with personal care	Exposure but low risk of splashing	Gloves and plastic apron
Escorting a client to the toilet; supporting them with personal care when they have vomiting and diarrhoea	High risk of splashing	Gloves, plastic apron, and eye, nose and mouth protection

Key terms

MRSA: methicillin-resistant staphylococcus aureus; it is a serious infection that is difficult to treat using normal antibiotics

Reflect

Reflect on a time when you have had to use protective clothing and equipment. How did it protect you?

Investigate

Investigate the use of protective clothing and protective equipment in your work place. What information is available?

Discuss

Discuss with your manager or supervisor the types of infection, and how risks of infection are minimised in your work setting.

Figure 14.5 Correct procedures for hand washing

Preparation:	Washing and rinsing:
1. Remove wrist and hand jewellery.	5. Use a liquid soap to all parts of the hands.
2. Cover cuts with plasters.	6. Rub hands together.
3. Remove nail extensions.	7. Make sure ends of fingers and between fingers are cleaned.
4. Wet hands under warm running water.	8. Rinse thoroughly.

Case study

Raqia works in a residential home for older people. Mr Francis and Mrs Wheeler require support with personal care while using the toilet. Mr Francis is helped to sit on the toilet, but can manage to clean himself and only needs support arranging his clothing and to be escorted back to the day lounge. When helping Mr Francis, Raqia wears a disposable plastic apron and disposable plastic gloves. When Mr Francis is back in the day lounge she removes the disposable apron and gloves and puts them in the correct bin, and puts on a fresh pair of gloves and a clean apron. She then helps Mrs Wheeler to use the toilet. On the way to the toilet Mrs Wheeler says she feels unwell and is suddenly sick. Raqia summons help from another carer and asks her to bring goggles and a face mask. Mrs Wheeler is sick again as Raqia helps her through the toilet door.

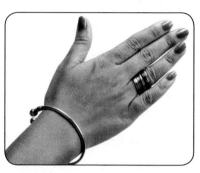

All wrist and hand jewellery must be removed before hand washing

1. What protective clothing does Raqia use when supporting Mr Francis, and why?
2. What protective clothing does Raqia ask for when supporting Mrs Wheeler, and why?
3. Reflect on the use of protective clothing in your work setting.

Practical Assessment Task   2.1   2.2

In this practical assessment task you must demonstrate your ability to provide support for personal care. You must make sure you have the permission of your line manager and the consent of the individual in your care before carrying out this task.

1. Explain the reasons for hygiene and safety precautions at a time when you are providing support for personal care.
2. Demonstrate appropriate use of protective equipment, protective clothing and hygiene techniques to minimise the risk of infection.

Your evidence must be based on your practice in a real work environment and must be witnessed by, or be in a format acceptable to, your assessor.

Reporting concerns about safety and hygiene

What to do if you have concerns

Every member of staff is responsible for maintaining hygiene and safety. Any concerns must be reported to your supervisor or line manager. There might be concerns about the safety and hygiene of equipment or facilities used for personal care. Issues might include:

- ▶ dirty toilets or hand-washing basins
- ▶ unclean baths
- ▶ soiled aprons
- ▶ unavailability of suitable gloves
- ▶ risks of infections spreading.

Your assessment criteria:

2.3 Explain how to report concerns about the safety and hygiene of equipment or facilities used for personal care

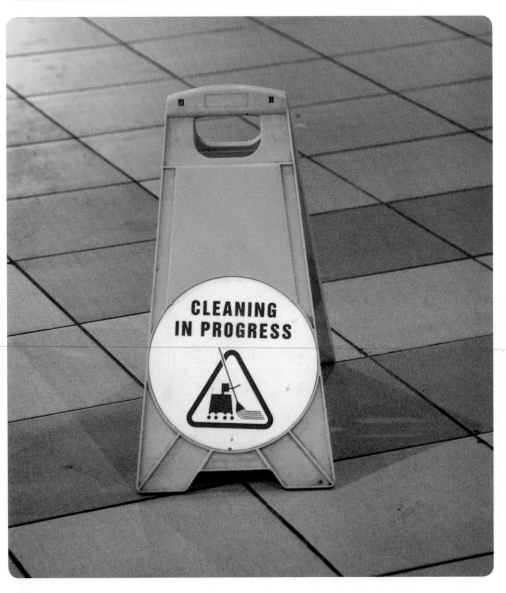

Case study

Raqia works in a residential home for older people. Mrs Wheeler is sick as Raqia escorts her to the toilet. Raqia summons assistance from another carer, Mary, by calling her across the room, and asks her to bring goggles and a face mask.

Mrs Wheeler is sick again as Raqia helps her enter the toilet area. Mary hurries in after them saying that all the face masks and goggles have been used already because of the recent outbreak of diarrhoea and vomiting in the home. Sitting on the toilet, Mrs Wheeler has diarrhoea.

When Mrs Wheeler feels a bit better and has been cleaned she is taken to her room for a lie-down. Raqia and Mary wash the floors and then dispose of their contaminated gloves and aprons. They then report the unavailability of face masks and goggles to their supervisor who immediately checks the stock and orders more. They also make a note in the reporting book so the next shift will know.

Finally, the manager asks Raqia to help her look at all the equipment and facilities to make sure that they are all in good order, and to draw up a list of ways for people to report concerns about safety and hygiene.

1. How did Raqia report the unavailability of goggles and face masks?

2. Discuss with your manager or supervisor how to report concerns about safety and hygiene for personal care.

Reflect

Reflect on your experience of reporting safety concerns.

Investigate

Investigate the ways in your work setting that concerns can be reported. Are they all reported directly to the manager or is there another means of reporting?

Discuss

Discuss with your line manager or supervisor how they have responded to any concerns about safety and hygiene.

Practical Assessment Task 2.3

In this practical assessment task you must demonstrate the ability to report concerns about the safety and hygiene of equipment or facilities used for personal care.

1. Write a memo to your line manager or supervisor in which you outline the ways that concerns about the safety of equipment and facilities used for personal care can be reported.

2. Explain to your assessor how concerns are reported in your workplace and how you have or would use them in practice.

Your evidence must be based on your practice in a real work environment and must be witnessed by, or be in a format acceptable to, your assessor.

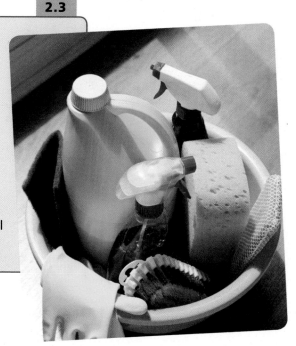

When and how do individuals summon help?

In health and social care individuals are sometimes unable to manage their own personal care. They may have to summon help for support:

▶ to begin a personal care activity

▶ during personal care

▶ at the end of a personal care activity.

How can they summon help?

Individuals can summon help by speaking, signing, using electronic call systems or personal alarms. These means of summoning help are used in the following ways:

▶ personal alarms can be worn as a wrist band, hooked to a belt or as a pendant

▶ voice intercoms can be used as two-way communication between one room and another

▶ ceiling pull cords can be tugged on to summon help

▶ speaking or calling out, when others are nearby

▶ signalling, when others are in sight.

Reflect

Reflect on a time when you wanted to summon help. How did you do it?

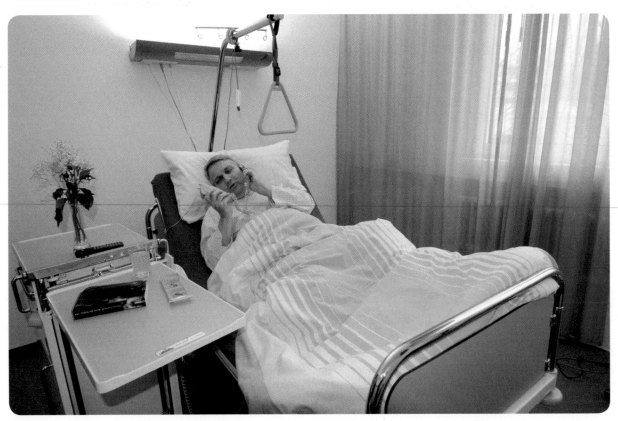

Personal alarms and other electronic means of summoning help are increasingly used

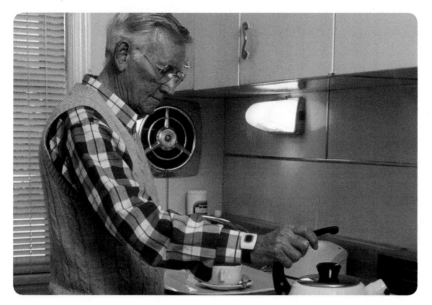

Investigate

Explore the internet for ways individuals might summon help in your workplace. What suitable electronic means are available?

Wrist band alarms are quite unobtrusive, resembling ordinary wrist watches

Case study

Albert Streep lives alone. He has rheumatism, which affects his balance. At night he has to get out of bed to use the toilet at least twice due to a prostrate problem. He is at risk of falling. As he lives alone there is nobody there to summon help from, so he uses a call system which is installed in his bathroom. If he falls in the bathroom he need only tug on the pull cord and a care agency will be alerted and visit him to see if he is alright. His friend, Chandler, who also lives alone at the other side of town, uses a personal alarm system which he wears as a wrist band. When, on one occasion, Chandler falls on his way to the bathroom he simply presses a button on his wrist and help is summoned. On Saturday afternoon they meet up at the pub and talk about their means of summoning help. They also know of another way they saw advertised in the newspaper, where an intercom is used that enables a person to speak to another person in another room.

1. What three ways of summoning help do they discuss?

2. What other ways of summoning help can individuals use?

3. Discuss with your supervisor or manager how individuals in your work setting can summon help.

Key terms

Rheumatism: a medical disorder affecting the joints

Practical Assessment Task   2.4

As a health or social care practitioner you should always risk-assess care situations and ensure that the people you provide care or support for are safeguarded from hazards and harm. In this practical assessment task you must describe ways in which you ensure that the individuals for whom you provide support during personal care activities can summon help in your work setting.

Your evidence must be based on your practice in a real work environment and must be witnessed by, or be in a format acceptable to, your assessor.

Safe disposal of waste materials

What is meant by waste materials?

There are different types of waste materials likely to be found in health and social care settings:

- ▶ bodily fluids
- ▶ food
- ▶ linen
- ▶ sharps
- ▶ clinical waste.

How are they disposed of?

All waste material must be disposed of safely, taking into account health and safety laws and local policies where you work (see figure 14.6 for examples). Wear gloves and an apron when dealing with waste materials, and make sure spillages are wiped up immediately.

Your assessment criteria:

2.5 Ensure safe disposal of waste materials.

Key terms

Sluice: a water channel used for disposing of waste materials

Figure 14.6 Disposal of waste

Type of waste	Examples	Waste disposal
Bodily	Saliva, sputum, blood, seepage from wounds, vomit, urine and faeces	These should be cleaned up, flushed down a sluice or toilet and the area cleaned with a disinfectant.
Food	Leftovers from meals and surplus food	These should be placed straight away in a special bin in the kitchen.
Linen	Soiled bed sheets, towels and clothing.	These should be placed in a bag reserved for soiled linen, and not mixed with other items.
Sharps	Used razors and other blades, and injection needles	These are placed in a yellow bin which is sealed before being incinerated.
Clinical	Dressings, bandages and swabs	These should be disposed of in marked clinical waste bins.

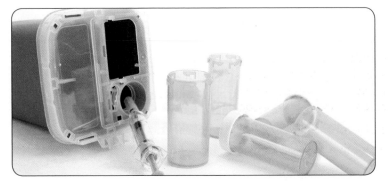

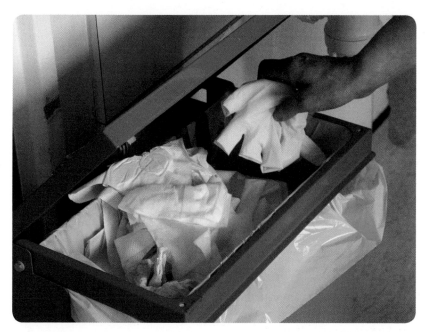

Safe disposal of waste and used protective equipment is essential to prevent and control infection in care settings

Case study

Imelda is asked to let a new care worker, Sherin, follow her about the care home during the morning shift and show her how to dispose of waste products. During the course of the morning they dispose of dirty towels, soiled sheets, bandages from a dressing and leftover food. Before lunch they remove their used gloves and aprons and talk about the morning over a cup of coffee. Then Imelda asks Sherin to check in the bathrooms to make sure none of the residents are there. In the bathroom Sherin finds a plastic dentures pot containing sputum left on a shelf. She disposes of the sputum by flushing it down the toilet and then rinses the pot out under running water. She then goes in to the dining room to help out with lunch.

1. Does Sherin dispose of the sputum correctly?

2. What else should she have done to maintain safety and hygiene?

3. Reflect on how you dispose of waste materials.

Practical Assessment Task   **2.5**

Safe disposal of waste is a key infection control activity in care settings and is often a part of personal care activity. In this practical assessment task you must demonstrate the ability to dispose of a waste materials safely and discuss what you do with your assessor.

Your evidence must be based on your practice in a real work environment and must be witnessed by, or be in a format acceptable to, your assessor.

Supporting individual to use toilet facilities

What type of support?

Sometimes it is necessary to provide support to individuals to use toilet facilities. This level of support can include helping them make themselves clean and tidy. This should be done in ways that are sensitive and respect the individual's dignity. Toilet facilities include:

- ▶ toilets
- ▶ bedpans
- ▶ urine bottles
- ▶ commodes.

Care workers should try to promote the individual's independence and encourage them to manage their own personal care as much as possible. Some people will need minimal assistance and others will need full care.

How is support assessed?

An assessment of the level of support is required. This assessment is based on the following questions:

1. What is the person's usual toileting habit?

2. Does the person have a problem with mobility?

3. Can the individual adjust their clothing?

4. Can the person wipe and clean themselves afterwards?

5. Can the person wash their hands?

6. Is the person affected by an illness or disability?

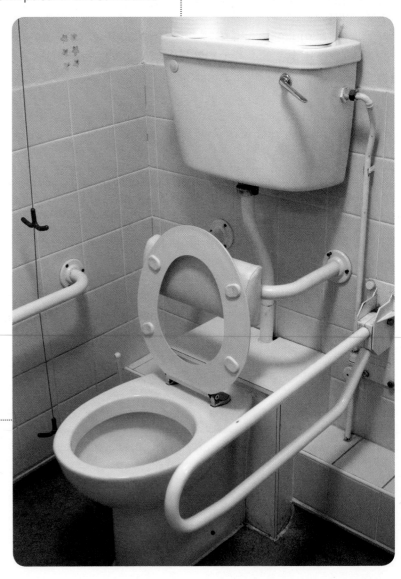

Case study

Ruth and Danny are helping Gemma use the toilet at the resource centre, which she attends to learn skills to become more independent. Gemma, who has a severe learning disability, is very dependent on her parents for most activities of daily living. She is being encouraged to manage her own personal care in the toilet to see how much she can do unsupported. Ruth and Danny explain what they are doing as they support her to take her trousers and pants down and make sure she is sitting on the toilet safely.

When Gemma has finished, they show her toilet paper and put it in her hand so she can wipe herself clean. This is successful and they decide that next time they will see if she can take the toilet paper herself. After the activity Ruth and Danny discuss how effective it was. They also discuss the ways in which they tried to respect Gemma's dignity. They decide that they respected her dignity by: closing the door; explaining what they were doing; giving her the opportunity to do things herself; keeping their voices quiet; addressing her politely.

1. How did Ruth and Danny support Gemma in using the toilet?

2. How did Ruth and Danny respect Gemma's dignity? Can you think of what else they could have done?

3. Reflect on what 'dignity' means to you.

Reflect

Reflect on your how you would like to be treated if supported in using toilet facilities.

Investigate

Investigate your employer's policies (if any) on respecting dignity.

Discuss

Discuss with you line manager or supervisor how they respect dignity when supporting individuals using toilet facilities.

Practical Assessment Task   3.1 3.2

In this practical assessment task you must demonstrate that you are able to support an individual to use the toilet. With the permission of your manager or supervisor, and with the consent of the individual, you need to show you can:

▶ support the individual in using toilet facilities

▶ make sure that the individual's dignity is respected

▶ support the individual in cleaning and tidying themselves after using toilet facilities.

Ask your manager or supervisor to write a testimony that you have demonstrated the above.

Discuss with your assessor the support you gave with using toilet facilities.

Supporting individuals to maintain personal hygiene while bathing and washing

How is the environment important?

When supporting an individual to wash and bath, the environment is very important. Individuals have differing needs. These different needs depend on their:

- ▶ disability
- ▶ preferences
- ▶ other needs (not related to their disability)
- ▶ required level of support.

Environmental factors include:

- ▶ water temperature
- ▶ room temperature
- ▶ toiletries
- ▶ materials
- ▶ equipment.

When is the environment right?

The environment is right when the individual's needs and preferences are met to help them with personal care. They will have access to their personal toiletries, materials such as towels and flannels, and any equipment and support they require.

Equipment and toiletries must be within easy reach of individuals so that they can be used safely and comfortably.

Your assessment criteria:

4.1 Ensure room and water temperatures meet individual needs and preferences for washing, bathing and mouth care.

4.2 Ensure toiletries, materials and equipment are within reach of the individual.

4.3 Provide support to carry out personal hygiene activities in ways that maintain comfort, respect dignity and promote active participation.

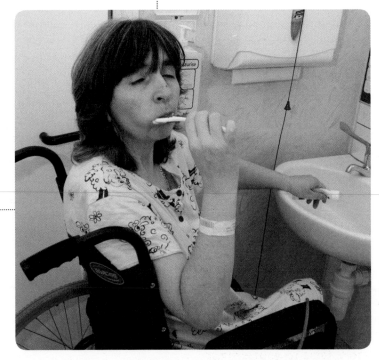

Supporting personal hygiene means that preferences are met, equipment is easily reached and active participation is encouraged

Case study

As part of her practical assessment task, Caroline, who works for a home care agency and is a candidate on a health and social care diploma course, prepares the bathroom for Angus. Angus lives in his own home, which has been adapted after he lost both legs in an accident. She discusses Angus's needs and preferences with him, and learns that he likes his bathroom warm and the bathwater hot. She checks the radiator is on, and that the window is closed. She checks the water temperature with a thermometer and by placing her hand in it. She then asks Angus if the water is the temperature he likes.

Angus can use the bath with the aid of an appliance that lifts him in and lowers him into the water. Caroline makes sure the appliance is in the correct position and that his toiletries and soap are within easy reach when he is in the bath. She then leaves Angus to bath and waits for him to call that he is ready to get out of the bath. She has put a towel near the appliance so that he can cover himself. After he dries himself, Caroline places his toothbrush and toothpaste next to him.

1. How does Caroline ensure that the room temperature and water temperature meet Angus's needs and preferences?

2. Does she ensure that Angus's toiletries, materials and equipment are within his reach?

3. How does she help maintain his dignity?

Reflect

Reflect on times when you have supported individuals with personal care needs. How did you ensure their needs and preferences were met?

Investigate

Investigate any policies and procedures in your workplace about meeting needs and preferences with personal care.

Discuss

Discuss with a friend or colleague what you like in your own bathroom.

Practical Assessment Task   4.1 4.2 4.3

In this practical assessment task you must demonstrate that you are able to support an individual to maintain their personal hygiene. With the permission of your supervisor or manager, and with the consent of the individual, you need to show you can:

▶ discuss the needs and preferences for personal care regarding bathing, washing and mouth care with that individual

▶ ensure any toiletries, materials and equipment are within reach of the individual

▶ provide support to ensure personal needs and preferences are met

▶ provide a testimony from your supervisor or line manager that you have met the assessment criteria

▶ discuss with your assessor how you provided support and maintained the individual's comfort, respected their dignity and promoted active participation.

Your evidence must be based on your practice in a real work environment and must be witnessed by, or be in a format acceptable to, your assessor.

Supporting individuals in maintaining their personal appearance

Some individuals who use health and social care services require support with their personal appearance. They might have a condition in which

▶ they are not aware of how they appear to others

▶ they are not able to look after their appearance.

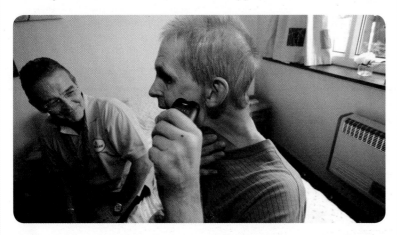

There is a wide range of activities that an individual might perform, and equipment they might use, to manage their personal appearance:

▶ hair care products and equipment

▶ nail care products and equipment

▶ cosmetics

▶ skin care products

▶ shaving products and equipment

▶ prostheses

▶ orthoses.

Bear in mind that individuals can be sensitive about their appearance. Provision of support should be handled carefully.

What support can be provided and why?

Support is provided to enable individuals to manage their appearance in ways that respect their dignity. It might be necessary to encourage individuals to keep their clothing and personal care items clean, safe and secure. The active participation of the individual should be encouraged, because:

▶ appearance has an effect on the individual's self-esteem

▶ participation encourages the individual to make choices and become more independent.

Investigate

Investigate on the internet how health conditions and disabilities can affect an individual's appearance.

Key terms

Orthoses: devices to control movement; for example, shoe inserts to support the heel

Discuss

Discuss with a friend or colleague how people value their appearance.

Case study

Zilla has learning disabilities and has been given two weeks' respite care in Northward House so that her parents, who are her usual carers, can go on holiday. Maxine works in Northward House and is Zilla's key worker. Before she goes home Zilla wants to surprise her parents. After breakfast she asks Maxine to help her with her appearance. Maxine agrees and together they make a list of what they plan, so that Zilla can say what she wants.

In the afternoon, Maxine supports Zilla in washing her hair, cutting and filing her nails, applying hand and face cream, and finally putting some make-up on. Zilla is very pleased with the results, and says it makes her feel very happy and beautiful. Afterwards Maxine reminds Zilla that she should look after her things, and helps her put her toiletries and nail care set away safely.

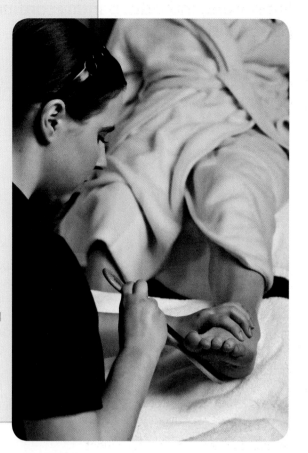

1. How did Maxine help promote Zilla's dignity and active participation?
2. How did Maxine encourage Zilla to keep her things tidy and safe?
3. Reflect on how important your appearance is to you.

Practical Assessment Task   5.1   5.2

In this practical assessment task you must demonstrate your ability to provide support to an individual to manage their personal appearance. With the permission of your supervisor or manager, and with the consent of an individual, you need to show you can:

▶ provide support to that individual in managing their appearance

▶ encourage the individual to look after their belongings

▶ obtain a testimony from your manager or supervisor that you maintained the individual's dignity and promoted that individual's active participation while providing support

▶ discuss with your assessor how you encouraged the individual's active participation.

Your evidence must be based on your practice in a real work environment and must be witnessed by, or be in a format acceptable to, your assessor.

Monitoring, reporting and recording personal care functions

Feedback is information about care activities that have been completed. On completion of personal care activities you will seek feedback from:

▶ the individual you support

▶ members of the care team

▶ others involved with the individual, such as family or specialist healthcare professionals.

Why seek feedback?

Feedback provides information on how well the support provided for personal care meets the individual's needs and preferences. This includes: meeting needs and preferences that are identified in the individual's care plan; adapting the care plan as new preferences and needs are discovered. You seek feedback on personal care so that care can be monitored, recorded and reported, in accordance with agreed ways of working.

What are 'agreed ways of working'?

Agreed ways of working are ways of carrying out tasks that are controlled by law, and by the local policies and procedures where you work. Individuals often attend to particular personal care activities at certain times of the day. Men might shave in the morning. Some people prefer to bath at night.

Health and social care settings often have agreed ways for monitoring, recording and reporting (see figure 14.7).

Your assessment criteria:

6.1 Seek feedback from the individual and others on how well support for personal care meets the individual's needs and preferences

6.2 Monitor personal care functions and activities in agreed ways

6.3 Record and report on an individual's personal care in agreed ways

Key terms

Agreed ways of working: ways of working that are controlled by law, and by the policies and procedures of organisations

Figure 14.7 Monitoring, recording and reporting on personal care

	Example of personal care activity
Monitor	An individual with a urine infection may need to use a commode during the night. Care workers can monitor how often an individual uses a commode at night by counting the number of times they get out of bed to use toilet facilities.
Record	Care workers can record the frequency that the individual uses the commode at night in the individual's care file.
Report	Information from the care file can be reported to colleagues, such as the doctor, who may be treating the urine infection.

Case study

At the beginning of his night shift at the respite centre, Colin is asked to support Simon, who has learning disabilities and a mental health problem. He has been sent to the centre under mental health law for a month. Since being there, Simon has been restless in the evening. Colin and Simon decide that Simon will feel better if he has a bath before going to bed. Colin supports Simon in preparing the bath. After the bath, Colin accompanies Simon to his room and asks him how he feels. Simon likes the bath because it reminds him of what he does at home before going to bed.

When Simon is in bed, Colin records the activity in his care file and notes that Simon liked the bath and says it makes him feel better. The next nights they do the same thing. Colin monitors how well Colin sleeps, seeking feedback at handover from his colleagues. It is the policy at the centre that all care activities are recorded in the individual's file, which means that Colin can also see a written record of Simon's sleep. Since bathing at bedtime, Simon has been more settled in the evenings.

1. Who did Colin seek feedback from about Simon's sleep?
2. How did Colin record and report on Simon's personal care in agreed ways?
3. Reflect on your personal care routines.

Practical Assessment Task   6.1   6.2   6.3

For this practical assessment task you must demonstrate your ability to monitor and report on support for personal care. With the permission of your manager or supervisor, and with consent of an individual, you need to show that you can:

▶ provide support for the individual's personal care
▶ seek feedback from the individual and others about the personal care
▶ monitor an individual's personal care in an agreed way
▶ record and report on an individual's personal care in an agreed way
▶ discuss with your assessor ways in which feedback was sought.

Your evidence must be based on your practice in a real work environment and must be witnessed by, or be in a format acceptable to, your assessor.

Reflect

Reflect on what it means to individuals that they are asked how their personal care meets their needs and preferences.

Investigate

Investigate in your workplace what personal care activities are monitored.

Discuss

Discuss with a friend or colleague how sensitive and private personal information should be recorded and reported.

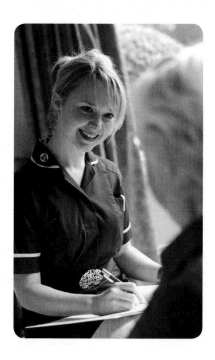

Are you ready for assessment?

AC	What can you do now?	Assessment task	✓
1.1	Encourage an individual to communicate their needs, preferences and personal beliefs affecting their personal care	Page 361	
1.2	Establish the level and type of support and individual needs for personal care	Page 361	
1.3	Agree with the individual how privacy will be maintained during personal care	Page 361	
2.1	Support the individual to understand the reasons for hygiene and safety precautions	Page 365	
2.2	Use protective equipment, protective clothing and hygiene techniques to minimise the risk of infection	Page 365	
2.3	Explain how to report concerns about the safety and hygiene of equipment or facilities used for personal care	Page 367	
2.4	Describe ways to ensure the individual can summon help when alone during personal care	Page 369	
2.5	Ensure safe disposal of waste material	Page 371	

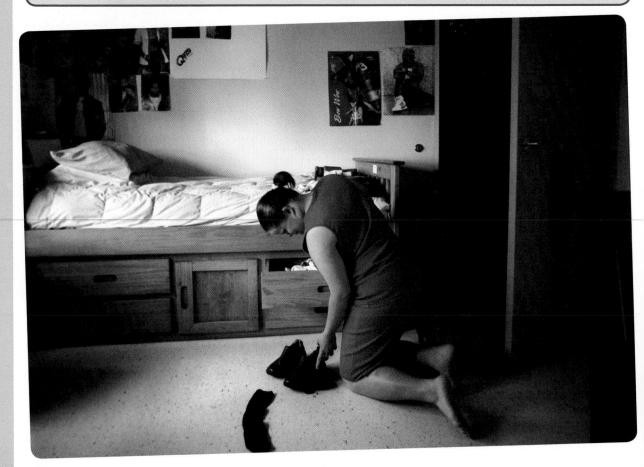

3.1	Provide support for the individual to use toilet facilities in ways that respect dignity	Page 373	
3.2	Support individuals to make themselves clean and tidy after using toilet facilities	Page 373	
4.1	Ensure room and water temperatures meet individual needs and preferences for washing, bathing and mouth care	Page 375	
4.2	Ensure toiletries, materials and equipment are within reach of the individual	Page 375	
4.3	Provide support to carry out personal hygiene activities in ways that maintain comfort, respect dignity and promote active participation	Page 375	
5.1	Provide support to enable individuals to manage their personal appearance in ways that respect dignity and promote active participation	Page 377	
5.2	Encourage the individual to keep their clothing and personal care items clean, safe and secure	Page 377	
6.1	Seek feedback from the individual and others on how well support for personal care meets the individual's needs and preferences	Page 379	
6.2	Monitor personal care functions and activities in agreed ways	Page 379	
6.3	Record and report on an individual's personal care in agreed ways	Page 379	